The Artificial Knee

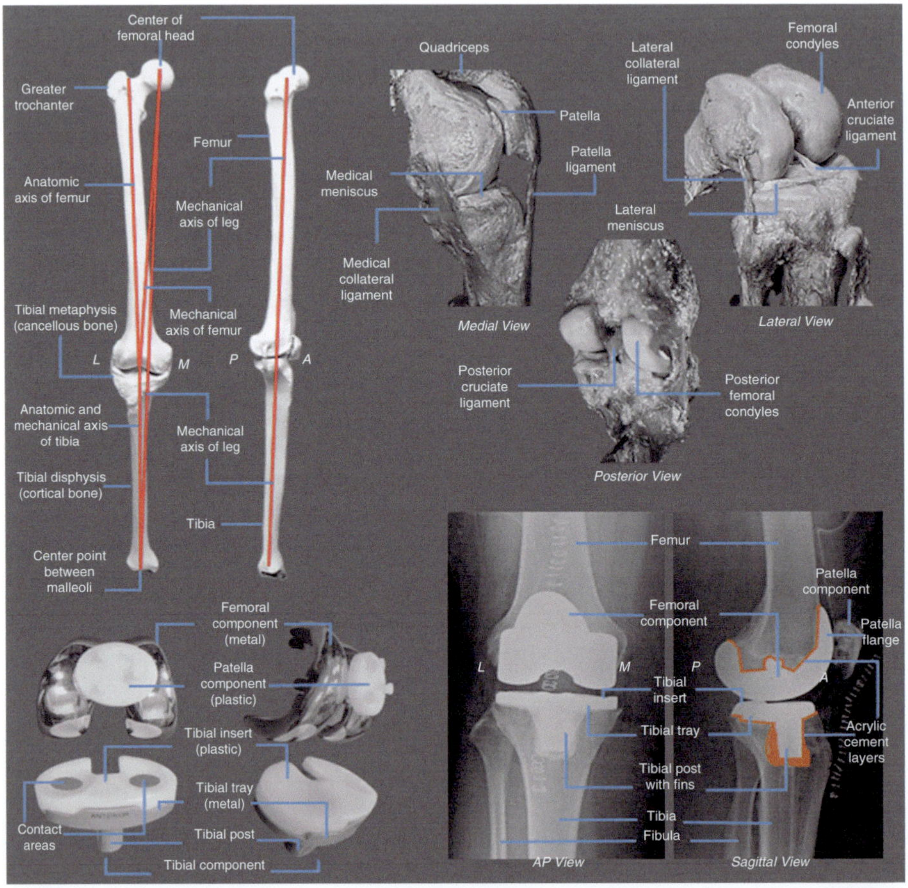

Top left, the overall alignment of the femur and tibia in frontal and sagittal views; top right, the anatomical structures of the knee, excluding the muscles; bottom left, a typical artificial knee, with the three different components, femoral, tibial, and patella; bottom right, AP and ML radiographs of an artificial knee, showing the cement mantle (orange) in the sagittal view. (Figure compiled by Jamie Liu)

Peter S. Walker

The Artificial Knee

An Ongoing Evolution

Springer

Peter S. Walker
Department of Orthopedic Surgery
New York University
New York, NY
USA

ISBN 978-3-030-38170-7 ISBN 978-3-030-38171-4 (eBook)
https://doi.org/10.1007/978-3-030-38171-4

This Springer imprint is published by the registered company Springer Nature Switzerland AG
The registered company address is: Gewerbestrasse 11, 6330 Cham, Switzerland

Contents

About the Author

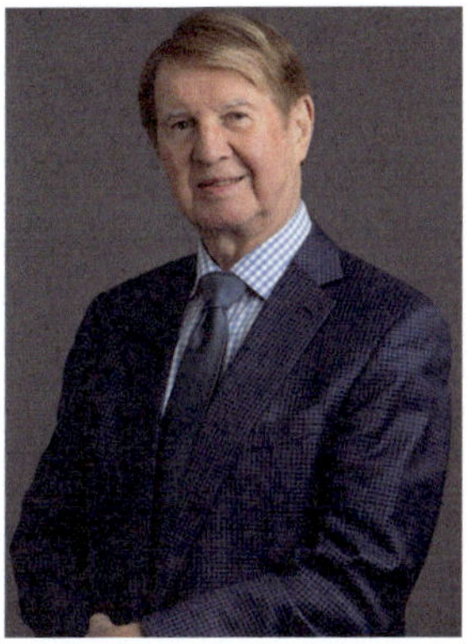

Peter S. Walker was educated in England at the Royal Grammar School, Newcastle, England, and then at the University of Cambridge. After a 3-year engineering traineeship in industry, he completed his PhD at the University of Leeds (1966–1969) under Professors Duncan Dowson and Verna Wright. Since then, he has been an active participant in the field of biomechanics of joints and the design of joint replacements, with a major emphasis on the knee. He worked for 18 years in the USA, 13 years in England, and then a further 20 years in the USA up to the present. He has collaborated with surgeons and bioengineers at renowned institutions, including the Hospital for Special Surgery; Howmedica (Stryker); Brigham and Women's Hospital, Harvard Medical School; Royal National Orthopaedic Hospital, University College London; and, currently, New York University Langone Orthopedic Hospital and NYU Tandon School of Engineering. He has coauthored over 300 articles with 12,000 citations. His basic research has included innovative ideas for total knee design, while many of the test machines and methodologies have been emulated by other labs. He has been a co-designer of several successful total knee systems; the Total Condylar, Graduated Knee System, Kinematic & Kinemax, Smiles Bone Tumor System, NexGen, and most recently the Persona, a leading knee system today. He has received several awards from various societies, the most notable being the Lifetime Achievement Awards from ISTA in 2004 and from The Knee Society in 2018.

1 Introduction

Key Questions, Overview, and Layout

While playing tennis recently, I was struck by how well my opponent moved around the court. At the end of the game, he remarked: "not bad for a couple of mechanical knees." He later explained that he had to follow a strict rehabilitation program to reach the activity level he had before his arthritis but that it was definitely worth the effort. After an artificial knee, most patients return to a normal everyday lifestyle free of pain and discomfort, while participation in active sports is not uncommon. Since the first artificial knees were implanted in the late 1960s, over 50 years ago, the quality of the outcomes has steadily progressed until the present day. This has been due to the concerted efforts of the surgeons and engineers who invented the artificial knees, to the companies who produced them, and to the countless patients who tried them, especially in the early days.

Historically, devices for relieving pain and restoring function to the arthritic knee were implanted as far back as 1891 although these failed due to inadequate materials and non-sterile surgical technique (Brand et al. 2011). In the 1940s and 1950s, metallic resurfacing components for the distal femur and more commonly the proximal tibia were used with reasonable success. These devices were mainly used in the less severe arthritic cases with modest functional demands and had the effect of realigning the lower limb and reducing pain. At the other extreme, metallic hinges with long intramedullary stems for fixation were used for the more severe cases, but reservations about the need for resection of the major ligaments, the large amount of bone removal, and the invasion of the intramedullary canals, limited their widespread adoption. It was not until the late 1960s that artificial knees similar to those in use today were invented. The author was working on his PhD at Leeds University in England from 1966 to 1969 on the subject of human joint lubrication, at the same time as the start of the artificial knee, and has worked in the latter field until the present time.

A major aim of this book is to show how artificial knees reached the stage they are today and what makes them work well in the majority of cases. This requires explaining the basic principles of the designs, how the designs originated and evolved, and the interactions between the many individuals who participated. The

P. S. Walker, *The Artificial Knee*, https://doi.org/10.1007/978-3-030-38171-4_1

starting point occurred in the mid-1960s when the artificial hip had become successful. It was realized that the success was due to the combination of bearing materials with a high wear resistance and a biocompatible cement which would fix the components rigidly to the bones. But there was quite a difference between the structure and function of the hip and the knee. The hip was relatively simple, being a ball-in-socket with a fixed center of rotation. The knee on the other hand was far more complicated, relying on many structures for its stability, and capable of more movements than just a simple hinge. It was not surprising that the early designers reached several different solutions for an artificial knee. The first designs ranged from unicompartmental knees where small components resurfaced the femoral and bearing surfaces but all of the ligaments were preserved, to large components which resurfaced the entire bearing surfaces and where the cruciate ligaments were resected. Other designs were intermediate to these two extremes.

A striking observation is that the large majority of the artificial knees used today are of two design types which originated in the 1970s, just about 10 years after the very first designs. These two types are the cruciate retaining (CR), which retains only the posterior cruciate ligament, and the posterior stabilized (PS) where a cam provides stability but the cruciate ligaments are resected. The key question addressed in this book is: Why do these two types dominate the market, when it might be thought that, particularly since 1980, superior designs would have emerged and

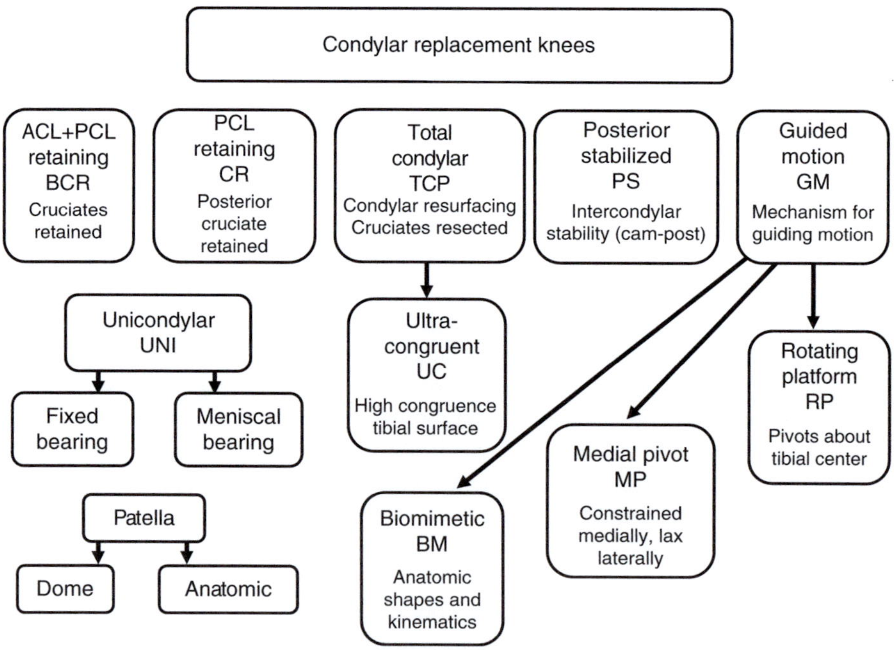

Fig. 1.1 The different types of condylar replacement artificial knees. ACL anterior cruciate ligament, PCL posterior cruciate ligament, BCR bi-cruciate replacement, CR posterior cruciate retaining, TCP Total Condylar prosthesis, PS posterior stabilized, GM guided motion

replaced the original ones? Could it be that the artificial knee had reached its limit such that the performance could only be improved incrementally? That would be surprising considering that since 1980 there has been a dramatic expansion in the knowledge of the biomechanics of the knee, major advances in materials and surgical techniques, and a vast number of follow-up studies on the functional outcomes, kinematics, wear, durability, and surgical technique. It is certainly true that this body of work has led to numerous improvements. Possibly the most important development has been polyethylene formulations which have substantially reduced the wear. Other developments have included refinements in component shapes, multiple sizes to provide a more accurate fit for each patient, and bearing surfaces with improved stability. Nevertheless the fact remains that the fundamental configurations and mechanics of the designs used most frequently today have not changed significantly since 1980.

While this book concentrates mainly on artificial knee design, the instrumentation and technique is also discussed, because this has a major effect on the outcomes. A similar observation as for artificial knees can be made about the instrumentation and technique; the majority of surgeries are performed with mechanical instruments which are based on the same principles of alignment as in 1980 and where the construction of the instruments is similar although allowing for greater adjustability. Computer-assisted surgery, which has been available for over a decade, is still used in only a small percentage of cases. That may be changing

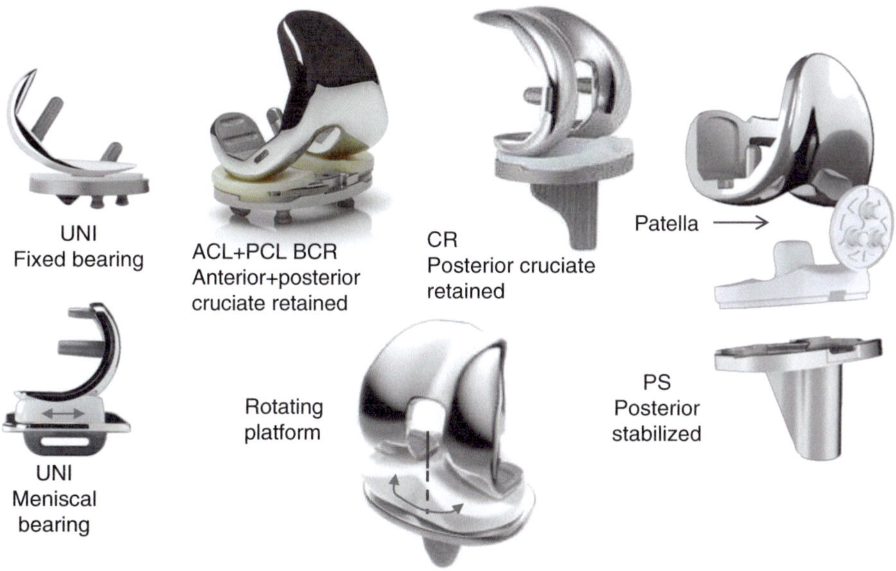

Fig. 1.2 The main types of artificial knee which had been developed by 1980. All designs, with the exception of the unis, have plastic patella components (arrow on the right). The medial pivot and the ultracongruent knees (not shown here) were developed after 1980. From 1980 to the present time, the majority of artificial knees used have been the CR and the PS

now that robotic equipment has been introduced, but adoption is still slow despite the advantages of accuracy of the bone cuts and soft tissue balancing.

Today, artificial knees are used in large numbers for the treatment of arthritis. According to a recent study, 966,000 cases were performed in the USA in 2017 (Idata Research 2017). While the large majority of the cases were primary artificial knees, revisions and unicompartmental knees were included. The numbers continue to increase year after year due to the increasing number of individuals with arthritis, particularly the "baby boomers" born between 1946 and 1964 who make up 29 percent of the population. There is also a great deal of emphasis today on the benefits of an active lifestyle, which increases the demand for artificial knees. The more widespread availability of the procedure is also a factor. This increased usage would not occur if the procedure was not successful. Based on joint registries from several countries, the failure rate of artificial knees is now very low, only about a half a percent per year on average. The failure rate is likely to become even lower due to the steady improvement in design, materials, surgical technique, and rehabilitation, as well as the education and specialization of orthopedic surgeons. In parallel with the improvements in durability, the functional results have improved also. Based on an extensive literature of follow-up studies, the majority of those with artificial knees are pain-free or experience only mild pain in certain activities and can carry out activities of everyday living. Many individuals can perform more strenuous activities including sports, although this is understandably related to overall condition, particularly muscle strength. A large percentage of individuals report that most of the time they forget that they have an artificial knee, but not to the same extent as for artificial hips.

This is not to say that the artificial knee procedure is without its problems. The most serious is infection, fortunately occurring in only a fraction of a percent of cases and which can usually be treated without removing the components. Instability is experienced in some cases, usually soon after the procedure, and if serious enough may require a component to be changed. Component loosening or fracture is a late failure mode, requiring revision surgery. Wearing out of the bearing surfaces, a common mode of failure in the early days of knee replacement, is now likely to be rare due to the much higher wear resistance of the new polyethylene bearing materials. The most common functional limitation of an artificial knee is that the range of flexion is not as high as in a normal knee, but is sufficient for most activities. Nonetheless getting in and out of an automobile and rising from low chairs may not be easy. Another limitation is that, while many patients can return home 1–2 days after the procedure and can walk shortly after, recovery can be uncomfortable and can take several weeks or even months.

Hence it can be claimed that about 50 years after they were first invented, artificial knees function well from a mechanical point of view. One of the early design principles was to minimize the stresses between interfacing surfaces which are loaded together, whether between the femoral and tibial components or between the components and the bone surfaces. This was emphasized by Alan Swanson, a Professor of Mechanical Engineering at Imperial College London, who worked with Michael Freeman, an orthopedic surgeon at the London

Hospital, on one of the first artificial knee designs in the late 1960s. A small pebble in a shoe causes pain due to the high local stresses. High heels can make an indentation in a soft surface. Everyone has experienced the discomfort of sitting on a hard flat surface for a long period of time. Reduce the stresses by removing the pebble, by wearing rubber-soled shoes, or by sitting on a cushion, and the problem is solved. In an artificial knee, if the contact stresses between the femoral and tibial components are too high, the plastic material will eventually fail due to deformation and wear. If a component is too small in area, the underlying trabecular bone will be overstressed causing it to gradually fail, leading to component subsidence. A principle such as minimizing stress needs to be incorporated into any type of artificial knee design.

The artificial knee itself consists of femoral, tibial, and patella components. Some components can have more than one separate part. For example, a tibial component usually consists of a polyethylene bearing fixed into a metal tibial tray, which is termed modularity. Each component has a bearing surface and an interface surface which connects to the bone. These surfaces can be further subdivided, an example being that the femoral component has a bearing surface that interfaces with the tibia, an area that interfaces with the patella, and a small area in between which interfaces with both. This description highlights another principle that the sliding surfaces must have the correct balance between stability and laxity. The stability must be sufficient to prevent excessive sliding movements which the patient would feel as instability. The laxity must be sufficient to allow sufficient rotation and flexion movements and to prevent a feeling of stiffness.

As well as the design of the artificial knee itself, the means of implanting the components must be considered. Principles apply just as much to the instrumentation and the technique as to the design itself. If the components are oriented to the bones incorrectly or if the components are not securely fixed to the bones, the knee may not function well or may prematurely fail. Hence the design of the instrumentation, the sizing and orientation of the components, and the way in which the fixation is implemented are all subject to satisfying certain principles if the artificial knee is to succeed. One example is that at the interface between the component and the bone, during loaded conditions, there must be minimal relative interface motion, or micromotion as it is called. The maximum micromotion tolerated is about one twentieth of a millimeter.

Finally, the patient is part of the equation. Although many aspects of the patient are outside of the control of the designer and the surgeon, the maximum functional level of the artificial knee and the time taken to achieve that stage can be strongly influenced by the instructions given to the patient and how well the patient follows those instructions. The quality and speed of recovery after the surgery can also be enhanced by the preparation in the weeks or months prior to the surgery. For example, reducing weight, stopping smoking, and strengthening muscles by exercise or physiotherapy prior to the surgery all benefit rehabilitation.

While sound principles are the basis of any design, they are not by themselves sufficient to guarantee success in practice. Before being able to confirm that a new design will be successful in a large population of patients, a field trial must be carried out. This applies to every new invention or product whether in medicine or in engineering. An automobile has numerous separate parts and systems, each of which will have been rigorously analyzed and tested prior to the model being released to the consumer. An essential part of the testing involves driving the vehicle under many conditions of road surfaces, climates, and driving styles. Because of this process, modern automobiles have few major flaws although some problems may emerge after product release, sometimes serious enough that a product recall is necessary. With an artificial knee joint, trials on a specified number of patients for a sufficient period of time are equivalent to testing an automobile on the open road.

In the early 1970s, a manufacturer could introduce a new artificial knee design to the market with few restrictions. Inevitably this led to early failures of some designs due to inadequate preclinical testing in the laboratory or lack of controlled clinical trials. Today the situation is completely different. For a total knee to be approved for clinical application, FDA requirements have to be met, consisting of an extensive menu of tests for wear, strength, and function, to demonstrate safety and efficacy. Nevertheless, even during the 1970s, when there was a proliferation of new designs and few controls, there was a progressive improvement in their performance, while unsuccessful design features were for the most part quickly weeded out. Even without regulations, it was in nobody's interest if a design performed poorly. The end result was that even before the end of the decade, several basic design forms had been developed that appeared to provide adequate function and showed no major problems, at least in the short term.

Not surprisingly, some failure modes took several years to become apparent. Wear of the polyethylene was one of these problems. It had been thought that because of the low wear rate in artificial hips, the same would apply to knees. What was different however was that in some knee designs, there was low conformity between the femoral and tibial bearing surfaces leading to high contact stresses. This led to accelerated wear, in some cases completely through the plastic layer. Another failure mode that took several years to recognize was component loosening due to inadequate bonding between the acrylic cement and the trabecular bone. This was due to insufficient penetration of cement into the spaces between the trabeculae, caused by not removing fluids and trabecular debris, applying the cement when it was too "doughy," and not applying enough pressure to force the cement into the bone. A further reason was that offset loading conditions could actually produce tensile stresses across part of the interface, pulling the cement out of the trabecular spaces.

Looked at from today's perspective, some of the deficiencies in the early designs may seem obvious. But at that time, personal computers were not yet invented, nor software for design, analysis, and modeling. Not only that, but biomechanical knowledge such as the forces acting in activities, the kinematics and what controlled it, and the geometry and mechanical properties of the tissues of the knee, was basic and fragmentary. Designing a component which became an integral part of an anatomical structure such as the knee was unfamiliar territory. The shapes of the implants and the instruments for an artificial knee needed to account for the anatomy, the boundaries imposed by the tissues, and the exposure at surgery. Many surgeons were not familiar with engineering principles, such as the concepts of stress and strain, forces and moments, elastic modulus, and tensile and compressive strength, although possibly so in a conceptual or intuitive way. Finally, relatively few testing methods had been developed for the evaluation of new design concepts.

Those challenges were steadily overcome, particularly where there was close collaboration between surgeons and engineers. A number of the early artificial knee designs were surprisingly successful due to the application of engineering, anatomic, and surgical principles. The process typically started with design ideas which originated from discussions between the surgeon and the engineer. These ideas would then have to satisfy both engineering and surgical principles at the same time. A component that could not be easily inserted into the knee would be rejected, as well as a means of fixation to the bone which would overstress certain areas of the bone. There would be agreement that surgical instruments needed to produce correct lower limb alignment for uniform force distribution and ligament balancing. Certain decisions had to be deferred pending the results of analysis or experiment, for which the methodologies had to be devised.

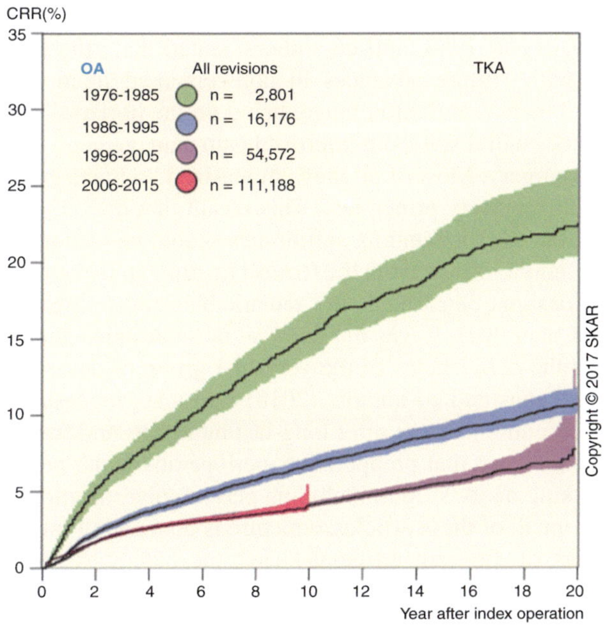

Fig. 1.3 Cumulative revision rates for artificial knee joints (not including unicompartmental) for four periods of 10 years. The revisions are for any reason. The revisions for the two latest 10-year periods are much less than for the first periods. The solid colors indicate the confidence intervals. Most of the cases were for osteoarthritis. Female/male ratios were about 60/40. Seventy hospitals participated. Infection accounted for just less than 1% of revisions. There were small percentages of cases where the patella was resurfaced and where uncemented components were used. Three designs of condylar replacement knees from major companies dominated the usage. (Reprinted with permission from the Swedish Knee Arthroplasty Registry, Otto Robertsson et al. 2017)

The history of the development of the artificial knee has been described in a number of well-illustrated articles and book chapters (Riley 1976; Murray 1991; Ranawat and Ranawat 2012; Robinson 2005; Amendolo et al. 2012; Papas et al. 2018). It is interesting to compare the authors' appraisals of the current status of the artificial knee and predictions for the future, with due regard to the dates of the articles. Lee Riley (1976), co-designer of one of the first metal-plastic total knees, stated that "cobalt-chrome alloy and high-density polyethylene were acceptable materials….and could be firmly fixed with methylmethacrylate. A wide range of prosthetic units are available which will provide acceptable clinical results if used within their design limits." David G Murray (1991), co-designer of an early rotating knee, thought that current techniques for primary knees will provide excellent results in 90% of cases. "An understanding of what has gone before is essential in planning effectively for the future." Raymond Robinson (2005), in a thorough review, charted the time sequence of the different designs and demonstrated the interplay between the inventors. Robinson interviewed numerous individuals who were involved with these early developments. He concluded that collaboration between specialists in different areas had produced successful artificial knees which preserved cruciates or which substituted by a cam mechanism, each type with mobile bearing options. Chitranjan Ranawat (2012), who organized the foundation of The Knee Society in 1983, and co-authors, stated that "the future of TKA is indeed bright," with "future advances in non-cemented fixation, wear-resistant polyethylene, and increased flexion range, being on the horizon." They considered that better outcomes will result from improved pain management, computer navigation, and robotic surgery. Most of all they emphasized "refined surgical techniques based on sound arthroplasty principles." This meant that not only should the bone cuts be accurate, but the surrounding soft tissues should be well preserved and balanced. Luca Amendola (2012), from the Rizzoli Institute in Bologna, focused on the most successful designs, illustrated with remarkable semi-transparent images produced by Fabio Catani MD. It was implied that these designs emerged by learning the lessons from the deficiencies of the very first group of designs from the early 1970s. Recently, Papas and co-authors (2018) said that "modern arthroplasty has evolved into a procedure that can offer long-lasting results and functional improvements." They pointed out that preoperative, perioperative, and postoperative management was making major strides, including periarticular injections to reduce pain and swelling. From all of these articles, a picture is obtained of interaction between multiple inventors of different artificial knees, the outcomes steadily improving over time, leading to the successful designs available today.

Moving now to the organization of the book, the chapters are written as a progression from one topic to the next, although each chapter can be read individually. For that reason, there is a certain amount of repetition in the different chapters, but this has been kept to a minimum. References are cited at the end of each chapter, so that the chapters are self-contained. The number of references has been kept to a minimum to avoid too much distraction from the text itself, and if preferred, the reader can go through the text without stopping to look at any of the references themselves. Today, there is a voluminous body of literature on almost every topic, and an exhaustive listing would have been prohibitive. The selection basis for the early work was to search out the first articles dealing with the design and clinical evaluation. For longer-term evaluations, recent reviews or meta-analyses were favored, together with a selection of the highest-quality individual articles. In an effort to avoid bias, articles with different conclusions were also selected.

On the question of "who invented things first," unless clear-cut, there is no attempt to specify this. The reason is that there was a great deal of interaction between early inventors, and while certain individuals can be credited with particular designs or ideas, the many exchanges and collaborations between those in the field were influencing factors. There were various time intervals between first originating a design, lecturing about it, publishing an article, and carrying out the first surgeries. In some cases, a design was produced by a manufacturer immediately; in other cases, the designer found it difficult to interest a manufacturer, resulting in a long delay.

An attempt has been made to be as objective as possible in presenting the material in this book. However there is inevitably more detail of work the author was personally involved with, simply because more detail was available. A lot of information about some of the early inventions is no longer available and hence could not be adequately covered. In addition, much of the early work was not fully described in publications. This is in marked contrast to today where there is a steady stream of publications to the point where it is difficult to absorb it all. One source of bias in the book may be that much of the work described is from England, particularly the early work, and then, later, from the USA. At the same time, there was a great deal of innovative work on artificial knees in Europe and Japan. Some of this work may be underrepresented. Indeed, one of the very earliest condylar knee designs was invented in Japan. In basic research, Scandinavia and Northern Europe are well-known for basic research in artificial knees, from the RSA method developed in Lund, Sweden, to the iterative finite element modeling from Nijmegen, in the Netherlands.

The figures are not referred to directly in the text, although they are placed in relevant positions. There are two reasons for this. Firstly, the text is written as a continuous narrative, not requiring any illustration. Secondly, the figures together with their explicit captions can be looked at individually without having to refer to the text. In this way, the figures provide additional perspective. Many of the figures are photographs of individuals in the field, almost all taken by the author, usually at conferences. Some of the pictures were taken in the 1960s, others very recently, providing a perspective of the extended timespan of the field of artificial knees. A number of figures were kindly provided by colleagues and are acknowledged. Permissions from publishers were received for all figures reproduced from articles.

Terminology is not easy in a book such as this. The usual word to describe an artificial knee is a total knee arthroplasty (TKA) or total knee. I have mostly used the term artificial knee, because it is more colloquial and it conveys any type from a unicompartmental to a hinge. Acronyms have been minimized in the text, although terms such as CR and PS quickly become used more frequently. At the end of the book, there is a detailed glossary, while at the front, there is a figure showing all parts of the knee.

The idea of writing a book on the artificial knee originated in late 2015. Because of the success of several different types of design, it seemed that an explanation of the engineering principles behind the designs would be a useful focus. Initially a lecture was created on this theme and first presented at the Insall Traveling Fellows annual meeting in 2016, organized by Norman Scott MD. From there, planning for the book commenced. To obtain the initial material, the author carried out personal interviews with early pioneers in the field or with those who were associated with them. These were (in alphabetical order) Bob Averill, David Blaha MD, Peter Bullough MD, Al Burstein PhD, Michael Freeman FRCS, Bill Krause PhD, John O'Connor PhD, Jim Pritchett MD, Chit Ranawat MD, Norman Scott MD, Bahaa Seedhom PhD, and Alan Swanson PhD. The first interview was with Alan Swanson in June 2017, at the Institution of Mechanical Engineers in London, England. The methodology for the interviews was to formulate questions derived from their early publications, or from direct knowledge of their work, and then to carry out a face-to-face interview which was recorded. Many other individuals were contacted by email or personally and provided valuable information on specific areas, for which the author is grateful. I particularly thank Thomas Einhorn MD who provided overviews about various aspects of the book and reviewed some of the material. Many new insights and information were uncovered during all of these exchanges such as the original ideas and how the ideas came about, factors often not well explained in early publications. The interviews were particularly revealing, especially as such a long time had elapsed since the time of the early work until now. Some of these pioneers are still active in orthopedics today, while others are pursuing endeavors in other areas.

The author is still involved with artificial knee experimentation and design, working in an academic setting. It needs to be stressed that the book is written from the perspective of a biomechanical engineer who has not performed any surgeries nor formally examined patients in a clinic. Surgeons who specialize in artificial knees will typically perform up to several hundred surgeries each year and over the course of several decades will follow up thousands of patients. This will result in a perspective that cannot be experienced by an engineer. Nevertheless, the material in this book has been accumulated since 1966 at the start of the author's PhD research work. Being supervised by Duncan Dowson and Verna Wright at Leeds University in England was a unique experience at a special time in the field of the biomechanics of joints. There was the opportunity for interaction with pioneers in the field in England, such as John Scales, Michael Freeman, Alan Swanson, John O'Connor, and Peter Bullough, but the person who stands out the most, understandably, was John Charnley. He, more than anybody else, started off the entire field of artificial joints. It was always a distinct honor to meet him at his Hip Center in Wrightington or at conferences in England or the USA.

In 1969, after completion of a PhD, the author had the privilege of being employed at the Hospital for Special Surgery in New York. I owe the deepest thanks to Harlan C Amstutz MD for this opportunity. Artificial hips were already being used at the Hospital, mainly through the efforts of Philip D Wilson Jr MD and Harlan Amstutz. This led to the interest in developing an artificial knee,

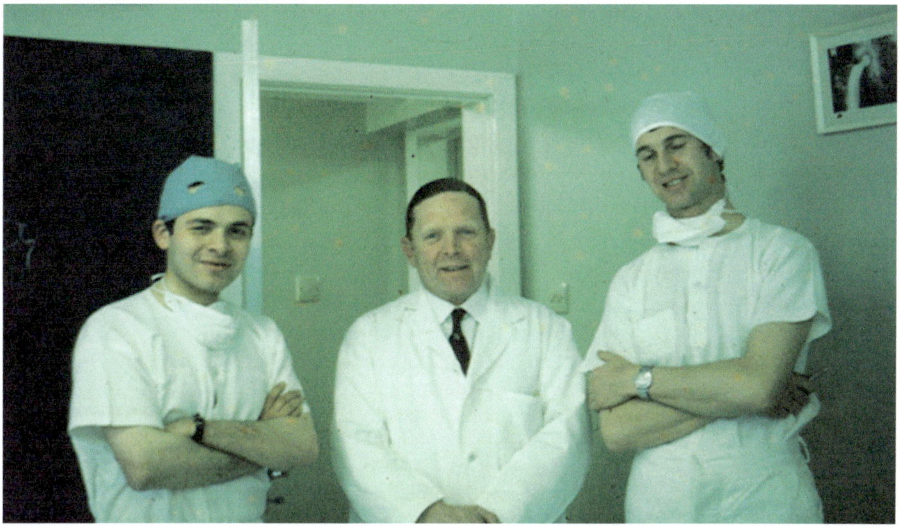

Fig. 1.4 John Charnley (center) welcomed visitors to his Hip Center at Wrightington Hospital in England and was interested in discussing all aspects of hip replacement and other orthopedic topics. In about 1967, Bahaa Seedhom (left) and Peter Walker (right) visited to observe a total hip operation, where the new laminar air flow unit was being used. The visit included a lab visit in which wear tests of materials were in progress, and new instruments were being developed. (©Peter S Walker)

work in this area already having started in England. Robert Lee Patterson MD and Philip D Wilson Jr MD, successive Chiefs of Orthopaedics, provided a supportive environment for the goal of developing artificial knees and other joints. The author worked primarily with Drs. Chit Ranawat, John Insall, and Alan Inglis on this endeavor, as well as with Fellows and Residents. After leaving the Hospital for Special Surgery, the author worked at Cintor in Boston (now part of J&J); Howmedica in New Jersey; Brigham & Women's Hospital in Boston, affiliated with Harvard Medical School and MIT; the Royal National Orthopaedic Hospital in Stanmore, affiliated with University College London; and finally New York University Langone Orthopedic Hospital where Joseph Zuckerman MD, Department Chairman, has provided a stimulating academic environment in which to work since 2003 for which I am grateful.

During all of this time, the author has participated in the Orthopaedic Research Society (ORS) and the American Academy of Orthopaedic Surgeons (AAOS) almost every single year since 1969. The Knee Society, founded in 1983, has been a constant source of education and insights through its distinguished members. Other notable society conferences have included the International Society for Technology in Arthroplasty (ISTA) and Computer-Assisted Orthopaedic Surgery (CAOS), as well as the European Society of Biomechanics (ESB) and the European Orthopaedic Research Society (EORS). But it has been the innumerable contacts and discussions with individuals in the field which has been the most valuable and provided the most personal pleasure.

I thank Minette Gorelik, my assistant, for typing the many revisions of each chapter; Albright Djokoto, a student at New York University, for navigating EndNote and RightsLink, as well as a lot of typing; and David DeSimone, librarian at NYU Langone Orthopedic Hospital, for advice on references and sources.

Most of all I thank my wife Wuliang for traveling with me to numerous conferences, for participating in every interview, for meticulously reviewing every chapter, and for making it possible for me to complete this book.

References

Amendola L, Tigani D, Fosco M, Dallari D. History of condylar total knee arthroplasty. In: Recent advances in hip and knee arthroplasty: InTechOpen; 2012. https://doi.org/10.5772/28203.

Brand RA, Mont MA, Manring MM. Biographical sketch: Themistocles Gluck (1853-1942). Clin Orthop Relat Res. 2011;469(6):1525–7.

iData Research. Total knee replacement statistics 2017: Younger patients driving growth. 18 July 2018.

Murray DG. In: Laskin RS, editor. History of total knee replacement, Total knee replacement. Basel, Switzerland: Springer; 1991. p. 3–15.

Papas PV, Cushner FD, Scuderi GR. The history of total knee arthroplasty. Tech Orthop. 2018;33(1):2–6.

Ranawat A, Ranawat C. The history of total knee arthroplasty. In: The knee joint: Springer; 2012. p. 699–707.

Riley LH Jr. The evolution of total knee arthroplasty. Clin Orthop Relat Res. 1976;120:7–10.

Robertsson O, Sundberg M, Lidgren L, W-Dahl A. The Swedish knee arthroplasty. Annu Rep. 2017.

Robinson RP. The early innovators of today's resurfacing condylar knees. J Arthroplast. 2005;20(1 Suppl 1):2–26.

Early Biomechanical Knowledge 2

What Was Known About Knee Biomechanics by 1970?

In the context of the advances which had been made in engineering technology in general, it may seem surprising that artificial joints for the hip and the knee were not invented until the 1960s. After all, these devices seem simple enough, consisting only of two main components which are fixed firmly to the bones, providing a low-friction and wear-resistant bearing. For thousands of years, simple journal bearings consisting of a rotating shaft in fixed bearings have been used in carts and carriages, while a basic form of rolling element bearings consisting of rows of logs was used for transporting enormous stones. Between 1498 and 1500, Leonardo da Vinci invented a ball bearing where spheres were captured in cages, producing continuous rotation by rolling rather than sliding, reducing both friction and wear. Successful bearings were routinely used in many types of transportation. The Stockton and Darlington steam trains started running in 1825, Ford's production line was assembling automobiles from 1913, while the first commercial airplane flight was in 1914. Treating arthritis of the joints was regarded as a medical problem, and it seems that there was little involvement of technical experts who could have contributed to devising practical solutions.

Joint Lubrication

The history of how different types of bearing evolved over time has been described in an epic book called the *History of Tribology* by Duncan Dowson (1998), tribology being the science of friction, lubrication, and wear. The book was a late project of Duncan Dowson, who from the mid-1960s was Professor of Tribology at Leeds University in England and a pioneer in elastohydrodynamic lubrication. In his book, Dowson included the topic of human joint lubrication because it was quite unlike anything which had been devised in engineering. The exceedingly low friction in animal joints was first measured in experiments performed in the

P. S. Walker, *The Artificial Knee*, https://doi.org/10.1007/978-3-030-38171-4_2

late 1950s (McCutchen 1962). The hypothesis was that in weight-bearing conditions, water in the cartilage will be squeezed out due to the high pressure, forming a thin film of water in between the opposing cartilage bearing surfaces. This water film will result in almost frictionless sliding, the mechanism being called "weeping lubrication." In addition, the slippery synovial fluid, which is present in the joint, will protect the bearing surfaces when the weeping mechanism was not operative. In the 1960s, stimulated by McCutcheon's work, experiments by other researchers led to alternate theories being advanced with esoteric names: squeeze-film lubrication, boundary lubrication, elastohydrodynamic lubrication, and boosted lubrication by synovial fluid entrapment and enrichment. All of these mechanisms could operate during the different functional conditions of human joints, augmented by complex macromolecular interactions at the surfaces (Jahn et al. 2016). However, the weeping lubrication theory, which can be likened to walking on a film of water, has considerable appeal. Its proponent, Charles McCutcheon, was convincing and persuasive in promoting it.

Dowson was intrigued by the extremely low friction which had been measured in human joints, together with the durability of the cartilage bearing material which lasted for a lifetime in the majority of people. This signified that the bearing surfaces were separated by a fluid film, but how could such a film be sustained in a bearing which operated at such low sliding speeds and where the sliding direction kept reversing? Dowson applied his theories to the problem and found that while fluid films were predicted under certain operating conditions, much of the time there would be boundary lubrication. It had been recognized that other factors were involved in protecting the bearing surfaces from damage: the porosity of the articular cartilage, the hyaluronate constituents of the synovial fluid, and macromolecular boundary effects. Could studies of human joints be applied in some way to the design of novel bearings, possibly for resurfacing the arthritic joint? In 1966 Duncan Dowson connected with Verna Wright, a Professor of Rheumatology at Leeds University, to establish the "Bioengineering Group for the Study of Human Joints." Among the first graduates were Peter Walker, Tony Unsworth, and Bahaa Seedhom. This was one of the early examples of a collaboration between engineering and medical departments, to conduct basic research and solve practical problems with a multidisciplinary approach. The activity was renamed as the Institute for Medical and Biological Engineering and directed from 1993 to 2016 by Professor John Fisher, who made the Institute into one of the leading centers on the tribology of artificial joints.

Failure of the joint lubrication was seen as one of the major causes of osteoarthritis of joints. For the knee, there were associated problems of instability of the joint and misalignment of the limb. The solutions for knee arthritis in the mid-1960s were debridement, osteotomy, tibial plateau replacement, femoral condyle resurfacing, patella resurfacing, and metal hinges. The material used for the implants was mainly cobalt-chrome-molybdenum alloy, trade name Vitallium. This material was well tolerated and had high strength and wear resistance. The main limitation of all these treatments was lack of complete pain relief and sometimes residual instability. Lack of rigid fixation of the implants to the bone was a frequent cause of failure, causing pain and bone resorption.

Joint Biomechanics

To design a successful artificial knee, knowledge of the biomechanics of the knee both in normal and arthritic conditions was needed. While in the hip joint, the ball-in-socket arrangement could be easily reproduced mechanically, for the knee, the mechanics were far from simple and were not well understood. Even though biomechanical studies had been carried out in Europe in the nineteenth and early twentieth centuries, this work was not widely known because of its being written in German and French and published in documents which were only accessible to specialists. Due to the efforts of Vera Pinskerova, Paul Maquet, Robert Furlong, and Michael Freeman, the content of much of this work was translated into English and summarized (Pinskerova et al. 2003). Many of the findings from this work could have been directly applied to artificial knee design.

Starting with the basic studies of the geometry of the joint surfaces, this would have application to the design of resurfacing components. The sagittal outline of the medial femoral condyle was described by a posterior-distal circular arc and a distal-anterior circular arc of larger radius, with a tangent point between the two arcs at about 30 degrees of flexion. On extending the knee, the anterior arc articulated against the distal-anterior tibial surface, elevating the femur on the tibia, acting as a gravity brake to hyperextension as well as tightening soft tissues. As the knee was flexed from a fully extended position, there was always an internal rotation of the tibia about its own long axis. This caused the lateral femoral condyle to displace posteriorly on the tibial plateau, whereas the medial femoral condyle remained at almost the same location on the tibial surface. The lateral and medial menisci moved with the femoral condyles. As seen on the upper surface of the tibia, the center of the internal rotation was located on the medial side. Hence there could be considered to be two simultaneous rotations as the knee was flexed, flexion of the tibia about a transverse axis through the center of the femoral condyles and an internal rotation of the femur about a medial vertical axis through the tibia. The role of the cruciate ligaments was described as a four-bar linkage, where at least some of the fibers of the anterior and posterior cruciate were taut at all flexion angles, thereby guiding the motion of the femur on the tibia. There was however little explanation of how the internal rotation of the tibia was guided. Had this early work been known when the first artificial knees were designed in the late 1960s and early 1970s, the designs may have been very different from what they were. In particular, it is likely that the artificial knees would have been asymmetric, with a more stable medial side and a more mobile lateral side and with some mechanism for causing the posterior displacement of the lateral femoral condyle during flexion.

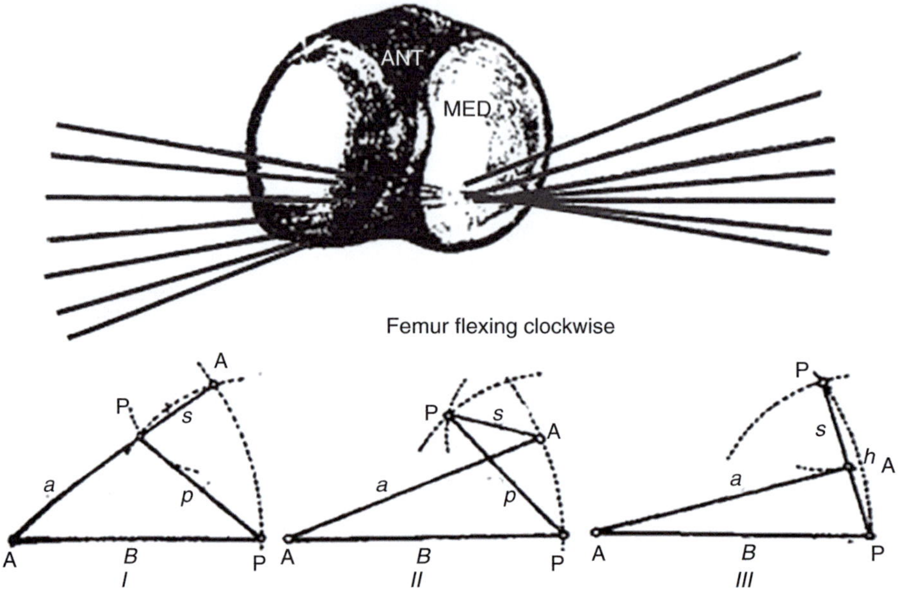

Fig. 2.1 Biomechanical studies in the nineteenth and early twentieth centuries. Top: Albert fixed the tibia, passed a rod through the femoral epicondylar axis, and, at 90-degree flexion, traced the rod as the femur was rotated internally and externally. A medial axis is seen. Bottom: Zuppinger proposed that the cruciate ligaments guided knee motion like a four-bar linkage. However it was later pointed out that this is an approximation because the ligaments do not remain uniformly taut throughout flexion (Pinskerova et al. 2003). (Reprinted with permission Clinical Orthopaedics & Related Research)

A landmark study was published in 1941 by Brantigan and Voshell from the University of Maryland School of Medicine. Although the paper was entitled "The Mechanics of the Ligaments and Menisci of the Knee Joint," rather than explaining the knee in mechanical terms, the authors focused on the anatomy first and how that controlled the mechanics. The authors were motivated to carry out this work due to the confusion in the field at the time: "a study of the literature on this subject leaves one bewildered." No less than 100 knee specimens were studied. One original aspect of the work was that the ligaments were treated as broad structures where different parts could loosen and tighten and where extremes of positions occurred gradually due to the strain-stiffening characteristics of the ligaments and menisci. The loosening of the lateral collateral ligament as flexion proceeded was noted, together with

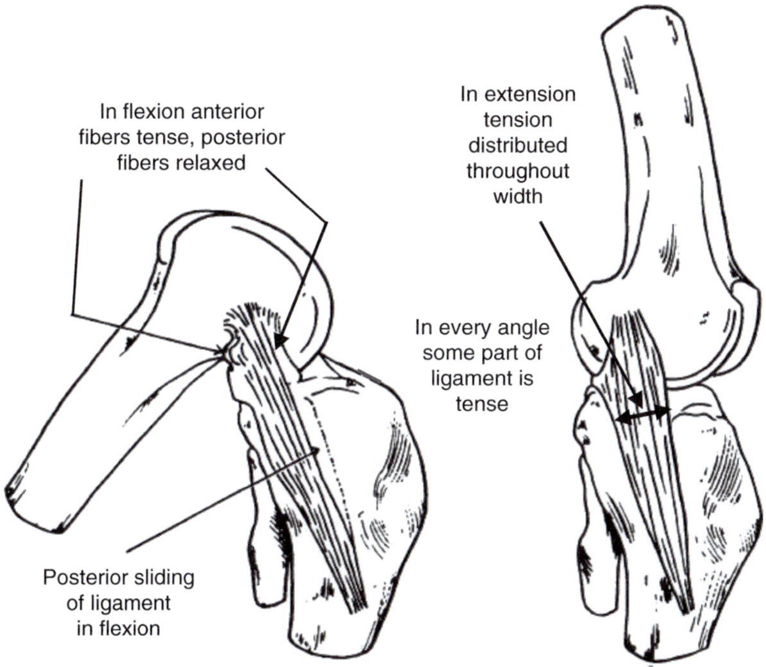

Fig. 2.2 Concepts of ligament function applied to the medial collateral ligament which consists of multiple fibers. The fibers are tensed by different relative amounts during the flexion range. This implies that the stiffness of the ligament varies with flexion angle. These concepts have important application to computer modeling of the knee (Brantigan and Voshell 1941). (Reprinted with permission from Journal of Bone & Joint Surgery A)

extreme posterior displacement of the lateral femoral condyle. In function, muscle and body weight forces restrained varus-valgus motion. The menisci were observed to cushion the contacts in hyperextension and in full flexion: "Motion of the menisci gave good evidence that the medial femoral condyle acts more nearly as the axis of rotation of the knee joint." "Some portion of the medial collateral ligament is taut in all places of extension and flexion." "It is hardly possible to give one or more separate or definite functions to any one ligament." These findings are remarkably consistent with those of the earlier European work described above, but with an additional perspective from an anatomic standpoint.

While an understanding of the anatomy and internal mechanics of the knee is essential, the functional aspects in activity are equally important. Outstanding research on the mechanics of locomotion was published in 1947, entitled

"Fundamental Studies of Human Locomotion and Other Information Relating to Design of Artificial Limbs." The work was supervised by Professor H. D. Eberhart, the Professor of Civil Engineering, University of California at Berkeley, and by VerneInman, Professor of Orthopaedics, University of California in San Francisco. The concept was to "bridge the gap between the engineering and medical phases." The work was commissioned by the National Research Council to advance the design of artificial limbs, for which there was a substantial need following the Second World War. The available designs of artificial limbs were not functioning well, and trial-and-error methods had failed to make substantial improvements. Much of the research consisted of motion analysis of level walking and stair climbing, where displacements and rotations in all planes were measured. For the knee during walking, it was found that there was a relative internal-external rotation between the femur and tibia averaging 9 degrees. A major conclusion of the study was: "Restrictions placed upon the normal transverse rotations will, to varying degrees, modify the synchrony and rhythm of walking. The awkwardness and

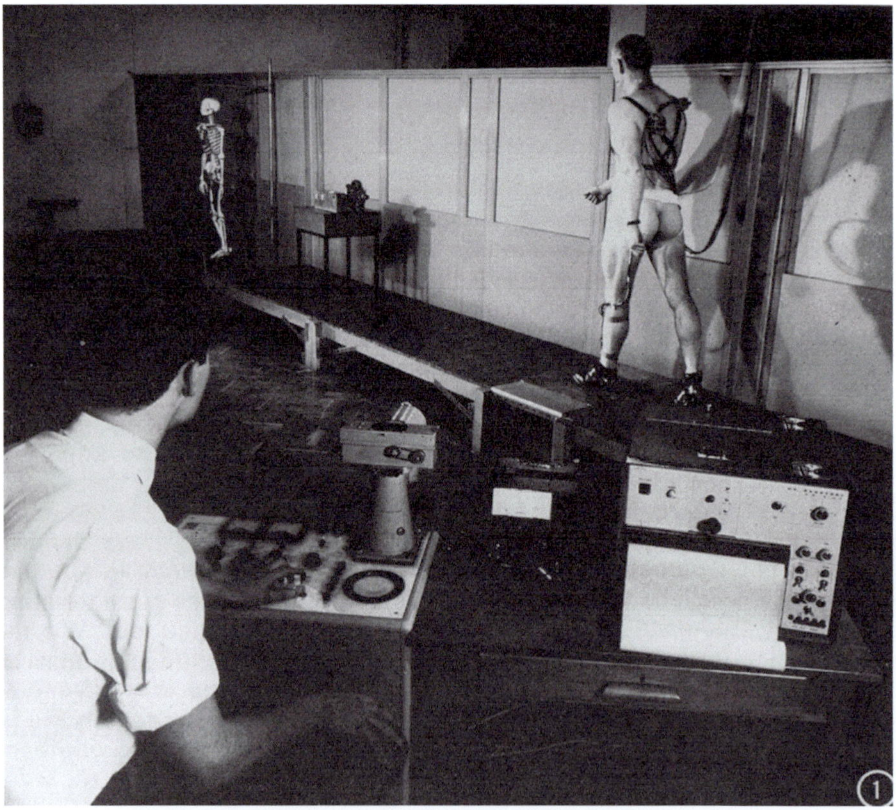

Fig. 2.3 An early gait laboratory developed in the Department of Mechanical Engineering at the University of California, Berkeley, by Professor HD Eberhart PhD and Dr. Verne Inman MD, PhD. The purpose was to study human locomotion with application to the design of prosthetics for lower limb amputees (Eberhart and Inman 1947)

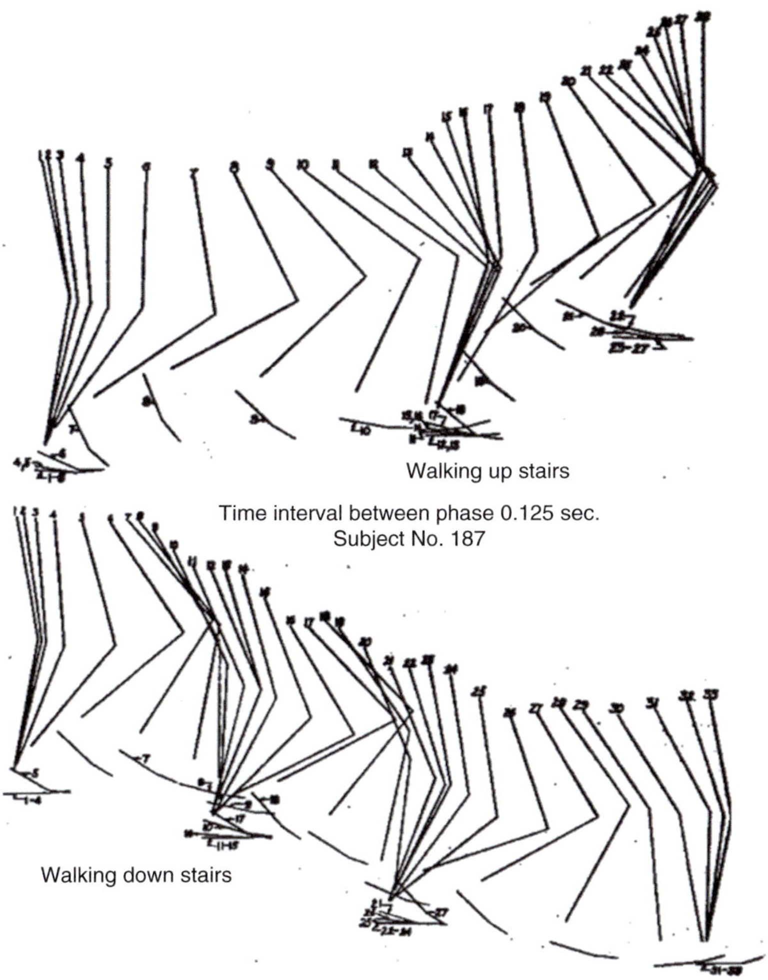

Fig. 2.4 Stick figures produced by Eberhart and Inman showing the successive angles of flexion in ascending and descending stairs. In both cases, the maximum flexion angles exceeded 90 degrees (Eberhart and Inman 1947)

discomfort of a subject required to wear a leg brace, which does not provide for rotations at the hip, knee, and foot, are no doubt due, in part, to the restriction of these motions." Ground-to-foot forces, both vertical and shear forces, were measured using specially designed force plates. Electromyography was used to determine muscle recruitment in the different phases of the activities. This data was used to estimate the peak forces in the knee during walking at twice body weight although details of the calculations were not provided. Some of the work was made available in a publication in 1953 (Saunders et al. 1953), but the full extent of the work was only published in a special report in 1947 to the National Research Council. Fortunately the work was continued over many years, and eventually the

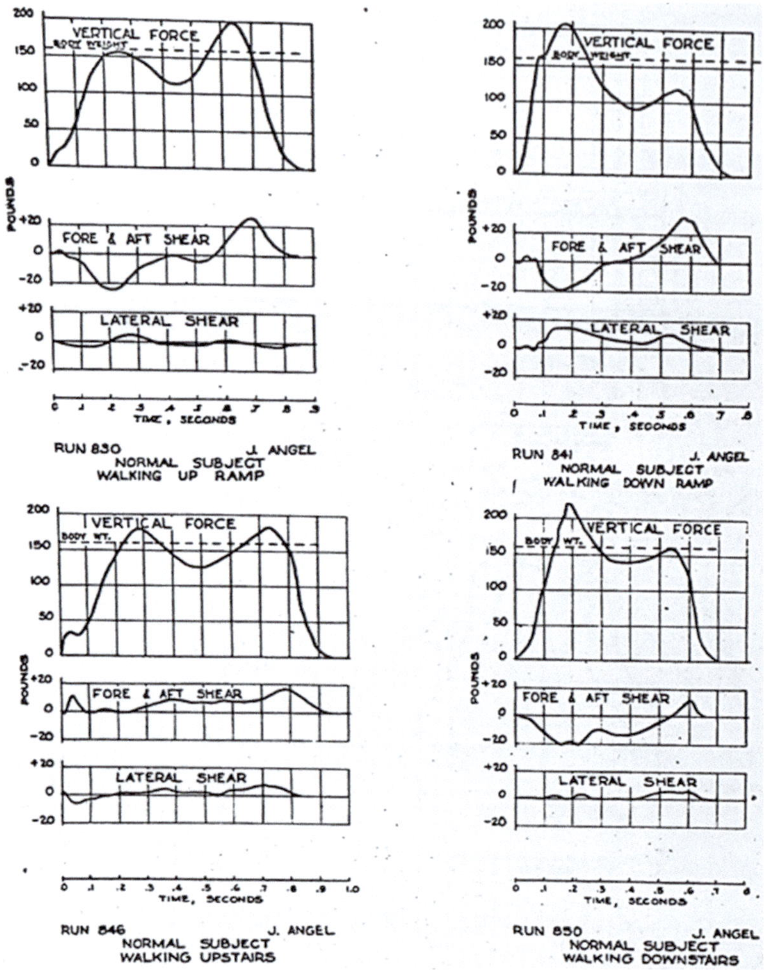

Fig. 2.5 Using advanced force plate design, Eberhart and Inman were able to measure the force components between the foot and the ground during different activities. Force peaks at heel strike and toe-off were clearly shown. The forces within the knee joint (estimated to be at least two body weights) are increased due to muscle forces. The fore and aft forces were small but still significant in that they are indicative of the shear forces within the knee joint (Eberhart and Inman 1947)

main findings were compiled in a book entitled *Human Walking* (Inman et al. 1981). The book contained superb mechanical depictions of the lower limb in various activities showing flexion angles and muscle action.

Only a few years later, in 1955, Arthur Steindler, Professor of Orthopaedic Surgery at the State University of Iowa (Buckwalter 2000), published a book entitled *Kinesiology of the Human Body* (Steindler 1955) where he described basic biomechanical principles of joint function. He defined rolling and sliding motions in the knee and pointed out that contacts were not points but areas of contact due to the deformability of the articular cartilage. He illustrated the structure of bones and joints and showed how muscles acted at certain lever arms from the joint centers. Motions of limb segments were described as open chain or closed chain depending on whether the foot was anchored to the ground or not. While Steindler did not reference any studies on these topics, it is clear that he used his intuitive knowledge based on insightful experience over many decades of orthopedic practice.

By the early 1960s, knowledge of the anatomy and properties of the major structures around the knee was sufficient to provide a general understanding of the mechanical function. The tubular structure of the long bones transmitted axial loads while providing adequate bending strength. At the knee joint, the expansions of the femoral and tibial condyles, composed of trabecular bone with a thin cortical shell, served several functions. In the frontal plane, the condyles were sufficiently wide such that varus-valgus moments could be supported with condylar lift-off occurring only under extreme conditions. The posterior projections of the femoral condyles provided enough clearance from the posterior tibial plateaus to allow for a high range of flexion. This is particularly evident during kneeling, when a flexion angle approaching 180 degrees can be achieved by some individuals. But even with the large surface areas of the femoral and tibial condyles and their smooth contours, the joint could not function as a bearing if the surfaces were bone. The contact areas would be too small due to the high modulus of elasticity of bone, leading to small contact areas and very high contact stresses. This would produce high bone-on-bone friction, high local temperatures, and stick-slip motion producing a jerky action. To prevent these problems, the bony condylar surfaces are covered with a material specialized as a bearing, articular cartilage. Remarkably, 3–5 mm layers of this material on the tibial and femoral condyles, as well as on the patella, provide smooth low-friction motion with minimal surface damage during multiple activities for the lifetime of most individuals.

But low friction itself would be insufficient in creating a long-lasting knee joint. In the hip joint, the ball-in-socket bearing surfaces are close to being fully conforming resulting in large contact areas and low contact stresses which are readily sustained by the articular cartilage (Greenwald and O'Connor 1971). However, in the knee, the lack of conformity between the femoral and tibial condyles would produce contact areas which were too small, producing high contact stresses which would eventually cause failure of the cartilage. It might be asked why the knee does not have closely conforming bearing surfaces as in the hip joint. The likely explanation is that the knee joint requires a high range of flexion as well as the ability for some internal and external rotation, to allow for maneuverability of the leg. A conforming uniaxial joint would not be adequate. Another requirement is that the knee needs to prevent side-to-side bending, which is not easy considering the knee is located at the center of a very long beam, the lower extremity. This is achieved by the large muscle forces across the knee which press the lateral and medial condyles of the femur against the plateaus of the tibia. A requirement in the knee joint itself is how to allow for high flexion and internal-external rotation while maintaining large areas of contact. The answer is the menisci which are interposed between the femoral and

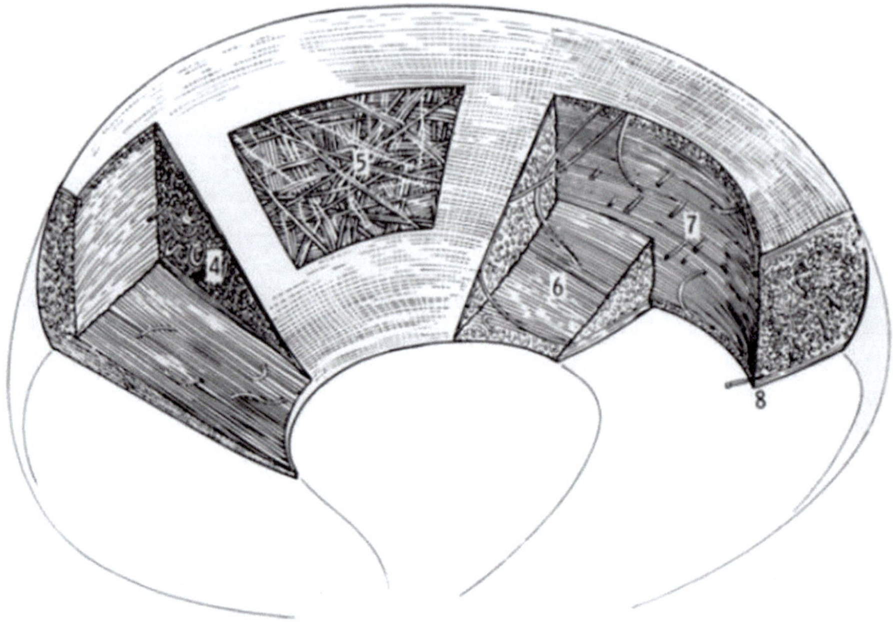

Fig. 2.6 Reconstruction of the fiber pattern of the meniscus. Histological sections of the meniscus in different planes were taken and viewed in polarized light, from which the directions of the collagen fibers were deduced. Because most fibers are circumferential and the high tensile strength of the material, it was suggested that the meniscus has a weight-bearing function between the femur and the tibia. Such forces would have the effect of radially expanding the meniscus, causing circumferential tension (Bullough et al. 1970). (Reprinted with permission from Journal of Bone & Joint Surgery B)

tibial condyles. Because of the deformability of the menisci and their loose peripheral attachments to the proximal tibia, they are able to change their shape and position according to the location of the femur on the tibia. This is particularly so on the lateral side where the femoral condyle slides over the convex surface of the tibia, in contrast to the medial side where the tibial surface is somewhat dished and limits the sliding motion.

The mechanical functions of the menisci were proposed as long ago as 1961 by Barnett, Davies, and MacConaill in their textbook dealing with the structure and functions of synovial joints:

- Shock absorption protecting the articular cartilage
- Increasing the congruity between the articular surfaces and increasing the stability of the joint
- Allowing a continuation of different movements of the joint
- Prevention of undue forward gliding of the femur on the tibia, analogous to a chock under a wheel

- Distribution of the weight across the joint by increasing the effective area of contact
- Assisting in the lubrication of the joint

These propositions were based mainly on anatomic studies. At that time, suitable experimental methodologies for determining the internal mechanics of the knee had not been developed. But the insights of the authors are remarkable in that they were all supported by subsequent experimental work after about 1970.

The first of such studies actually proposed that the menisci were weight-bearing because the tibial cartilage beneath them was always well preserved, which could only occur if the cartilage was loaded (Bullough et al. 1970). Additional support for this theory was that the collagen fibers in the meniscus were predominately circumferential indicating that the meniscus was resisting radial expansion. Meanwhile in the 1960s, it was common practice for surgeons to remove damaged menisci, in order to treat the pain and "catching," not realizing that there might be serious consequences (Smillie 1967). Surprisingly, degeneration of the cartilage surfaces due to the elevated contact stresses and the increased sliding on the bearing surfaces usually took several decades to become evident (Jackson 1968; Lanzer and Komenda 1990).

It was realized by designers of the early artificial knees that reproducing the complex structure and composition of articular cartilage and the menisci was beyond the capabilities of materials science at that time, which still holds true today. Nevertheless metal-on-polyethylene, already being used in artificial hip joints, could still provide a bearing with a low friction coefficient of about 0.1 compared with 0.01 of cartilage, as well as a low wear rate. It was interesting however that in the early 1980s, artificial knees with sliding meniscus components were designed, but using cobalt-chrome alloy and high molecular weight polyethylene, rather than materials with more deformability.

In the anatomic knee, if the cartilage surfaces provided almost frictionless sliding and the menisci reduced the contact stresses, the motion and stability were seen to be controlled by the major ligaments. During flexion-extension, at least some of the fibers in each ligament appeared to be taut, which led to the impression that the ligaments guided the motion in a well-defined and reproducible way. However, this was mainly conjecture, as up to the mid-1960s, there had been no controlled experiments carried out to measure the length-tension relations of the ligaments. Mechanical materials testing machines were only starting to be used in the field of orthopedic biomechanics. Nor was there any data of the forces acting across the knee, particularly the shear forces, in different activities. Consequently, ligaments were thought of as being of a fixed length, as evidenced by the depictions of knee motion where the ligaments were shown as bars of fixed length and single attachment points, controlling the motions. Furthermore, motion was considered primarily in the sagittal plane. Motions at the sliding surfaces themselves were described as either rolling or gliding (sliding) or a combination of the two. Along with this model of knee motion was the concept of instant centers of rotation. If a wheel is on a fixed axle and rotates, a point on the outside of the wheel will rotate about the axle. However if the axle moves anteriorly or posteriorly as the wheel simultaneously rotates, the center of rotation will either be above or below the level of the axle. It is noteworthy that the above descriptions of knee motion and the role of the ligaments assumed that the knee was flexed passively without the high forces and moments which occur in function. Test rigs for mechanical evaluation of knee specimens, or means of measuring the mechanics of the living knee during activities, had not yet been devised. Nevertheless in the field of gait analysis where the motion of limb segments was studied, spectacular stick figures were produced using stroboscopic photography by Muybridge, Edgerton, and others (Wing and Beek 2004), as well as by Eberhart and Inman (1947) in their locomotion studies, described earlier in this chapter.

Further research was carried out on the function of the ligaments in the mid-1960s by Hallen and Lindahl from the University of Umea in Sweden. They built on the earlier work of Brantigan and Voshell by carrying out laxity experiments and measuring displacements and rotations. The authors considered the ligaments not as bars of fixed length, but as extensible springs which allowed a wide range of femoral-tibial positions, while still providing restraints at the extremes of motion (Hallen and Lindahl 1965, 1966). They questioned the terminal external rotation of the tibia as the leg was brought into full extension, the "screw home mechanism," citing some of the early work from Meyer and Fick. An angular measuring device was used on 16 knee specimens and on 14 patients who had hip arthrodesis. In the latter, femoral rotation could not occur, thereby making the tibial angles an accurate indicator of rotation. While accepting that an average terminal rotation of 7 degrees occurred in the final 20 degrees of extension, in the case of the living subjects, they found that the subject could actively rotate the tibia such that "the outward rotation can be more or less prevented by will power." Even for the specimens, "depending on the position of rotation in 20 degrees flexion and full extension, it was possible to obtain passively an outward or an inward rotation or no rotation at all." However they made the important observation that when the knee was flexed through its neutral path of motion at any flexion angle, rotational laxities occurred when axial torques were applied. Hallen and Lindahl also measured the laxities after serial sectioning of different ligaments such that by calculating the laxity increases, they deduced which structures were important in controlling the rotation. These authors also pointed out that full extension of the knee was a special situation where the soft tissues of the posterior capsule tightened, applying high forces across the condyles and hence producing varus-valgus stability. They recognized that when compressive forces were acting due to soft tissues, body weight, or muscle action, large varus or valgus moments were required to produce condylar lift-off. Even today, full extension is not easy to define, because the end point depends upon the extension moment which is applied. Furthermore, the angle of flexion can be defined either by the long axes of the entire bones or relative to the centerlines of the femur and tibia in the 10–15 cm adjacent to the knee.

Considering now the forces at the knee due to the ground-to-foot force, the medial-lateral force distribution will depend upon the overall alignment of the lower

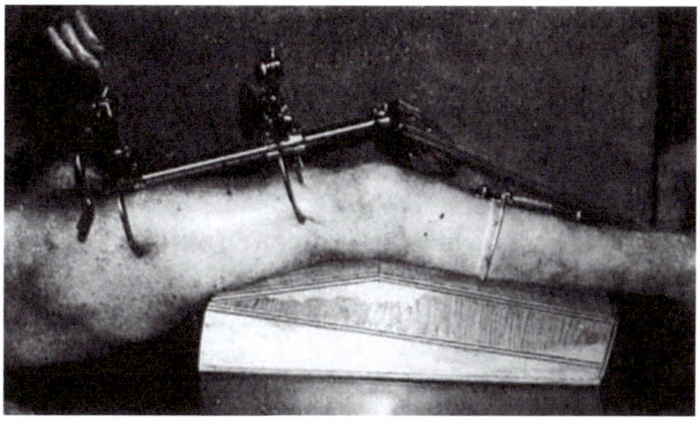

Fig. 2.7 Hallen and Lindahl carried out experiments in knee specimens to determine the laxities including varus-valgus and internal-external rotations. The bones were fixed with external prongs and the angular measurements measured with protractors. They carried out serial sectioning of ligaments, a novel idea at the time, to determine the relative contributions to stability (Hallen and Lindahl 1965, 1966). (Reprinted with permission from Acta Orthopaedica Scandinavica)

limb. In knees with a varus deformity, the forces on the medial side of the knee will be higher than on the lateral side. This can then cause damage to the medial meniscus and cartilage, leading to yet more varus and even higher medial forces, which is a common pathway of osteoarthritis. A common treatment for varus osteoarthritis was osteotomy (Jackson 1968) whereby the force balance across the knee was corrected by realigning the proximal tibia by removing a wedge of bone or creating a wedge-shaped gap or even making an arc-shaped cut and rotating the proximal tibial fragment. This had a sound biomechanical basis in that by reducing the medial forces, pain relief and even restoration of cartilage were achieved. Mark Coventry MD from the Mayo Clinic was a proponent of osteotomy and presented a number of valuable guidelines on the technique, indications, and long-term results (Coventry 1965; Coventry et al. 1993). Another way of realigning the knee was to interpose metal plates between the medial condyles using either MacIntosh or McKeever tibial plateaus. The insertion involved creating a horizontal cut across the medial plateau. There was no direct bonding between the lower surface of the implant and the exposed trabecular bone, but shear stability was provided by a textured surface or by keels. The metal bearing surface was smooth for articulation with the medial femoral condyle. Clinical studies showed a correction of alignment with pain relief, but similar failure modes as for osteotomy could occur, namely, pain or recurrence of the deformity (Scott et al. 1985).

Returning to the question as to why it was not until the 1960s that artificial hips and knees were introduced, the answer may lie in the traditions of orthopedic surgery and the way in which advances were made. There was little serious collaboration between surgeons and engineers, even though some surgeons may have had engineering expertise. Prior to about 1960, collaboration was generally between surgeons and the technical staff of orthopedic manufacturing companies on the aspects of design and materials for implants, but the companies did not have the background or resources for in-depth analysis or testing. However during the early 1960s, a revolutionary development occurred. John Charnley, an orthopedic surgeon from England, developed a successful artificial hip joint. Charnley was a unique individual who worked at Wrightington Hospital, not far from Manchester in northwest England. Wrightington itself was a small village, while the hospital was a collection of single-story buildings originally for the treatment of tuberculosis.

Charnley's artificial hip consisted of an intramedullary stem with a polished sphere at the top, articulating in a high-density polyethylene socket to provide a low-friction and wear-resistant bearing. The components were fixed to the femur and acetabulum using acrylic cement which hardened on application at surgery. This material had been used by Edward Haboush in 1957 at the Hospital for Joint Diseases in New York, to fix a cap over the arthritic femoral head and neck in several cases of hip arthritis (Haboush 1958). Mechanical problems prevented Haboush's work from progressing further. However, Charnley had seen this work on a visit to New York and, when he returned to England, consulted with Dennis Smith, a Professor of Dentistry at Manchester, about applying acrylic cement to the Charnley hip. Acrylic was already in widespread use for dental applications (Smith 2005). The principles underpinning the fixation method were that the fixation material would act as a grout between the components and bone rather than as an adhesive and that the cement would be pressurized on insertion to provide a complete interlock with the interstices of the trabecular bone. A crucial advantage was that the rigid fixation of the components to the bones had the effect of eliminating the pain.

The development work was carried out in Charnley's biomechanical laboratory set up in the hospital. The laboratory was run on a very limited budget with used machines donated by local factories. Who could have known what was about to be produced! By the mid-1960s, it was evident that the artificial hip design was working well and was likely to be a successful solution to the treatment of osteoarthritis of the hip. It might have seemed a simple matter to apply the same principles to the design of an artificial knee joint, and while this may have been the case in terms of the materials, it transpired that a great deal of work was needed on the design of the artificial knee itself to make it work as well as the hip.

We now consider the further understanding of knee biomechanics and the functions of the different structures, which was needed in order to design a successful artificial knee. A notable void in the knowledge was the magnitude and direction of the forces acting through the knee during everyday activities. In the mid-1960s, there had been a major breakthrough in this area for the hip joint by John Paul, a Professor of Bioengineering at Strathclyde University in Glasgow, Scotland. By using a combination of gait analysis, ground-to-foot force measurement, electromyographical data, and anatomical measurements, Paul used equilibrium equations to solve for the forces acting across the hip during walking and other activities (Paul 1969). The most important finding in the force analysis was that in the frontal plane, the ground-to-foot force caused a moment about the center of the femoral head, which had to be equilibrated by the abductor forces. But the moment arms were such that the abductor force had to be twice that of the ground-to-foot force, so the total force across the hip joint was about three times body weight, much higher than expected.

This force analysis was a landmark achievement in biomechanics, which allowed researchers and designers to carry out analysis and testing which had previously been impossible. For example, Seth Greenwald at Oxford University immediately used the data as input for his experiments on the contact areas in the hip (Greenwald and O'Connor 1971). Following the hip work at Strathclyde University, James Morrison, a PhD student of John Paul, applied similar methods to determine knee forces, the results being published in 1968 and 1970. (It was surprising that Morrison's publications were not co-authored by Paul, who was the originator of the methodology and supervisor of Morrison.) Applying the hip concepts to the knee, it was apparent that in the sagittal plane, the line of action of the

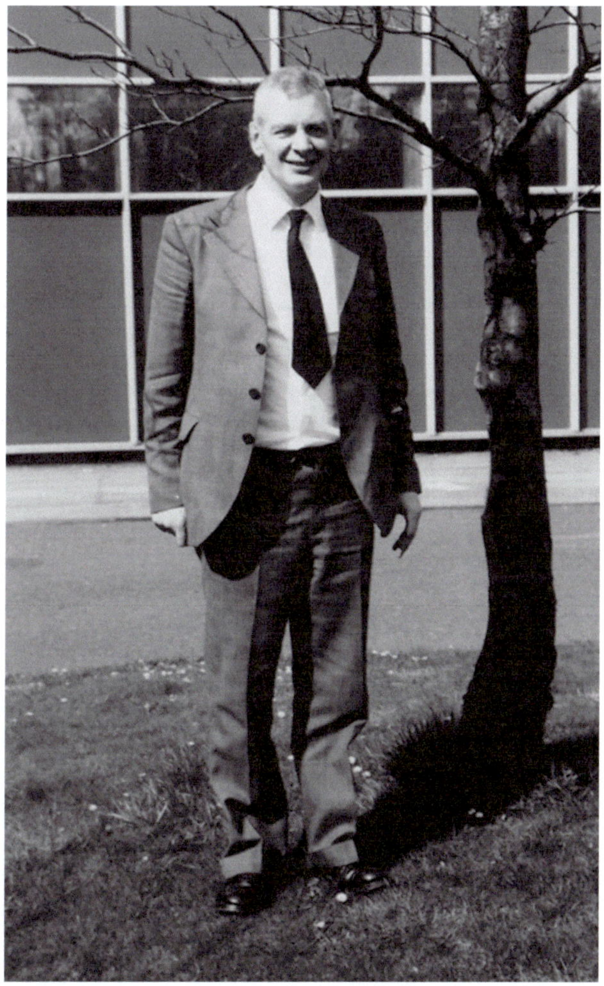

Fig. 2.8 John Paul PhD, Professor of Bioengineering at Strathclyde University in Glasgow, Scotland. He was a pioneer in the methodology of calculating the forces in the hip joint in the mid-1960s. The method was then applied to the knee joint in the late 1960s. Over several decades, he chaired committees in the International Standards Organisation and the Institution of Mechanical Engineers in formulating standards for the testing of artificial hips and knees. (Photo taken at his university c 1975) (©Peter S Walker)

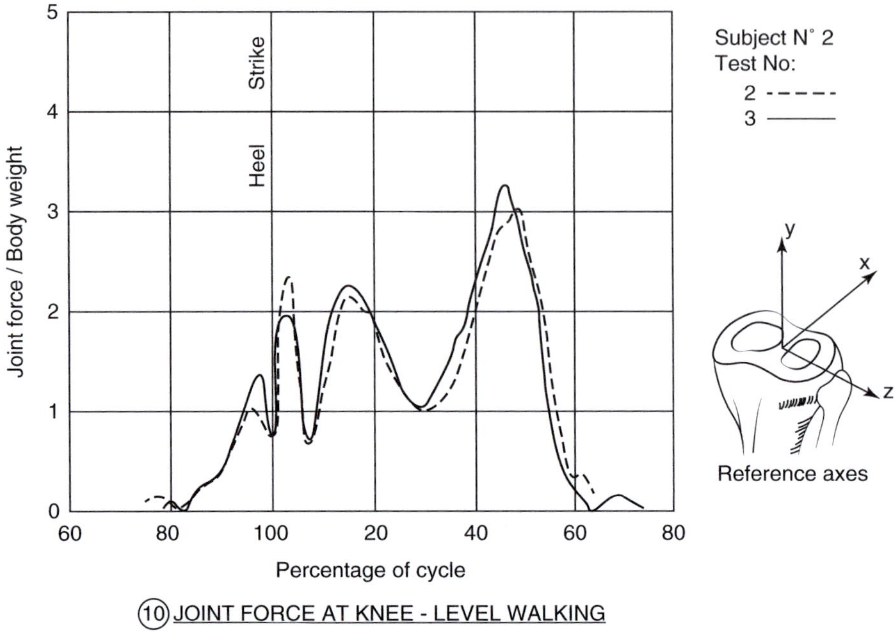

Fig. 2.9 The forces across the femoral-tibial bearing surfaces, calculated from gait analysis, ground-to-foot forces, electromyography, and a model of the knee containing the geometry and the ligaments. There were two force peaks just after heel strike and then a larger force peak at toe-off. The work was carried out at the University of Strathclyde by James Morrison, supervised by John Paul, and published in 1968 and 1970. (Reprinted with permission from Journal of Biomechanics)

ground-to-foot forces was at a distance from the femoral-tibial contact points such that either the quadriceps or the hamstrings muscles would need to apply larger forces than body weight to equilibrate. As for the hip, this would produce peak knee joint forces in the region of three times body weight. These peaks occurred at heel strike and toe-off in the stance phase of walking. In addition to these vertical forces, anterior-posterior shear forces and internal-external torques occurred between the femur and the tibia, although of much smaller magnitude than the axial force.

It is against the above backdrop that the first artificial knees were invented. However, further background is needed to put into context the emergence of the modern-day artificial knee. Metal on polymeric bearings was already in widespread use in engineering applications. To determine a suitable polymer for the hip, Charnley had carried out wear studies on specially designed wear machines on numerous polymeric materials to identify those with sufficient wear resistance. After initially choosing Teflon, which showed excessive wear in patients within 1–2 years, high-density polyethylene was subsequently found to have an acceptably low wear rate. As well as low wear, Charnley also emphasized low friction to minimize the shear stresses at the interfaces. He demonstrated the effectiveness of metal-on-polyethylene combined with a small-diameter femoral head, using a pendulum machine. The longer the time before the swinging ceased, the lower the frictional torque. Charnley's design had far lower friction compared with the McKee-Farrar metal-on-metal hip being used at the time. Hence polished metal against high-density polyethylene seemed the best choice for an artificial knee.

During the 1950s and 1960s when the artificial hip was being developed, hinged knees were being used, mainly in Europe. The uncemented type such as the Walldius were used in salvage situations and undoubtedly served a useful purpose. The cemented systems, such as the Shiers and the Stanmore, provided immediate stability and a useful range of flexion. However there was considerable reticence for widespread application due to the large amount of resection of the distal femur and proximal tibia necessary and the major problem of revision due to the long cemented intramedullary stems, in cases of revision. Today, hinged designs requiring less bone resection and with rotational freedom, and an anatomic patella flange, provide a useful fallback solution for severe arthritis or after previous revisions of conventional condylar replacement knees.

Hence, the late 1960s saw the transition from the previous treatments of osteotomy, metal spacers, and hinges to cemented metal-on-plastic condylar replacements. This represented a major landmark in the treatment of knee arthritis. The impetus for this transition was undoubtedly the success of the total hip which by then was being used in increasing numbers in many countries other than England. While many of the principles of the artificial hip could be directly translated to an artificial knee design, it was not immediately obvious how best to design an artificial knee as evidenced by the widely different configurations of the early designs.

It was not surprising that one of the very first knee designs was produced at Wrightington by a visiting Fellow, Frank Gunston from Winnipeg, Canada. The Hip Center at Wrightington was an ideal place for this initiative due to the presence of a biomechanical laboratory where the hip development had been carried out. The knee that was designed, called the Polycentric, could be developed and manufactured in the laboratory. The surgical instrumentation was simple yet accurate because the femoral components, being half-circular metal discs, were designed to be inserted into slots in the femoral condyles, while the plastic tibial components were to be similarly positioned in the tibial condyle. This was an innovative and fundamental concept in design which has stood the test of time to this day: reproduce the original contours of the bearing surfaces and preserve all of the ligaments. In parallel with this work was that of Michael Freeman at the London Hospital and Alan Swanson at Imperial College London. They were given the go-ahead to form a bioengineering unit in order to start work on an artificial knee design. It was considered that surgeon-engineer collaboration supported by a major technical university was necessary for such an enterprise. These two early beginnings of artificial knee design were the starting points for an immense expansion in the design and use of artificial knees, in England, in Europe, in Japan, and then in the USA.

In parallel with this expansion, there was a need for methods of evaluating the function of patients other than by simply taking radiographs and measuring the flexion angle. When problems such as component loosening, instability, or polyethylene wear occurred, biomechanical experimental studies were needed to address these problems. Gait analysis was one of the methods used. Ed Chao PhD, who joined the Mayo Clinic in 1971, established an advanced laboratory for the purpose of

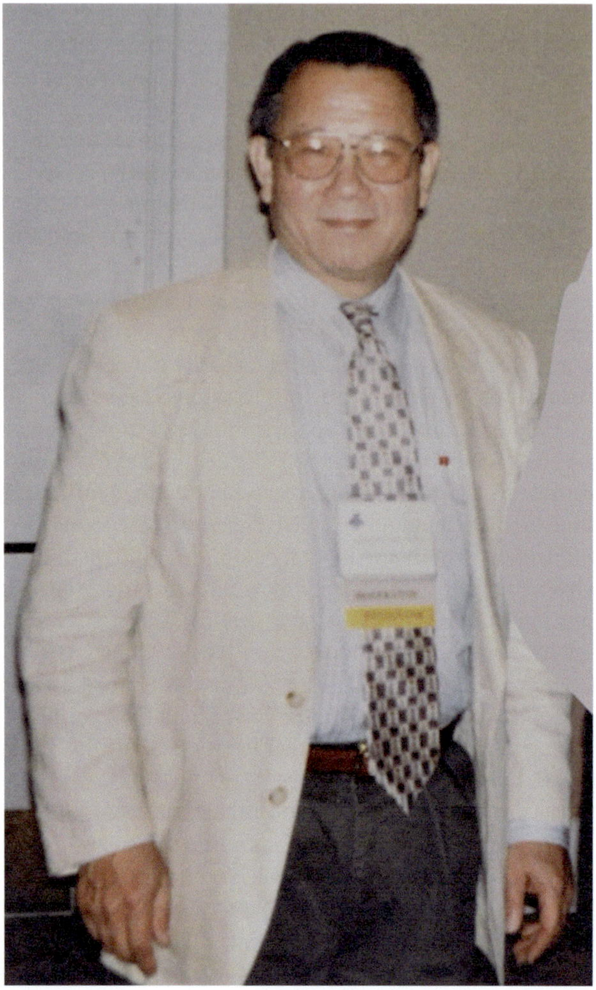

Fig. 2.10 Ed Chao PhD became Director of Bioengineering at the Mayo Clinic in Rochester, NY, in 1971 and served in that position for 20 years before moving to Johns Hopkins University. Ed's rigorous analytic, design, and teaching abilities enabled him to mentor hundreds of engineering and medical students in his lab and introduce innovative biomechanical methodologies. The achievement that he is the most proud of is the design of bone tumor implants for adult and juvenile patients, making the implants both functional and durable. He was a dedicated member of the International Society of Limb Salvage (ISOLS). (Photo taken c 2004) (©Peter S Walker)

evaluating the Polycentric and Geometric artificial knees which were starting to be used by Mark Coventry, Richard Bryan, and others. Chao analyzed the data from the motion capture system and the force plate data by defining numerous mathematical parameters and was able to compare the function of the artificial knee patients with that of normal subjects of a similar age range (Chao and Stauffer 1974).

In parallel with the invention of many new artificial knee designs, the 1970s saw an overall expansion in activities relating to human joints and their artificial replacements. At Case Western Reserve University in Cleveland, Ohio, Victor Frankel MD and Albert Burstein PhD were running courses to educate surgeons in biomechanics and even developed an instrumented tibial component to measure the knee forces in vivo, although this work was cut short due to lack of funding. Orthopedic and biomechanics societies were featuring this popular new area in their programs. Many special courses and conferences were organized. At Columbia University in

New York, Van Mow PhD was formulating mathematical models for the behavior of articular cartilage and for soft tissues such as ligaments and tendons. This work was the foundation for further advances by researchers such as Savio Woo PhD and Gerard Ateshian PhD. Peter Walker PhD and Keith Markolf PhD devised experimental methods for measuring the laxity and stability of the knee and attempted to match the behavior of artificial knees with that of the normal intact knee. At the University of Leeds in England, the focus was primarily on friction and wear of materials, for which new testing regimens were developed. Towards the end of the 1970s, finite element techniques were becoming available, which found an application in the analysis of tibial component fixation, by Jack Lewis PhD, Roy Crowninshield PhD, and others. Manufacturing companies played an important role in the processes needed to produce the anatomic shapes of the implant components as well as the instruments and in ensuring a high quality of materials to avoid failure in service. In this way design and research in artificial knees expanded, fueled by the increasing demand from patients and the generally successful results that were being achieved.

What Was Known About Knee Biomechanics by 1970?

Studies on the biomechanics of the knee, which could have been applied to artificial knee design, were carried out in Europe well before 1970, but the publications were not available in English and were unlikely to have been widely known. Likewise, a major study of knee motion carried out in the 1940s, which clearly showed axial rotations, was only documented in a report to a government agency. Studies of ligament function published before 1970 were available but do not seem to have influenced artificial knee design. The only work that may have had an influence was the determination of the forces in activity, carried out at Strathclyde University. For the most part, the development of artificial knees from 1970 was carried out without the benefit of much background knowledge. However a number of studies of knee biomechanics in the 1970s were applied to design and in some cases provided crucial design ideas and concepts. Almost no background work on instrumentation had been carried out, other than by using the concepts of osteotomy, but even then, it does not seem to have been directly applied to an appreciation of alignment and force distribution.

References

Barnett C, Davies D, McConaill M. Synovial joints their structure and function. Charles C Thomas: Springfield; 1961.

Brantigan OC, Voshell AF. The mechanics of the ligaments and menisci of the knee joint. J Bone Joint Surg Br Vol. 1941;23(1):44–66.

Buckwalter JA. Arthur Steindler. Orthopaedic scholar, teacher, and clinician. Clin Orthop Relat Res. 2000;374:171–82.

Bullough PG, Munuera L, Murphy J, Weinstein AM. The strength of the menisci of the knee as it relates to their fine structure. J Bone Joint Surg. 1970;52(3):564–7.
Chao EYS, Stauffer RN. Biomechanical evaluation of geometric and polycentric knee arthroplasty. Conference on Total Knee Replacement, Institution of Mechanical Engineers, London, 16–18 September 1974.
Coventry MB. Osteotomy of the upper portion of the tibia for degenerative arthritis of the knee. J Bone Joint Surg Am. 1965;47:984–90.
Coventry MB, Ilstrup DM, Wallrichs SL. Proximal tibial osteotomy. A critical long-term study of eighty-seven cases. J Bone Jt Surg. 1993;75(2):196–201.
Dowson D. History of tribology. London: Professional Engineering Publ; 1998.
Eberhart HD, Inman VT. Fundamental studies of human locomotion and other information relating to design of artificial limbs. Report to Committee on Artificial Limbs, National Research Council, Washington DC. 15 July 1947.
Greenwald AS, O'Connor JJ. The transmission of load through the human hip joint. J Biomech. 1971;4(6):507–28.
Haboush EJ. A new operation for arthroplasty of the hip based on biomechanics, photoelasticity, fast-setting dental acrylic, and other considerations. 1958 [classical article]. Bulletin (Hospital for Joint Diseases (New York, NY)). 1996;55(2):95–111.
Hallen LG, Lindahl O. The lateral stability of the knee-joint. Acta Orthop Scand. 1965;36(2):179–91.
Hallen LG, Lindahl O. The "screw-home" movement in the knee-joint. Acta Orthop Scand. 1966;37(1):97–106.
Inman VT, Ralston HJ, Todd F. Human walking. Baltimore: Williams & Wilkins; 1981.
Jackson JP. Degenerative changes in the knee after meniscectomy. Br Med J. 1968;2(5604):525–7.
Jahn S, Seror J, Klein J. Lubrication of articular cartilage. Annu Rev Biomed Eng. 2016;18:235–58.
Lanzer WL, Komenda G. Changes in articular cartilage after meniscectomy. Clin Orthop Relat Res. 1990;(252):41–8.
McCutchen CW. The frictional properties of animal joints. Wear. 1962;5(1):1–17.
Morrison J. Bioengineering analysis of force actions transmitted by the knee joint. Bio-med Eng. 1968;3:164–70.
Morrison J. The mechanics of the knee joint in relation to normal walking. J Biomech. 1970;3(1):51–61.
Paul JP. Loading on the head of the human femur. J Anat. 1969;105(Pt 1):187–8.
Pinskerova V, Maquet P, Freeman MA. The anatomic literature relating to the knee from 1836 to 1917: an historic note. Clin Orthop Relat Res. 2003;410:13–8.
Saunders JB, Inman VT, Eberhart HD. The major determinants in normal and pathological gait. J Bone Jt Surg Am. 1953;35A:543–58.
Scott RD, Joyce MJ, Ewald FC, Thomas WH. McKeever metallic hemiarthroplasty of the knee in unicompartmental degenerative arthritis. Long-term clinical follow-up and current indications. J Bone Joint Surg Am. 1985;67(2):203–7.
Smillie IS. The current pattern of internal derangements of the knee joint relative to the menisci. Clin Orthop Relat Res. 1967;(51):117–22.
Smith DC. The genesis and evolution of acrylic bone cement. Orthop Clin North Am. 2005;36(1):1–10.
Steindler A. Kinesiology of the human body. Springfield: Publ Charles C Thomas; 1955.
Wing A, Beek P. Motion analysis: a joint centenary. Hum Mov Sci. 2004;23(5):iii–v.

The Design Process

3

Has a Systematic Design Process Been Applied to Artificial Knees?

In this chapter, a systematic methodology for designing a new product will be described. The product could be simple or complex, large or small, a completely new product, or a variation of an existing product. The description of the process will be related to the artificial knee. The development of the early artificial knee designs will then be examined to determine if a systematic design process had been applied.

Every object which has been invented has involved a design process of some sort, even if that process has not been explicitly defined. Yet it might seem that whatever design process has been used, it has often been deficient based on the number of products which are delayed in their completion, experience cost overruns, are difficult to operate, do not look attractive, or do not work as intended. But considering the large numbers of products which are streaming out into the market, the deficient ones are a small percentage. To obtain a successful design solution and avoid problems, care is needed in selecting the design process most applicable to the product being designed and in implementing the process systematically (Cross 2008).

Following a design process is valuable for a number of reasons:

- It requires a clear definition of the need, what the invention is required to do, followed by a listing of the specifications and the constraints, called the design criteria.
- It is a systematic process that should result in a final product which best satisfies the defined need and design criteria.
- Many projects are complex, involving different components and technologies, and hence require a rigorous process to maintain an ordered progression of the design over an extended time period.
- In an increasingly competitive world, it is essential that a design be completed in a practical period of time, at an acceptable cost, and with a result that will satisfy the needs of the end user.
- Adhering to a set of rules should maintain objectivity in decision-making and minimize the possible negative effects of human factors.

P. S. Walker, *The Artificial Knee*, https://doi.org/10.1007/978-3-030-38171-4_3

An essential first step in the design process is to specify why something should be designed at all, identifying a need. An example is the requirement to cross over a river to access the territory beyond. It is easy to jump to the conclusion that a bridge is needed. However, it is more logical to first consider different solutions. This would then open up the solution to a boat, a catapult, a zipline, a crane, a cable car, a helicopter, a tunnel, or even damming the river. Every solution can have a number of variants. For example, a bridge can range from a simple suspended footbridge to an elaborate arch carrying trains, automobiles, and pedestrians. The choice of the most appropriate solution will be facilitated by specifying a set of design criteria. These criteria can include the required usage such as pedestrians only or vehicles as well, the volume of the usage, the cost constraints, the timetable, the durability expected, the time to make the crossing, and aesthetics.

The above concepts can be applied to the artificial knee. The need for a treatment for osteoarthritis of the knee has been recognized for centuries. However, it was only in the late nineteenth century that a practical solution was formulated. The inventor was a German surgeon, Theophilus Gluck, who proposed some type of hinged joint which was fixed into the hollow intramedullary canals of the femur and tibia using cement (Gluck 1891; Brand et al. 2011). Gluck stated design criteria for a device which would treat the arthritis, a remarkable step which indicated Gluck's systematic way of thinking:

- The components must be secured rigidly to the bones.
- A minimum volume of bone must be removed.
- It must provide complete stability.

The device which Gluck designed was a narrow hinge made from ivory which fitted into the intercondylar region, with stems which were cemented into the intramedullary canals. In his original article, Gluck does not indicate if he considered various solutions, but he only described the solution which he chose for application to patients. While the design may have been mechanically sound, it failed due to infection when used in patients. Even though all of the design criteria may have been met, the need for sterility was unknown at that time. Another criterion not directly stated was durability. It was probably assumed that the materials were sufficiently strong and rigid, and there would not be an issue with mechanical failure. This was a reasonable assumption because the material was ivory, successfully used in demanding mechanical applications in the wild. Another mechanical factor which was not stated was the wear of the interfaces under repetitive sliding over a long period of time, but the material strength and the smooth surfaces were probably thought to provide adequate wear resistance.

To illustrate the influence of specifying the design criteria on the design solution reached, exactly the same design as Gluck's was reinvented 82 years later (Walker and Shoji 1973). In the Biomechanics Laboratory at the Hospital for Special Surgery in New York in 1970, Peter Walker; two orthopedic fellows, Hiromu Shoji and David Mendes; and a veterinarian, Fernando Figarola, had been studying the center of rotation of the knee as it was flexed and extended. It was found that a fixed-axis

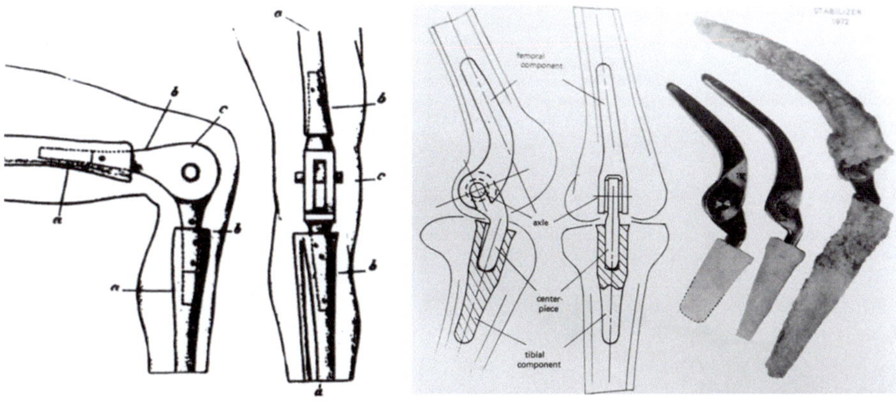

Fig. 3.1 The remarkable similarity between the intercondylar linked knee designed and used in a patient by Themistocles Gluck in 1891 (Gluck 1891; Brand et al. 2011) and a design tested in animals at the Hospital for Special Surgery in 1973 (Walker and Shoji 1973). The similarity is attributed to the identical set of design criteria specified prior to formulating the designs. (Reprinted with permission from Arch fklin Chir and from Clinical Orthopaedics and Related Research)

hinge would be a reasonable approximation provided it included some freedom of motion. An intercondylar hinge was designed and implanted in both dogs and sheep such that the hinge axis coincided with the average axis of rotation of the knee. However, because all of the load across the knee joint was transmitted by the hinge and the intramedullary stems, the femoral and tibial condyles were unloaded. As a result, the cartilage became degenerate, and the trabecular bone within the condyles became porotic, which would probably result in later mechanical failure and would compromise a revision. The research group at Special Surgery was not aware of Gluck's design, and their new design was arrived at completely independently. The important point is that the reason for the similarity in designs was that the same design criteria were used.

The degeneration of the condyles is an example of a phenomenon termed "unintended consequences," an undesirable outcome which was not predicted. In the case of the design produced in the 1970s, it could have been predicted from the research on disuse atrophy from Oxford University in England by Joseph Trueta and Peter Bullough, who showed that areas of joints that were habitually unloaded became degenerate, because chondrocytes and osteoblasts need mechanical loading to maintain healthy tissue. While thinking outside of the box is usually easier in hindsight, it is probably true in general that the further an artificial system diverges from the anatomical geometry and mechanics, the more likely there is to be some unintended consequence.

While an intercondylar hinge fulfilled the design criteria, other solutions could also have been formulated. For example, curved rails to resurface the femoral condyles together with resurfacing components for the tibial plateaus would fulfill the criterion of minimum bone resection and would also provide stability if the ligaments were still intact and functional. In the above example, if a choice had to be

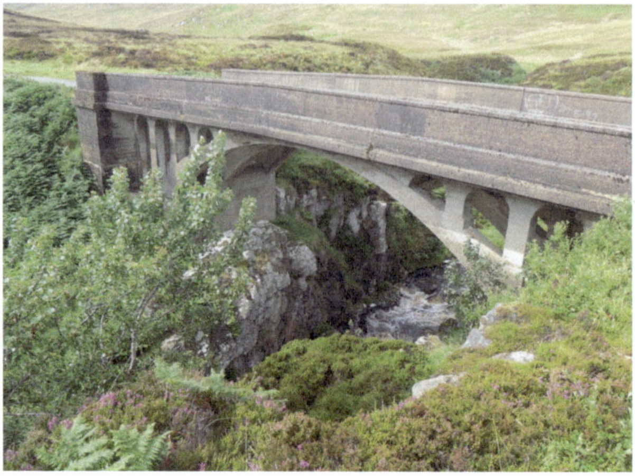

Fig. 3.2 The Garry Bridge – Bridge to Nowhere. There was a need to connect the northeastern corner of the Isle of Lewis, Scotland, to the main southern part. A reinforced concrete bridge was designed and constructed from 1918 to 1923. The height was 50 ft, the span 100 ft, and the width 15 ft, and 140 workers were engaged in the construction. By the time the bridge was completed however, the need was no longer there. But today, the bridge serves to reach the northern footpath from which there is spectacular coastal scenery. (©Peter S Walker)

made between a linked intercondylar device and a condylar replacement, how would a decision be made of the best solution? The obvious method would be to assess how well each design satisfied the design criteria. Based on Gluck's criteria, the intercondylar hinge would be chosen on the basis of rigid fixation, minimum bone removal, and complete stability. However, today, other design criteria would be added, which would tip the decision in the other direction. Not the least of these criteria would be to avoid invasion of the intramedullary canal due to the serious consequences of infection, loosening, or femoral fracture.

Simplified Design Process

From the various steps which are necessary to progress from the design criteria to a final product, a basic model of a design process can be specified and conveniently described with a flow chart. The first step is to define the need or the problem to be solved. This is the first creative step in design, perceiving something that is amenable to a solution. In a holistic framework, the need can be defined as "a treatment for osteoarthritis of the knee," because this would allow for a range of solutions including nonsurgical. On the other hand, if a company wanted a product in the already-established artificial knee market, the need would become "an artificial knee to treat osteoarthritis," which would limit the solution to different configurations of artificial knees. In a field such as this, where there are already a number of design solutions on the market, the need can be defined more narrowly. For example, how did the meniscal bearing and rotating platform designs originate? For the Oxford

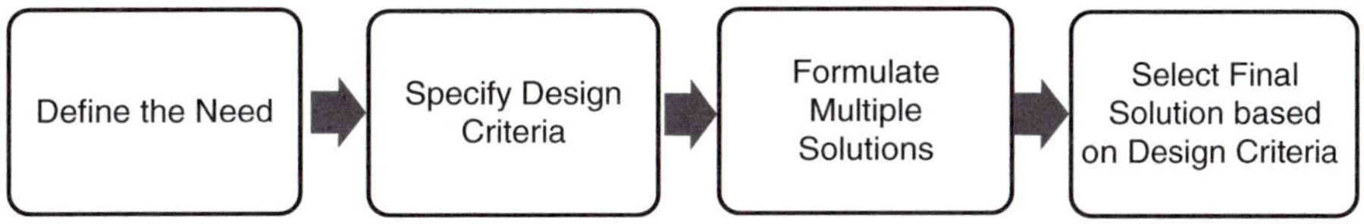

Fig. 3.3 A basic model for the design process, progressing from a definition of the need to the final solution

unicondylar knee, the need was for a bearing which would be unconstrained anterior-posterior to be consistent with the four-bar mechanism of knee motion, but which would have low contact stresses on the plastic (it might seem that the two requirements are incompatible, but a solution was found); for the low contact stress (LCS) rotating platform, the need was for an artificial knee which would have conforming bearings to reduce wear, but would not be constrained in internal-external rotation. To give more recent examples, the vitamin-E infused highly cross-linked polyethylene was based on a need for a material which would have exceptional wear resistance but which would not oxidize in the long term. The instrumented tibial trials used for balancing at surgery were based on the need for a soft tissue balancing technique where the surgeon could obtain quantitative values with the femoral and tibial trials in place. Such narrow definitions of the need are both creative and valuable in that they can initiate a completely new design or way of doing something.

Having established the need, the next step is to specify design criteria. These are intended to provide guidelines for the proposed solutions and are the means for comparison. The design criteria must be framed in a way that is useful both for formulating and for evaluating design solutions. Assuming a company assembled a group of experts in different fields as a design team, it is likely that the design criteria would fall into four categories: function, durability, surgical, and commercial viability. It is not sufficient to state that function must be "normal," because the level and type of function, as well as the kinematics, vary for every individual. Instead, some type of stability criterion needs to be defined and whether this should vary for each separate case. Durability relates to strength of the components, the fixation to the bones, and the wear, each needing specific criteria. The surgical aspects relate to the alignments, which require the actual values and the allowable tolerances. Soft tissue balancing is another factor which requires definitions and tolerances. The time factors and ease of surgery also need to be specified in some way. Commercial factors include the costs of the implants and inventory, as well as the instruments, and whether there are identifiable advantages over other designs or systems.

The next step is to formulate multiple design solutions. To illustrate how this might work in practice, assume that a need is defined as "to enable a person to traverse along a pavement or roadway much faster than walking." The solution could be a bicycle, a scooter, a skateboard, roller skates, a wheelchair, a Segway, a hoverboard, a motorcycle, an electric unicycle, or a jet-powered pack, and there will be others. How would it be decided which of these was worth further consideration and which should be eliminated? Assume that two of the design criteria were that the solution had to be self-powered and easy to transport when not in use. This would eliminate all powered vehicles, while the solution would have to be foldable and lightweight. In practice, given the design criteria, it would have been unnecessary to put forward powered vehicles at all, but at the initial stage, it is better to be broader. For example, if a battery-powered device could be easily recharged by body power rather than by plugging it in, it might be acceptable.

It can be asked if there is any systematic method of formulating design solutions. At one extreme it can be regarded as a creative process that is more evident in certain individuals than in others. Such an ability can even be seen at an early age where some children can draw imaginative pictures, make complicated Lego constructions, or create intriguing stories. At the other extreme, it can be regarded as a process which is amenable to a logical or systematic process. For example, the bearings which nature has evolved, the history of bearings in engineering, and the artificial knees already designed could be systematically searched. Most of the new ideas of artificial knee design and technique have originated from individuals who introduced new insights or concepts, without much explanation of how the design was arrived at. Undoubtedly some of these ideas were made possible by first carrying out experimental studies on the knee itself, for example, to determine the mechanisms of stability, the function of ligaments, the effects of muscle actions, the motion patterns, and so on. Carrying out such studies provides a perception of the knee as both a structure and a mechanism. An obvious way to proceed is to imitate the knee itself, a "biomimetic" approach. Biomimetics (or biomimicry) can be looked at in two ways. Firstly, to reproduce the actual structural forms, to make the shape of the artificial knee components exactly the same as anatomic and, if any ligaments or menisci are deficient, to replace those also. This raises the question as to how exactly to mimic the normal anatomy. Does it involve shape only, or are mechanical properties included, such as modulus of elasticity, tensile strength, wear resistance, and friction coefficient? These factors would be dealt with later in the design process, where each solution would be subject to an evaluation of its practicality. A cautionary note is that a project should not be sidetracked in solving a problem such as developing a new material. A second approach to biomimetics is to say that the shape of the biological structures per se does not need to be reproduced, but the solution must perform the same function. The simplest solution for a knee joint is a uniaxial hinge, which provides the most predominant motion, and this is certainly an acceptable solution for some knee conditions. However, for arthritic knees in general, a more sophisticated solution is needed which would include the laxity and the stability behavior. In this case, the cruciate ligaments may not need to be retained if the bearing surfaces provide the same function.

Having formulated several design solutions, the next step is to compare the solutions to determine which most closely satisfies the criteria. It is useful to subdivide the design criteria into "musts and wants." For example, the solution must be self-powered (a must), but it has to be lightweight (a want) and low cost (a want). Hence, solutions which do not satisfy the "musts" are eliminated immediately, and the comparison of the remaining solutions is based on how well they satisfy the "wants."

This can be accomplished by assigning scores to the different "wants," using a ranking between 1 and 10. The scores for the "wants" can also reflect their importance, such that weight could have a maximum score of 5, but cost a maximum of 10. During the analysis of each solution, some solutions could be modified to increase their score. At the end of this process, the solution with the highest score can be selected and the others eliminated.

How best can the different steps in the design process be achieved? The early knees were usually designed by a single individual or by a surgeon working with an engineer. This served the need of formulating a completely new design. Today, when the need is usually to improve an existing system, a team of individuals with different specialties is more appropriate. Whatever the case, there are certain aspects of any new project where creative ideas are required, either in the artificial knee itself or in the instrumentation and technique. The most efficient way to accomplish that is for the larger group to define the need and the design criteria, but a small subset of individuals assigned for the design itself. These individuals would be creative and motivated and would require days or weeks to reach satisfactory solutions.

In this simplified model of the design process, analysis and testing are not included. However these are critical steps in order to quantitatively evaluate and compare each design. There is often confusion between designing something and evaluating it. It is often considered that when the final design is reached, it should then be subjected to a set of tests to verify its safety and effectiveness under service conditions. Instead, it is more appropriate to regard the testing as a part of the design process itself, such that a design can only be finalized after the evaluations have been carried out. Today, with the availability of analytic software such as finite element analysis for stress determination, and dynamic simulation for kinetics, designs can be rigorously analyzed in a number of ways, including optimization. However even after such a process, the final design would still need to be manufactured and physically tested to account for materials and manufacturing factors. Such testing is still regarded as falling within the design process because the results of the test may require or suggest changes to the design itself.

Controlled Convergence Design Model

With the analysis and testing embodied within the design process, the simplified model can now be extended to what has been termed a controlled convergence model (Pugh 1991). Pugh's model was derived from many years of industrial design experience of both individual components and large assemblies. Later in his career, Pugh became a Professor at Strathclyde University in Glasgow, Scotland, which allowed him to disseminate his design knowledge further. Pugh recognized that after initial brainstorming to produce several design solutions, after working on these solutions for a period of time, new solutions would frequently emerge. Why these solutions did not emerge initially is an interesting question. Part of the answer is that once the designers start to make prototypes and analyze initial designs, it

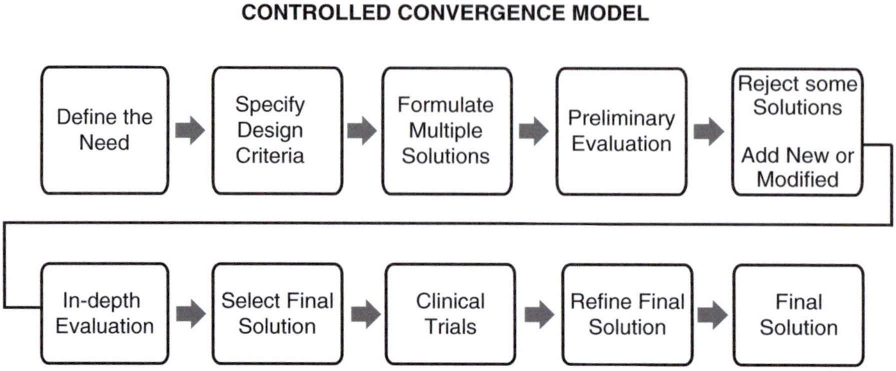

Fig. 3.4 A model for the design process based on the controlled convergence model from Stuart Pugh. The final three steps concerning a clinical trial have been added to make the model applicable to an artificial knee or any implantable medical device

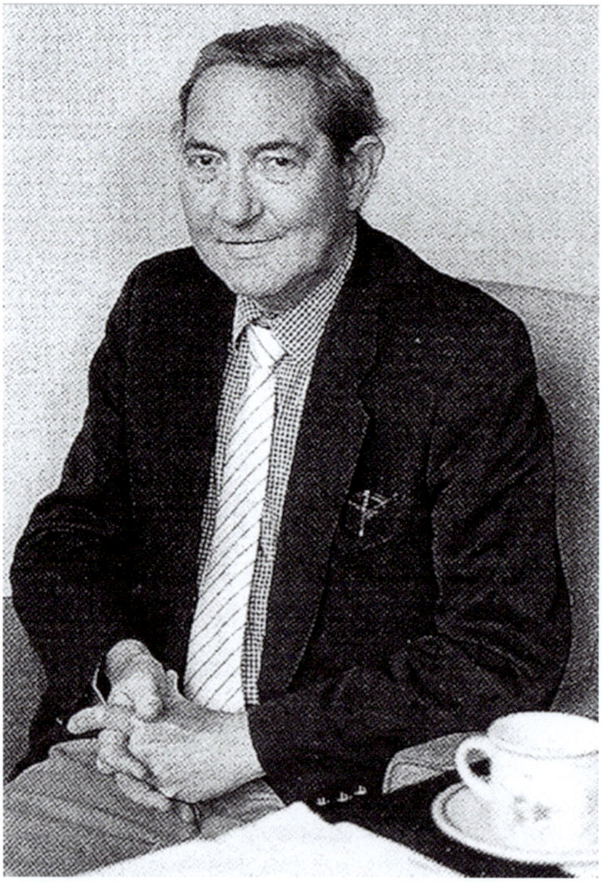

Fig. 3.5 Stuart Pugh had a varied career in industry and academia. In his faculty position at the University of Strathclyde, Scotland, he expounded his ideas on the design process in a book called *Total Design: Integrated Methods for Successful Product Engineering*, published in 1990

stimulates the mind to generate yet newer ideas. The end result is that at each step in the design process, the number of solutions under consideration will reduce because some ideas will be found to be inferior, but other ideas will be added. So long as the number of the former is greater than the latter, eventually only a single solution will remain, hence the term used by Pugh, controlled convergence. This gradual process is fueled by the analysis and testing which is carried out at the different stages.

Analysis and testing typically start from simple mechanical calculations, to analysis using software packages, to testing using purpose-built simulating machines. In the case of artificial knees, shape and size will be formulated using databases of bone shapes from MRI or CT scans. Stress analyses of the contact areas on the bearing surfaces and on the underlying trabecular bone will be performed using finite element analysis (FEA). Kinematics will be assessed using test machines or software. Fatigue strength will be investigated with cyclic load machines. Wear and friction will be measured with elaborate multichannel knee simulating machines, wear being a process that is materials dependent and which cannot yet be predicted by computer models.

However all of these analyses and tests are but models of reality. No amount of testing in a computer or on laboratory test machines can completely predict the performance in the patient. Today this statement has to be interpreted in the context of the 50 years of experience of artificial knees in patients, with a wide range of design types, surgical techniques, material variations, and patient activities. Nonetheless, whenever any new aspect of a design, material, or technique is introduced, there are unknown and unpredictable outcomes that might occur. The design changes can be initiated to correct some known deficiency or to take advantage of a new idea or technology.

When a design is considered complete, it needs to be verified by a further extension of the design process, namely, field trials. Most engineering products are tested in this way before final release to the market. Automobiles are tested in all types of weather and road surfaces, on the open road and in cities, with slow and aggressive driving, and with different load distributions. Yet even after such testing, and corrective measures taken to remedy problems, many recalls are reported in the media, for deficiencies relating to accelerator pedals, air bags, braking systems, cruise controls, and so on. The reason why so many of these problems were not detected when the vehicles were field tested is that they only later occurred on a very small percentage of the total vehicles sold or under an unusual set of conditions. There is a parallel situation with artificial knees today. Considering that around 900,000 are used each year in the USA alone, it would be surprising if rare and unpredicted modes of failure did not occur. Despite product deficiencies occurring even after field trials, there would be even more deficiencies if a product was released to the market without carrying out such field trials. Hence, it has to be accepted that no matter how rigorously a product is designed and tested, there still exists the possibility of problems in service.

The controlled convergence model explicitly includes field trials, or clinical trials, as applicable to medical devices. Because of the multifaceted nature of the entire design process, each stage requires input from a group of individuals of different specialties and abilities. In the case of artificial knees as well as with most other medical devices, there are a number of different facets of the design, in which case the design process can be applied to each facet separately. For artificial knees, these facets include:

- The femoral component: the shape of the bearing surfaces and patella flange
- The tibial component: the shape of the bearing surfaces and the means of fixation to the tibial bone
- Interaction between the femoral and tibial components: contact area, laxity, and stability
- The materials for the components: fatigue strength, friction, and wear
- The surgical instruments for preparing the bone to fit the components: ease of use and accuracy
- The surgical technique itself: alignment, accuracy of fit of components, soft tissue balancing, and fixation methodology

For each facet, specific testing methods can be used. For example, an orthopedic company was recently developing a multi-size system of components. For the tibial component, the optimal size and shape of the tibial fixation peg were required. One criterion was that the peg would not impact the posterior cortex of the tibia on insertion. A large database of tibial models derived from CT scans was used. In the computer, the proximal tibial cut was made, and the best size of tibial component was selected based on the peripheral fit. Variations in the posterior tibial slope and the depth of cut were tested. The end result was a peg shape which would not impinge except in rare conditions. Embodied in the analyses was a statistical model. In recently introduced artificial knee systems, such bone databases have also been used to define the dimensional parameters for the multiple components.

Over time, a set of tests has been defined as a final check on the safety and efficacy of artificial knees. As a result of the accumulated experience of artificial knee design over the past several decades, testing methods have been specified by the American Society for Testing and Materials (ASTM) and the International Standards Organization (ISO). In the USA, these tests are required by the Food and Drug Administration (FDA) prior to using new designs in patients, while similar schemes are used in other countries. Over time, new standards emerge, while others are updated or abandoned. Whether or not all of the tests have been carried out prior to design finalization, they are mandatory for a design to proceed to clinical application. At this time, formal clinical trials are not required by the FDA for devices that closely resemble prior clinically used devices, a 510 K designation. However it is common practice for manufacturers to restrict the use of a new product to a limited group of surgeons to detect if there are any deficiencies, prior to general release. This precautionary step has obvious benefits: it avoids a large number of patients at risk, and if a design modification was necessary, it would be expensive to implement if there was a large inventory in the field. To the credit of the field of artificial knees, over the past decade or more, apart from some instances of inconsistent fixation of certain tibial component designs, there have been no major clinical problems with artificial knees.

Design Process for the Early Artificial Knees

What was the design process used for producing the earliest knee designs? From the late 1960s, when artificial knees were first designed, Charles Townley MD, from Port Huron in the USA, had for many years been designing and using metal resurfacing components for the femur and the tibia (Townley 1988). He also made drawings of complete artificial knee designs, but these were not implemented due to the lack of suitable materials. Jim Pritchett reported that Townley showed his ideas to John Charnley in the early 1960s (Pritchett 2009). This may have been a cue for Charnley to assign Gunston a short time later as a visiting Fellow to work on the knee. Townley did not have the benefit of working in a university setting where he might have found collaborators and technical support, but rather he worked mainly by himself and made his own models. He did specify design criteria for his designs however, the most important being to restore the anatomy as closely as possible, to remove as little bone as possible, to preserve all ligaments, and to ensure correct limb alignment at surgery. His design fulfilled all of these criteria, and by the late 1960s, when suitable materials became available, he was able to interest DePuy in producing his knee system, the Townley Anatomic knee. As well as carefully developing his design over many years, other attributes led to its success. Prior to his surgical training, Townley had spent a year at an engineering school. When he turned to orthopedics, he carefully studied the anatomy and mechanics of the knee and evaluated several ideas of implant designs for treating arthritis. He made numerous models and carried out surgical testing on knee specimens. He was a highly accomplished surgeon able to achieve accurate component placement with only basic instruments (Pritchett 2009). It can be concluded that Townley took a biomimetic approach to artificial knee design, reproducing the geometry of the knee joint and the alignment as closely as possible, in order to obtain normal functional results.

The second example of artificial knee design in the late 1960s was the work of Frank Gunston, a trainee surgeon from Winnipeg, Canada, who was a Fellow with John Charnley at Wrightington Hospital in England. He was assigned to solve the "difficult problem of the painful and unstable knee in rheumatoid polyarthritis" by applying "the biomedical principles and experience gained from total hip arthroplasty combined with an analysis of normal knee movement" (Gunston 1971). It is notable that Gunston did not seem to have applied the work on knee anatomy and mechanics carried out in Europe up to that time, for the reason explained in Chap. 2. Background, the inaccessibility of this work in the English literature. Instead Gunston made some basic observations of knee motion from radiographs and concluded that there was both rolling and sliding at the condylar surfaces, calling this polycentric motion, which gave the name to his implant design. Gunston's design criteria were to allow for this motion, to be able to correct the level of the bearing surfaces on each condyle, to provide rigid fixation of the components, and to avoid invasion of the patellofemoral bearing surfaces. Charnley, having initiated the project and encouraged the work as it proceeded, did not become involved in a major way due to his involvement with his hip designs. Gunston worked mainly with the technicians in the Bioengineering Laboratory where all of the development work on Charnley's hip was still taking place. Another design criterion which later emerged was ease of manufacture, as it was decided to make Gunston's knee components in the laboratory itself. This criterion was accomplished by designing components using stainless steel and high-density polyethylene, the same materials used in the total hip, in shapes which could readily be made using basic workshop equipment. No doubt minor modifications were made to the design and instrumentation based on implanting in specimens and on initial surgical cases. The Polycentric knee development was a result of a unique combination of factors: Charnley's development of the total hip, in that materials for the components and fixation were applicable to the knee, access to a Bioengineering Laboratory, and the skills and full-time dedication of Gunston who was educated in both engineering and orthopedic surgery. There was an interesting sequel to the design of the Polycentric knee. On Gunston's return to Winnipeg, Canada, in 1969, Lowell Peterson and Richard Bryan, from the Mayo Clinic in Minnesota, visited Gunston and asked if they could use his design. Gunston did not have any manufacturing organized, but he agreed that the Mayo Clinic could pursue the design on their own. They accordingly interested Howmedica in producing it, but first, Peterson, Bryan, and also Mark Coventry carried out design modifications, notably increasing the contact area of the components for improved fixation and wear resistance. Subsequently, these surgeons carried out well over a 1000 cases. More details will be given in Chap. 9.

There was a very different situation for the development of the Freeman-Swanson knee in London. In the interview the author held with Alan Swanson in 2017, Swanson explained the circumstances of the collaboration. In the mid-1960s, Michael Freeman was a recently appointed Registrar at the London Hospital and, having seen the success of the artificial hip, became interested in developing an artificial knee. However he realized that technical expertise would be required for which he had the idea of forming a biomechanics unit at Imperial College, University of London. This was an audacious idea considering his junior status at the time, but the end result was that the Professor of Mechanical Engineering introduced Freeman to Alan Swanson, a young lecturer at the time, and gave them permission to start a biomechanics unit to work on knee joints. The process started with a definition of the need: restoration of knees with severe arthritis to normal function. There is an important contrast here with Townley's approach which was to treat knees with arthritis severe enough to require surgery but not with the severe deformities that were described by Freeman. The reason was that in London and in Europe as a whole, metallic hinges were being widely used to treat knees with severe deformities, and the idea was to develop a more conservative resurfacing type of artificial knee to use instead of hinges. Freeman and Swanson formulated a set of design criteria which were based on engineering principles as well as on the surgical requirements. The principles included large surface areas for transmission of forces to the resected bone surfaces, as well as between the metal and plastic components themselves to minimize the wear of the plastic. Stability requirements were based on femoral-tibial conformity, but with a spinout limit to serve the dual purpose of setting a limit to the axial torque that could be transmitted while still allowing some rotational freedom. Freeman and Swanson held regular meetings, in between which models were made and ideas tested theoretically and experimentally. By carefully defining the design criteria, they were able to limit their design solutions to one design form with only a few minor variations.

For testing the design, they made fixtures to measure the strength of the fixation of the tibial component to tibial bone specimens and concluded that the torque to cause dissociation was much higher than would be encountered between the foot and the ground under any realistic conditions. They also built a cyclic motion machine to demonstrate that wear and deformation of the polyethylene were exceedingly small, of a similar amount to that seen in artificial hip joints. The first implantation in a patient was in 1970, after which the usage was expanded. In some cases, there was side-to-side instability between the femoral and tibial components, a degree of freedom which was unconstrained in their design. In other cases, the patella did not track smoothly across the anterior femur component as the knee was flexed and extended, but bumped over the projecting anterior part of the femoral component. Determining certain deficiencies in the clinical trials resulted in changes in the design which made the subsequent performance much more successful. Hence Freeman and Swanson followed a design process closely, including carrying out both laboratory evaluations and clinical trials.

The above designs involved only one or two principal designers, but with assistance from technical staff at hospitals, universities, and companies. Mention should be made of the Kodama-Yamamoto knee, designed by two orthopedic surgeons from Matsuyama, Japan. This knee was developed in the late 1960s although details of their design process are not available. Also in the late 1960s, there was a notable example where a team approach was initiated for the design of the Geometric knee. The team consisted of engineers who initiated the design, a group of surgeons whose role was to evaluate and modify the design and develop the surgical technique, and manufacturers to produce the components and the instrumentation. The details will be described in Chap. 9.

Progress in Design After 1970

While the late 1960s saw the emergence of only a few designs, from the early 1970s, there was a steady expansion. Starting mainly in England, design and manufacturing quickly spread to the USA, Europe, and Japan. Established orthopedic companies saw this new opportunity to expand their business. Many large companies developed several different knee designs at the same time and would compete to attract the most prominent surgeon designers. Many surgeons, often with the assistance of engineers, were motivated to produce their own total knee design. Orthopedic associations, such as the British Orthopaedic Association (BOA) and the American Academy of Orthopaedic Surgeons (AAOS), started to include sessions on total knees in their programs, while special conferences were organized by prominent institutions and also by companies.

One of the most important such meetings was arranged by the Institution of Mechanical Engineers (IMechE) and the British Orthopaedic Association (BOA), held in Birdcage Walk in London in September 1974. A wide range of early designs, most with short-term clinical results, was presented. Some of these designs were close replicas of the anatomic joint itself, while others embodied ingenious mechanical features to guide the motion and provide stability. Also, biomechanical data was presented of the forces in the knee, the principles of stability, and testing methodologies. Some designs with a sound rationale showed early clinical success, while other designs were already showing problems. At this conference, there was a battleground between the proponents of the well-established hinges and the "new-fangled" condylar replacements. Mr. Shiers FRCS was a distinguished surgeon who designed a cemented hinge in 1959 and used it on cases with very severe deformity, mostly with successful results. At the conference, he pronounced that "the knee is a hinge and the best way to treat a hinge is with another hinge." In the ensuing years, while the condylar replacements prevailed, hinged designs still continued to be used. For example, they played a crucial role at the Royal National Orthopaedic Hospital in Stanmore for the treatment of bone tumors, as well as for treating arthritis with severe deformities and for revisions of failed artificial knees (Wilson et al. 1974). That hospital was the leading center in the development of implants for enabling patients with bone tumors to walk after removal of long bone segments including joints. The design criteria for those hinges included durable fixation, especially because many of the patients were in their teens and 20s. Hinged design has evolved to this day, most designs now including rotational freedom to improve function and reduce component loosening. Their provision of immediate stability, correct alignment determined by the stems, and ease and speed of surgery have been their major advantages. The incidence of infection has been substantially reduced by improvements in operating room practices.

During the 1970s and beyond, some artificial knee designs were modified, some were withdrawn, and new designs emerged. The driving force behind this progression was the clinical experience itself but, just as importantly, the collective experience, ideas, and interaction between the different designers. For example, if a particular design was found to have component loosening problems, observation of other designs without such problems would result in modification by reducing the femoral-tibial constraint or by adding more substantial fixation pegs. Patella pain would prompt the design of a patella flange on the femoral component and a plastic patella resurfacing component. Entrapment of cement particles in the bearing surfaces, which accelerated wear and increased friction, led to improved cementing techniques and cement containment pockets in the components. The differences between designs were largely based on the severity of the arthritis, to differences in "philosophy," or simply due to alternate design configurations performing equally well up to that time. It was apparent that there were a number of design solutions which would fulfill the need and satisfy a set of design criteria. Hence while an engineering design process may have been followed in most cases, either explicitly or implicitly, an additional factor was the collective experience, interaction, and insights of particular designers.

It is also important to recognize that many new design features originated as a result of experimental studies. While a design of a total knee can be seen as a coherent model, it is composed of separate features or facets as noted previously. These facets can relate to the component designs themselves, to the materials, to the method of fixation, and to the instruments and surgical technique. The following chapters will deal with the different facets individually. In an exchange with Maury Hull PhD from University of California, Davis, he considered that the design process can be thought of as an "interactive evolutionary process" in that the interactions of the designers, new concepts or design features from particular designers, basic and applied research, and the accumulation of clinical results, led to a steady progress of the designs over time. By 1980 there had been a convergence in the shapes and design configurations. Posterior cruciate retaining (CR) and posterior stabilized (PS) were most widely used. There was also a following for unicompartmental knees, ACL + PCL retaining, and rotating platform. By and large, following a design process had led to this stage.

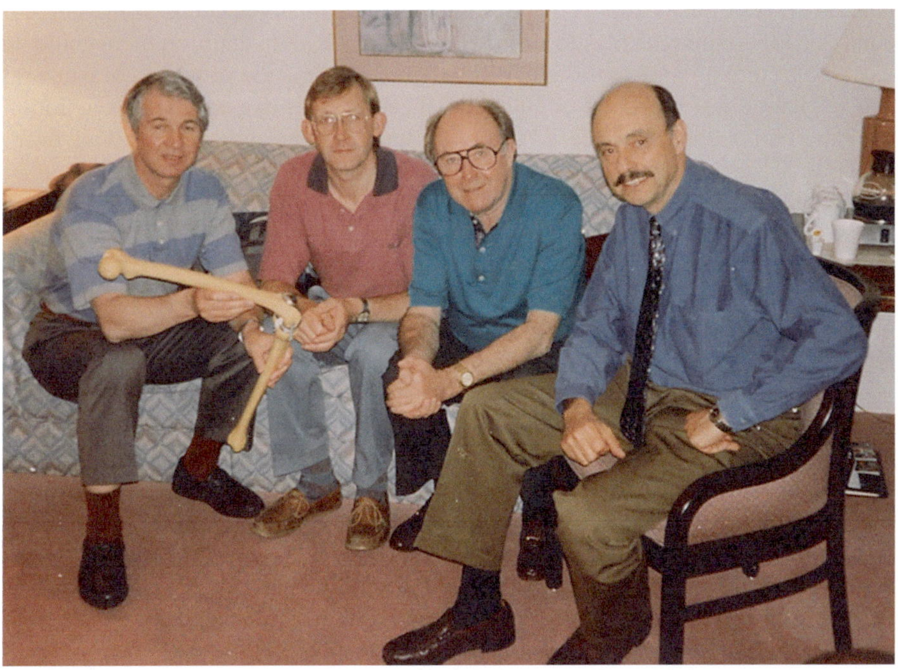

Fig. 3.6 A design meeting for the NexGen Knee System. Left to right: Peter Walker PhD, Design Consultant, John Insall MD, and Jorge Galante MD. Typical of the 1990s era, a large company would set up a design team of surgeons and engineers, together with their own staff. The team would be divided into several subgroups, as shown here, for dealing with specific design types. (Picture taken c 1990) (© Peter S Walker)

This chapter will be concluded with a brief description of robust design, a design concept formulated by Genichi Taguchi, a Japanese quality engineer (Taguchi and Clausing 1990). Taguchi's focus was how to improve the quality and reliability of products by determining the optimal design and manufacturing parameters so that the products would be of the highest quality with fewer problems during service conditions. His statistical methodologies for testing were widely applied in the automobile industry and led to the reputation of Japanese cars for their reliability and smooth performance. Applying the concepts to artificial knees, the design itself and the tolerances in the manufacture of both the components and instruments would lead to more accurate alignment, less loosening, and reduced wear. The performance would not be adversely affected by deficiencies of technique or by the type of activities of the patient.

As an example, in a condylar design with double-dished partially conforming bearing surfaces, the contacts will still be close to the "bottom of the dish," and there will still be adequate anterior-posterior and rotary stability, even if there is some misalignment. In contrast, if the tibial surface is shallow or even flat in the anterior-posterior direction, if the component is sloped too posteriorly on the proximal tibia, there could be excessive posterior sliding of the contact points. If the femoral and tibial bearing surfaces are close to being flat in the frontal plane, if there is lift-off of one condyle due to a high varus moment, the edge of the femoral condyle will dig into the plastic surface causing damage. In addition there could be unstable medial or lateral sliding. Yet another example is the provision of a central peg for fixation of the tibial component. If the cement has adequate penetration over the entire upper surface of the tibia, the component would be well fixed. However if substantial areas of the surface became debonded, overall loosening would occur. In that case, a central peg would act as an insurance in case of such surface loosening.

Has a Systematic Design Process Been Applied to Artificial Knees?

In most cases, a systematic process has been followed, in that the design criteria have been specified, tests carried out, and alternate configurations considered, with the design gradually reaching a conclusion until clinical trials were started. However the ideas for specific design features have evolved gradually over time, due to the results obtained and the interactions between those working in the field. The end result was a convergence of designs up to about 1980, when only two types of designs dominated, with a following for a few other designs. Since then, the design process had led to other design forms with the goals of optimizing functional performance, often using computer modeling for the analysis. Further advances can be made by specifying even more stringent design criteria, based on rigorous functional outcome measures.

References

Brand RA, Mont MA, Manring MM. Biographical sketch: themistocles gluck. Clin Orthop Relat Res. 2011;469:1525–7.

Cross N. Engineering design methods. London: Wiley; 2008.

Gluck T. Referat über die durch das Moderne Chirurgische Experiment gewonnen positive Resultate (Report on the positive results obtained by the modern surgical experiment). Arch fklin Chir. 1891;41:187–239.

Gunston FH. Polycentric knee arthroplasty. Prosthetic simulation of normal knee movement. J Bone Joint Surg. 1971;53(2):272–7.

Pritchett J. Obituary: Charles O. Townley. Clin Orthop Relat Res. 2009;67(1):308–9.

Pugh S. Total design: integrated methods for successful product engineering. Wokingham: Publ Addison Wesley; 1991.

Taguchi G, Clausing D. Robust quality. Harv Bus Rev. 1990:65–75.

Townley CO. Total knee arthroplasty. A personal retrospective and prospective review. Clin Orthop Relat Res. 1988;236:8–22.

Walker PS, Shoji H. Development of a stabilizing knee prosthesis employing physiological principles. Clin Orthop Relat Res. 1973;94:222–33.

Wilson JN, Lettin AWF, Scales JT. 20 years of evolution of the Stanmore hinged total knee replacement. Conference of total knee replacement, institution of mechanical engineers, London, 16–18 Sept 1974.

Laxity and Stability

4

How Has Laxity and Stability Been Incorporated into the Designs?

The principal motion of the knee is flexion-extension about a transverse axis, but because the femur and tibia are held together by extensible ligaments and the cartilage bearing surfaces are deformable, the knee behaves as a flexible hinge. This means that displacements and rotations can take place in all directions and at all angles of flexion, representing the laxity of the knee. Laxity is a fundamental property of the knee which has a number of functions and consequences. When the forces on the knee are small, the femur and tibia can be relatively positioned within a large envelope giving the limb maneuverability, useful in confined spaces. In function, laxity allows time for muscles to activate and stabilize the external forces before a stiff boundary is reached. If the knee was a rigid hinge, sudden external forces would cause very high impact forces against the anatomic structures resisting the motion.

Laxity is most commonly defined as the displacements and rotations which occur between the femoral condyles and the tibial plateaus when forces are applied. For example, in a seated position with the knee at 90-degree flexion, the foot can be twisted internally or externally, causing axial rotation of the tibia relative to the femur. If the upper part of the shank is pushed and pulled, there will be posterior and anterior displacement of the tibia relative to the femur. If the knee is in a normal relaxed state, that is termed a neutral position. If a force is applied to the tibia, laxity will easily occur, but as the force is increased, there will be less and less laxity until an end point is reached. The stiffness of the knee has steadily increased up to that end point. The laxity can be measured by various means and related to the applied forces. To describe the laxity quantitatively, the usual method is to define an axis system in the proximal tibia and distal femur. In the tibia the axes will be the same as the anatomic axis, with anterior-posterior and medial-lateral axes being mutually perpendicular. Axes are similarly set up in the femur. However the anatomic axis along the center of the femoral shaft is oblique to a line across the distal femoral condyles. For that reason, the vertical femoral axis is usually defined as a line between the center of the femoral head and the center of a line across the distal

P. S. Walker, *The Artificial Knee*, https://doi.org/10.1007/978-3-030-38171-4_4

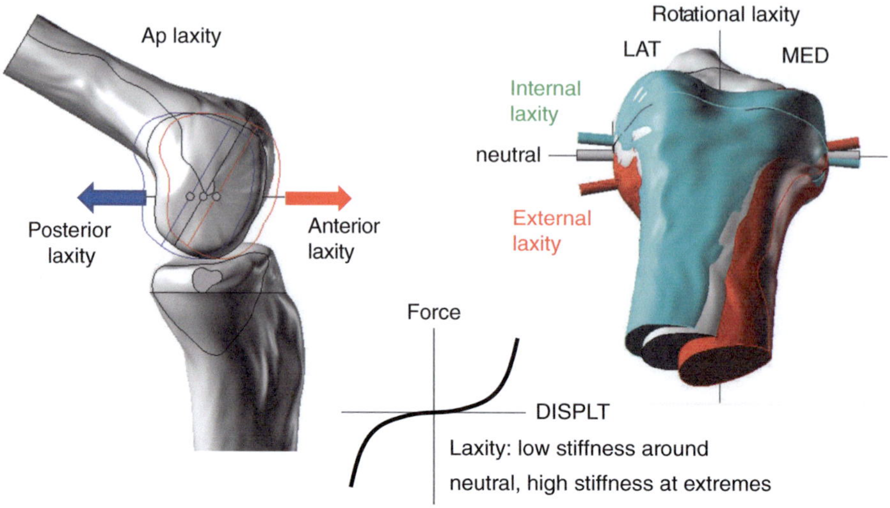

Fig. 4.1 Anterior-posterior (AP) and rotational laxity of the knee. AP laxity is produced by shear forces, rotational laxity by torques. The central region about the neutral position has a low stiffness where only small forces or torques are required to produce movements. As the femur moves away from the neutral position, the stiffness becomes progressively higher. The laxities reduce when there is a compressive force acting across the knee

femoral condyles. The displacements and rotations can then be described of the axis system of the femur relative to the axis system in the tibia, the latter being regarded as fixed.

Stability has no rigorous definition in that it is a clinical description rather than a measurable quantity. The knee joint is considered to be stable when the displacements and rotations during activity are within a normal boundary without any damage to the ligaments or menisci due to excessive elongation. If the displacements and rotations are increased further, soft tissue injury will occur. Due to the injury, the knee will then be unstable, able to displace beyond the normal boundaries even without excessive forces being applied. The three most important instabilities are anterior-posterior displacement, internal-external rotation, and varus-valgus rotation. These are caused by excessive stretching or tearing of one or more of the cruciate ligaments, collateral ligaments, and posterior capsule. In sporting activities, varus-valgus instability can be caused when there is a high enough force applied at one side of the knee. For example, an impact force on the outside of the knee will apply a valgus moment, causing lift-off of the medial condyles and, if the force is sufficiently high, a tear of the medial collateral ligament. If the valgus moment is accompanied by external rotation of the femur on the tibia, the anterior cruciate can be torn also. In the absence of any injuries to the ligaments, the knee will usually be stable to all types of loading within the normal laxity boundaries.

Another path to instability of the knee is when the cartilage bearing surfaces of the femur and tibia become worn, as occurs in arthritis. Normally the cartilage layers are about 3 mm thick on each surface. Even if only half of the layers become worn, this represents 3 mm of looseness of the main ligaments around the joint, which can cause instability. In anterior-posterior and rotation, the instability can be counteracted by the additional dishing due to the wear being restricted to specific areas. Up to the late 1960s when condylar replacement artificial knees were first designed, there had been little quantitative research on laxity and stability, although the concepts themselves were well recognized in sports medicine. In contrast there had been considerable attention given to the motion of the knee and the restraining role of the ligaments as far back as the nineteenth century (Pinskerova et al. 2003).

Remarkable work on ligament function was carried out by Brantigan and Voshell in 1941. In this work, they used beams and pulleys to apply known forces and moments and then measured the resulting laxities. Then in the mid-1960s, Hallen and Lindahl (1966) reported their work on the rotational behavior of the knee and what structures controlled it. As the knee was extended, the difference between maximum internal and external rotation was measured as torques were applied. They realized that it was difficult to define specifically what was internal and what was external due to the ambiguous neutral position. However they did find that the arc of rotational laxity moved progressively into internal rotation of the femur of the tibia as the knee reached extension. This was called the screw-home phenomenon. Hence by the time the first condylar knee designs emerged, there were the beginnings of an understanding of laxity and stability, shown to be a consequence of the ligaments, the shape of the bearing surfaces, and the menisci which provided a cushioning effect at the extremes of motion.

The designers of the prevailing hinged joints had no use for laxity, and deliberately avoided it. Their first priorities were stability and provision of flexion-extension. Even in designing the first condylar replacement total knee, Freeman and Swanson (1972, 1973) concentrated on providing stability and gave relatively little consideration to laxity. To provide stability, they decided to completely bypass the role of the cruciate ligaments in providing anterior-posterior and rotational stability, instead using the close conformity of the bearing surfaces. They took the dramatic step of making the bearing surfaces of the components provide all the necessary stability in both weight-bearing and non-weight-bearing conditions. Their decision to resect both of the cruciates was primarily for ease of surgery, an important design criterion. Cruciate resection was a radical step which had not been contemplated previously.

Knees with severe varus or valgus deformities were their main focus in designing an artificial knee for which correction of deformity using bone resections was easier with only the collateral ligaments present. The roller-in-trough configuration allowed for only flexion-extension motion about a single transverse axis, similar to the motion of a hinge. However Freeman and Swanson limited the depth of the trough such that some spin-out of the roller would occur when high torques were applied between the femur and tibia. The idea was to prevent excessive torques from being applied to the tibial fixation, but it had the dual effect of allowing for some rotational laxity. Another feature of the bearing surfaces was that in full extension,

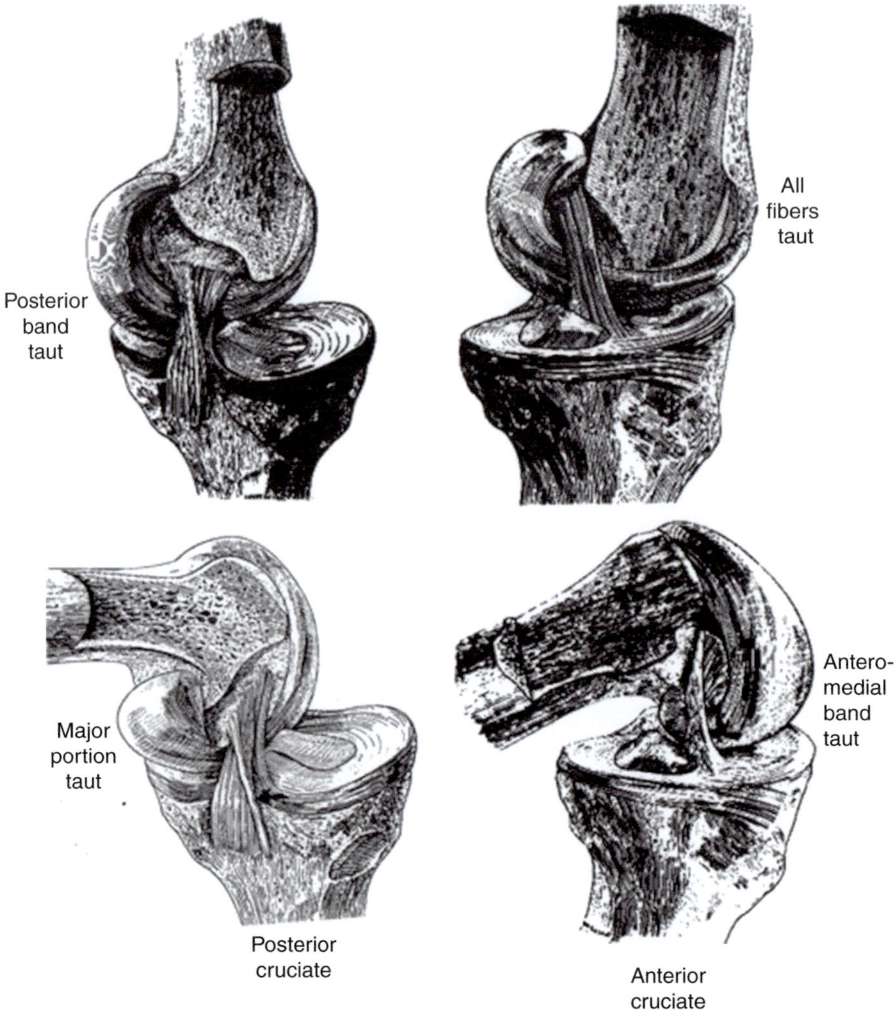

Fig. 4.2 From the examination of 44 knees, ligaments were shown to consist of bundles which were loose or taut at different flexion angles. With the knees mounted in an apparatus to control the motions and forces, serial sectioning of ligaments was used to determine their relative function (Girgis & Marshall 1975). (Reprinted with permission from *Clinical Orthopaedics & Related Research*)

a projection from the anterior of the femoral component articulated with a flattened region at the anterior of the tibial surface. The effect was to provide an anterior pivot point which would limit further extension by tensing the posterior soft tissues. This mechanism is similar to the action of the medial side of the anatomic knee, where the upward slope of the tibial bearing surface is augmented by the anterior horn of the medial meniscus.

A totally different approach to providing laxity and stability in a total knee was conceived by Gunston (1971). The idea was that an artificial knee could be designed using the same technologies that Charnley had developed for the hip. "The biomechanical principles and experience gained from total hip replacement arthroplasty were combined with an analysis of normal knee replacement." Many of the knee cases were rheumatoid arthritis with cartilage wear but without major deformities which likely accounts for the minimalist anatomic approach taken by Gunston. His idea was to resurface the femoral and tibial condyles where the sagittal contours were a close match to the original bearing surfaces. The means by which this was achieved on the femur was by an ingenious component design in the form of discs which were fitted in slots cut in the condyles. This gave a direct visualization of the parallelism of the component and the original bearing surfaces. With this strategy, the cruciate and collateral ligaments would be at their normal lengths, resulting in normal laxity and stability for that patient. "Lateral instability (varus-valgus) was eliminated by adjustment of the relative levels of the prosthetic articular surface." There is however some incompatibility of using discs which have a constant radius: the sagittal profiles of both lateral and medial femoral condyles show a larger radius distally than posteriorly. Due to this, the anterior of the disc component would be embedded below the surface, but this would avoid the potential problem of impaction of the patella in high flexion.

It is significant that these two earliest approaches to artificial knee design had totally different shapes of components and the means by which laxity and stability were achieved. The Freeman-Swanson design was a mechanistic approach relying on the components to provide reproducible and predictable mechanics, whereas the Gunston design was an attempt to preserve the normal laxity and stability characteristics of each individual knee. This defined the two extremes for the design of artificial knees. The mechanistic approach was particularly applicable to large deformities, while the anatomic approach was compatible with only mild-moderate degeneration and cruciate preservation.

Nevertheless the mechanistic approach could in principle be applied to all cases, and this idea was carried forwards in a different way by modifying the shape of the bearing surfaces. This approach started in the early 1970s, based on research studies on the factors which controlled laxity and stability. Limitations of the prior studies of laxity and stability of the anatomic knee were that the knees were tested without axial forces being applied, not representative of functional conditions. Moreover the previously applied forces to cause displacements and rotations were not measured, while it was assumed that the knees reached a relatively hard stop at the limits of the laxity range. In addition, around 1970, concepts of knee motion still focused on the sagittal plane. As an example, a key paper described the instant centers of rotation as the knee flexed and extended and showed how these centers changed during the flexion range (Frankel et al. 1971). The main point of the paper was to show that the smoothly changing instant centers in a normal knee were disrupted in pathological conditions. The idea of using instant centers was expanded upon in showing the anterior-posterior motions of the contact points which occurred, based on

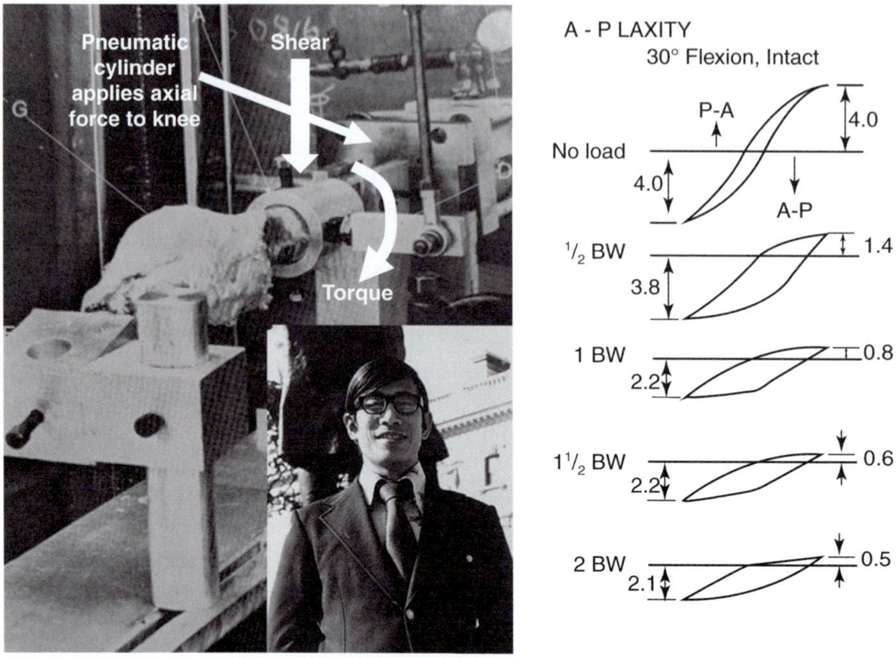

Fig. 4.3 Studies to measure the effect of an axial compressive force (long narrow arrow) on the laxities. The apparatus was mounted in an Instron machine which applied torque (curved arrow) or a shear force (straight vertical arrow). The laxity values reduced considerably with forces up to 2 body weight (Wang and Walker 1974; Hsieh and Walker 1976). The concepts were directly applied to the design of the Total Condylar knee. (Photo of Hua Hsieh taken in 1974 at the Conference on Total Knee Replacement, Institution of Mechanical Engineers, London, England) (Figures reprinted with permission from *Journal of Bone & Joint Surgery A*) (inset ©Peter S Walker)

radiographs taken at successive flexion angles (Walker and Shoji 1973). This had led to the proposition that tibial bearing surfaces in a condylar replacement type of artificial knee should allow some freedom of anterior-posterior motion, whereas the laxity was not accounted for.

Soon afterwards studies were carried out which showed the effect of axial forces on the laxity. These studies were carried out at the Hospital for Special Surgery in New York in the early 1970s (Wang and Walker 1974; Hsieh and Walker 1976). Knee specimens were fixed in a test rig, and an Instron loading machine was used to apply cyclic shear forces or torques between the femur and the tibia, while the displacements and rotations were measured. Tests were carried out with a range of axial forces applied to represent functional conditions. There were several important findings. The laxity was found to be nonlinear, with a very loose region for a small applied shear force or torque comprising most of the laxity, followed by a relatively stiff region at the extremes of the laxity. In the loose region, there was little resistance from ligaments, whereas at the extremes of laxity, the opposite was the case. The implication was that there was considerable freedom of motion when the knee was unloaded, whereas at the extremes of motion, the ligaments tighten and prevent further movements.

When axial loads were applied to simulate function, there were major differences in the laxity behavior. As the load was increased, the laxity steadily reduced. When the loads reached those typical of everyday activities, the laxities were reduced to only a few millimeters of displacement and a few degrees of rotation. These motions were well within the boundaries of the total laxities which occurred under small axial loading. This behavior had important implications; the ligaments themselves could not have been providing the constraint under loaded conditions, but some other factor was providing constraint due to the axial loads. One possibility was the friction between the cartilage bearing surfaces, but this was unlikely because with a friction coefficient of less than 0.01 in a healthy joint, an axial load of 1000 Newtons would provide a small shear resistance of only 10 Newtons. The factor considered to be the reason was an "uphill mechanism" caused by the dishing between the femoral and tibial bearing surfaces: "The mechanism proposed was the uphill movement of the femur, as the femur and the tibia were displaced or twisted relative to one another" (Hsieh and Walker 1976). The uphill movement would be due to the shape of the bearing surfaces and the increase due to the deformation of the cartilage caused by the loads. The medial meniscus was also considered to increase the effective dishing of the medial bearing surface in that it was peripherally attached and would be trapped between the femoral and tibial surfaces. Anatomic factors supporting the mechanism were that anterior displacement of the femur on the tibia was strongly resisted by the upward anterior slope of the medial tibial plateau, whereas axial rotation was reduced much less under load because the femur could pivot on the medial side of the tibia, with the generally convex lateral tibial plateau providing little resistance.

This uphill mechanism concept was later corroborated by Markolf et al. (1976, 1978). In the first of Markolf's studies, elaborate fixtures were applied to the knees of 50 living subjects to apply and measure anterior-posterior and varus-valgus laxities. When the subjects maximally tensed their muscles, laxities were reduced to 25–50% of the unloaded values. In the second study on specimens: "The stiffening of the knee (reduction of laxity) with applied joint load….suggests that there is a protective mechanism for ligaments of the knee…. We believe that joint congruency, which is a function of the contours of the tibial plateaus and femoral condyles, is a major contributing factor contributing to the stabilizing effects of the joint loading." In all of these studies, the constraints applied to the knee during the laxity measurements need to be defined. For example, if the tibia is fixed and the femur is displaced in an anterior-posterior direction, if the femoral and tibial condyles are to remain in contact, there must be freedom for a small amount of varus-valgus of the femur on the tibia. This is because the surfaces of the medial and lateral tibial plateaus are not parallel. The same applies to an internal-external rotation test. This is the concept of coupled laxities which was first recognized by Piziali et al. (1977). The consequence is that in a particular test, the other degrees of freedom should not be constrained. This principle applies to the design of all types of knee testing methods, whether in vivo or using laboratory machines.

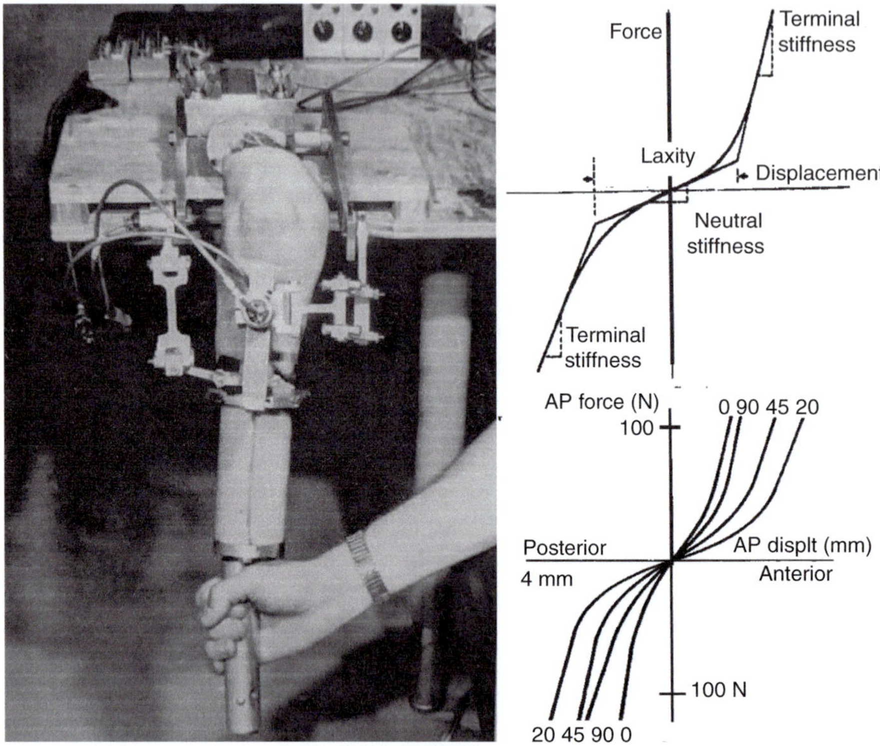

Fig. 4.4 Experimental apparatus used by Keith Markolf PhD to measure the laxities of the knee, both displacements and rotations. Motions in different planes were not constrained, giving more accurate laxity values. The authors defined the load-deflection graph with a loose central portion, and stiff portions at the extremes. The laxities and stiffnesses varied with the angle of flexion (Markolf et al. 1976). In an in vivo study, Markolf showed that when the subjects tightened their muscles, there was a 25–50% reduction in the AP laxity (Markolf et al. 1978). Markolf has continued to produce studies of the role of the knee ligaments in laxity and stability, working at the UCLA Biomechanics Laboratory in Los Angeles. (Reprinted with permission from *Journal of Bone & Joint Surgery A*)

The concept of laxity and stability was the basis of the Total Condylar knee designed in 1972 by Ranawat, Insall, and Walker and first used in patients in 1973 (Walker et al. 1974). The femoral component was the starting point. In the frontal and sagittal planes, radii similar to that of an average anatomic femur were chosen. The tibial radius values, larger than the corresponding femoral radii, were calculated to provide the required laxity and stability based on the laxity data. The result was femoral-tibial bearing surfaces which were partially conforming in both the frontal and sagittal planes. In the frontal plane, there was an added advantage of this scheme. If there was an applied varus or valgus moment sufficient to cause lift-off of one of the condyles, there would be a stable pivot point. This would prevent side-to-side sliding which would be felt as instability by the patient. The femoral

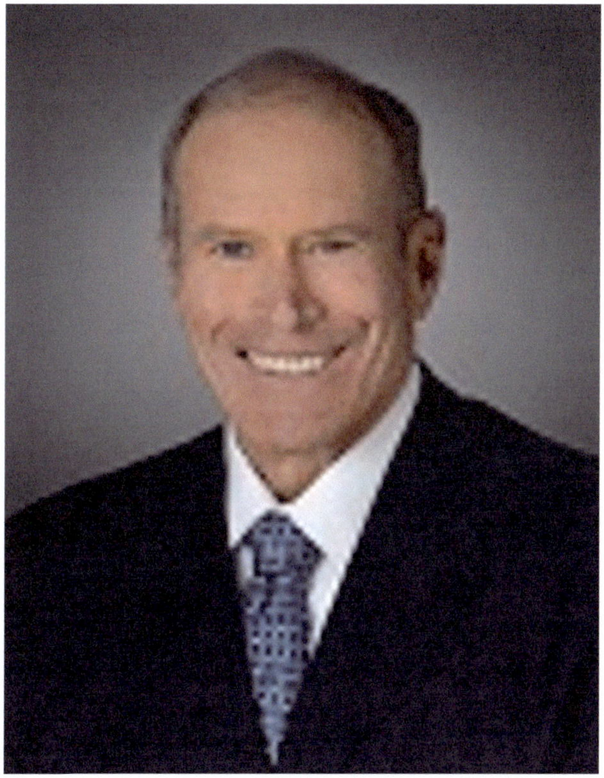

Fig. 4.5 Keith Markolf PhD started his career in biomechanics in 1970 with studies of the spine and then turned his attention to the hip and knee joints. In 1976, he published the first of several important and high-quality studies on the laxity and stability of the knee, work which had a direct application to artificial knee design. Since that time he has continued to carry out studies of the biomechanics of the knee and has published over 100 papers on the subject. He currently works at the UCLA Biomechanics Laboratory in Los Angeles. (Reprinted from *UCLA Biomechanics Lab Annual Newsletter 2014–2015*)

component also had an integral patella flange for which a plastic patella dome was designed (Aglietti et al. 1975). The combination of all of these features provided a combination of laxity and stability, with the laxity being reduced in weight-bearing conditions. The "partially conforming double-dished bearing surfaces" substituted for cruciate function and provided similar stability as if the cruciates were present. These stabilities included anterior-posterior displacement and internal-external rotation.

The principles of laxity and stability are embodied in most condylar total knees. As a generalization, designs where both of the cruciate ligaments are preserved (ACL + PCL type) usually have shallow tibial bearing surfaces on the basis that the anterior-posterior stability is provided mainly by the cruciates themselves. Some designs use shallow dishing or raised lips anteriorly and posteriorly to limit the extremes of motion, but up to these limits, there is considerable laxity possible between the femoral and tibial bearing surfaces. When the anterior cruciate is resected (CR type), the tibial surface usually has moderate dishing to substitute for the stability normally provided by the anterior cruciate. Ideally, this dishing should include an enhanced posterior lip to prevent the femur from locating at the posterior edge of the tibial surface, which would result in instability as well as damage to the

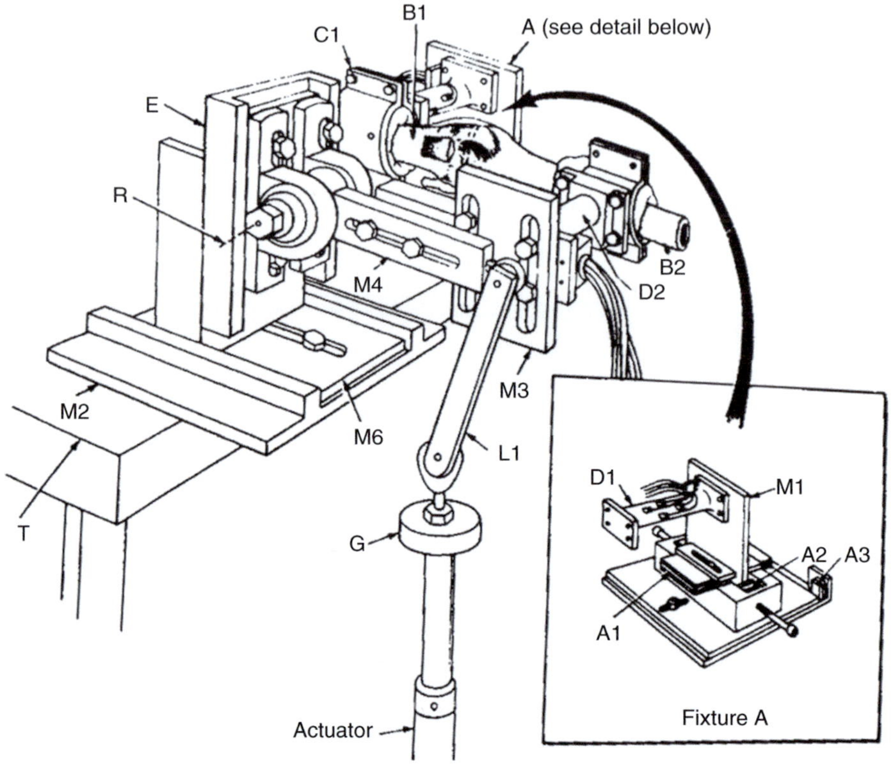

Fig. 4.6 Apparatus constructed to measure the nonlinear stiffness properties of the knee during different displacements and rotations. Coupled behavior was noted where anterior-posterior displacement produced internal-external rotation. Hence in testing, care is needed to not constrain the coupled motions (Piziali et al. 1977). (Reprinted with permission from *Journal of Biomechanics*)

plastic. For designs with resection of both cruciate ligaments (PS or UC types), even further dishing is provided on the tibial components in order to limit both anterior and posterior displacements of the femur on the tibia. In the ultracongruent designs, the tibial dishing can be extreme, restricting the laxity to only a few millimeters in the centers of each condyle. For all types of design, the condyles of the femoral component can be similar, averaging the anatomic values of the lateral and medial radii. The tibial radii are determined by which ligaments are present as explained above. Guidelines for the ideal tibial radii in the different design types were later specified in experiments carried out using a knee simulating machine (Luger et al. 1997). This study defined the ideal radii of the tibial bearing surfaces for the ACL + PCL, the CR and the PS types of artificial knees.

The posterior stabilized type (PS) is a special case in that the effect of the cam-post is superimposed on the stability provided by the femoral and tibial bearing surfaces. Near extension, the cam-post prevents posterior displacement of the femur on the tibia. In early flexion there is no contact. After about mid-flexion when the

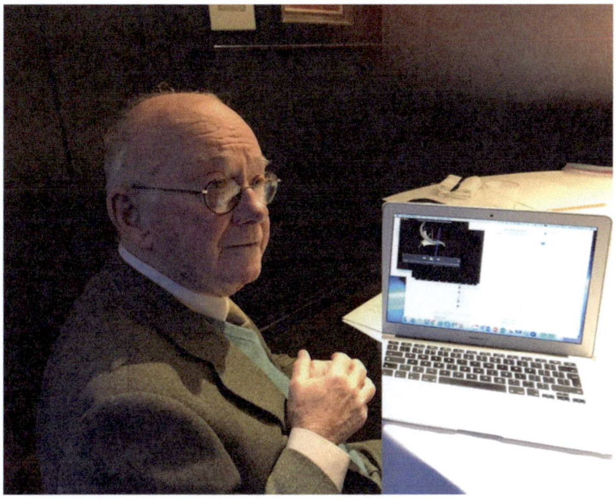

Fig. 4.7 John O'Connor PhD, a Professor of Mechanical Engineering at Oxford University, England, developed the Oxford meniscal knee, together with John Goodfellow FRCS of the Nuffield Orthopaedic Hospital. O'Connor published numerous studies of ligament modeling and knee kinematics, emphasizing the 4-bar linkage concept. The meniscal knee, allowing freedom of motion, was in tune with the cruciate ligaments which caused posterior displacements of the femur with flexion. (Photo taken at interview at Oxford 2017) (©Peter S Walker)

posterior surfaces of the cam-post come into contact, anterior displacement of the femur on the tibia is prevented. Other design intentions of the cam-post are to increase the range of flexion and the lever arm of the quadriceps. The cam-post does have the effect of reducing the anterior-posterior and rotational laxities in both extension and in high flexion.

It can be proposed that if artificial knees are to function in a similar way to the anatomic knee itself, the laxity and stability characteristics should be similar. The solution employed for off-the-shelf designs is to choose average values. However the laxity and stability values in anterior-posterior displacement or internal-external rotation vary considerably between individuals. To more closely match each patient, their laxity characteristics would need to be estimated in some way and then suitable radii for the bearing surfaces of the tibial component calculated. Alternatively there could be a simple choice between high or low laxity tibial components.

One important consideration is whether the laxity and stability of the medial and lateral sides should be different. In Chap. 2 Background, studies carried out in Europe were referred to which showed that during flexion, the lateral contact point displaced posteriorly much more than the medial contact point, resulting in axial rotation with the center of rotation on the medial side. This type of motion has been referred to as a "medial pivot." However a medial pivot concept was not considered for the early artificial knee designs for the two reasons explained; the European literature was not well known, and at that time knee motion was usually depicted in the sagittal plane only. Certainly there was recognition of the axial

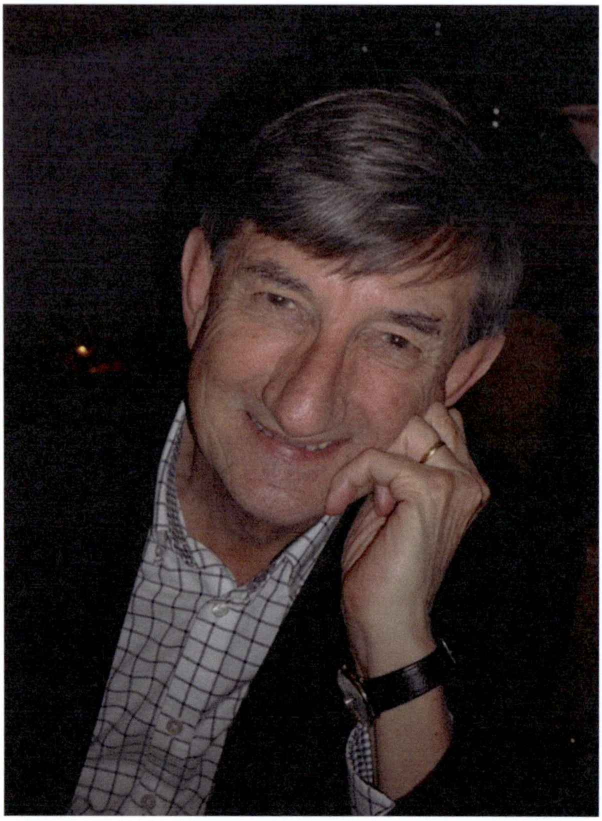

Fig. 4.8 Andrew Amis PhD was trained as an engineer at Rolls-Royce and then gained a PhD in Bioengineering at Leeds University, England, under Duncan Dowson PhD and Verna Wright MD. In 1979, he joined the Mechanical Engineering Department at Imperial College where he is still actively involved. During this time, he has carried out numerous insightful studies on the laxity and stability of the knee and the biomechanical functioning of artificial knees. In addition, he has worked with numerous surgeons on practical problems, often involving the solution of complex reconstructive problems. Amis has been a well-known participant in the European Federation of Sports Medicine Societies. (Photo taken in 2018) (© Peter S Walker)

rotation which occurred, but there was no consideration of asymmetry between the lateral and medial sides of the components. Such a scheme was eventually described in a 1992 patent (Tuke and Freeman 1993). Mike Tuke was an inventive engineer who joined Freeman and Swanson's Biomechanics group at Imperial College London in the 1970s. Tuke and Freeman devised a medial pivot type of knee replacement, as an advancement of the original Freeman-Swanson design: "…an improved knee prosthesis which will allow the patient to move his knee substantially in the same manner as though he had not had to undergo implantation of a knee prosthesis." This is an ideal design criterion for an artificial knee and is the essence of the PROM which has been introduced recently called the Forgotten Joint Score.

The medial pivot concept for an artificial knee was also being pursued by David Blaha in the USA. Blaha had been a Fellow with Freeman in the early 1980s. They had numerous discussions about the asymmetry of the lateral and medial motion, and did not accept the 4-bar linkage concept of knee motion which was described by John Goodfellow and John O'Connor at Oxford. Further details of the medial pivot knee will be described later in Chap. 11 Guided Motion Knees. However in the context of laxity and stability, the lateral and medial sides behaved quite differently in terms of the laxity and stability which they provided. The medial femoral condyle was a spherical surface, seated in a matching surface in the medial tibial plateau. This allowed no linear laxity but allowed unconstrained rotation about a vertical axis. In contrast, the lateral tibial plateau allowed freedom of AP motion without any constraint to rotation about the medial side. Hence the bearing surfaces would not provide both laxity and stability on the lateral and medial sides as in a typical condylar replacement knee, but preferential stability on the medial side. Constraints would still be provided by the collateral ligaments however. In an anatomic knee, the deformability of the medial bearing surfaces and the meniscus and the elasticity of the ligaments still allow some anterior-posterior displacements to occur on the medial side, so in that sense the medial side would not act as a fixed medial pivot, but rather as a "loose medial pivot." But the many studies on laxity up to about 1990 did not sufficiently describe the internal mechanics of the knee under a wide range of loading conditions simulating different activities. Nevertheless designing an asymmetric artificial knee was a very important step in that it defined a completely new type of design to the existing symmetric designs. Today, there has been renewed attention to designs with a differential between the laxities on the lateral and medial sides.

So far only anterior-posterior and internal-external laxities have been discussed, because this was the main focus of most of the studies. Markolf also measured varus-valgus laxity and was the first to point out that a certain moment had to be applied to cause lift-off of one of the condyles, after which one of the collateral ligaments supplemented by the cruciates would control the subsequent laxity. While anterior-posterior and internal-external are an inherent part of normal knee motion, varus-valgus is a mode to be avoided, because it indicates that the loading condition is such that ligament injuries could occur.

The laxity of the knee in axial compression is usually not referred to, yet it may have significance in that while the joint surfaces undergo deflections of several millimeters during functional loading, the materials used for artificial joints only experience small deflections. In load-deflection experiments of the anatomic knee, due to the deformability of the menisci, Krause et al. (1976) found that energy absorption was considerably reduced on the removal of the menisci due to their load-bearing role. The load-deflection curve will also depend upon the thickness of the articular cartilage on both the femur and tibia and the effective modulus of elasticity during the repetitive loading in walking. Shepherd and Seedhom (1999) compared the cartilage thickness in the hip, knee, and ankle and found that the thickness was greatest in the least conforming joint, the knee. Another important finding was that the modulus of elasticity in compression was higher the thicker was the cartilage. The thickness was averaged for the femoral and tibial condyles, the latter divided into the area which was covered or not covered by the menisci. The mean femoral thickness was 1.7–2.7 mm; for the tibia, the mean thickness ranged from 1.5 to 3.0 mm. Using MRI and stereophotogrammetry, the cartilage thicknesses were accurately mapped over the entire surfaces of the femoral and

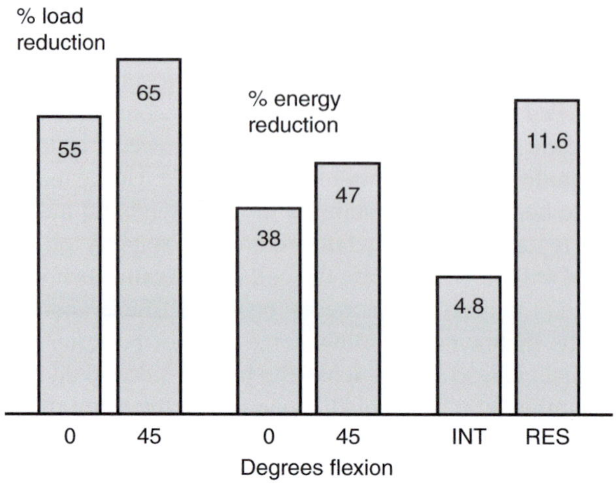

Fig. 4.9 Bill Krause carried out experiments showing the vital role of the menisci in attenuating the forces and in energy absorption during axial loading. Left, two pairs of bars: The percentage reduction in load and energy absorbed after removal of the menisci, for a given deflection value. Right pair of bars: The contact stresses for the intact knee before (INT) and after (RES) meniscal resection. Drawn from tabulated data (Krause et al. 1976)

tibial condyles (Cohen et al. 1999). The mean maximum thickness on the femur and tibia were as much as 4.0 and 4.5 mm, respectively. In two different studies, Guaon Li and colleagues from Massachusetts General Hospital in Boston used fluoroscopy to determine the deformations of the cartilage in living subjects. In a lunge activity, the cartilage deformation was 22–30% (Bingham et al. 2008; Liu et al. 2010). During a gait cycle, the percentage deformation had a maximum value of 23% compared with the resting thickness. When these values are related to the maximum cartilage thickness of the femur and tibia combined, in the region of 6–8 mm, the linear deformations were about 1.5–2.0 mm. While these are small amounts, they are significant in relation to the elongations of the cruciate and collateral ligaments whose stiffnesses are in the region of 60 Newtons/mm. In the resting position of the knee, the pretensions in the collateral ligaments have been measured at 50 Newtons in each ligament. This means that during an activity cycle, the ligament tensions could reduce to a small value. In this case the stability of the knee would rely to a large extent on the geometry of the bearing surfaces and the menisci, together with the stabilizing effects of the muscles themselves. Another factor related to the deformation at the knee is the accelerations when the foot impacts the ground. It was found that the vertical accelerations across the knee were higher in arthritic and artificial knees, compared with normal knees (Kahn et al. 2013).

An ideal design criterion for an artificial knee is that the laxity and stability after the artificial knee has been implanted are the same as when the knee was in its normal healthy state. If all of the soft tissues are retained, the bearing surfaces of the

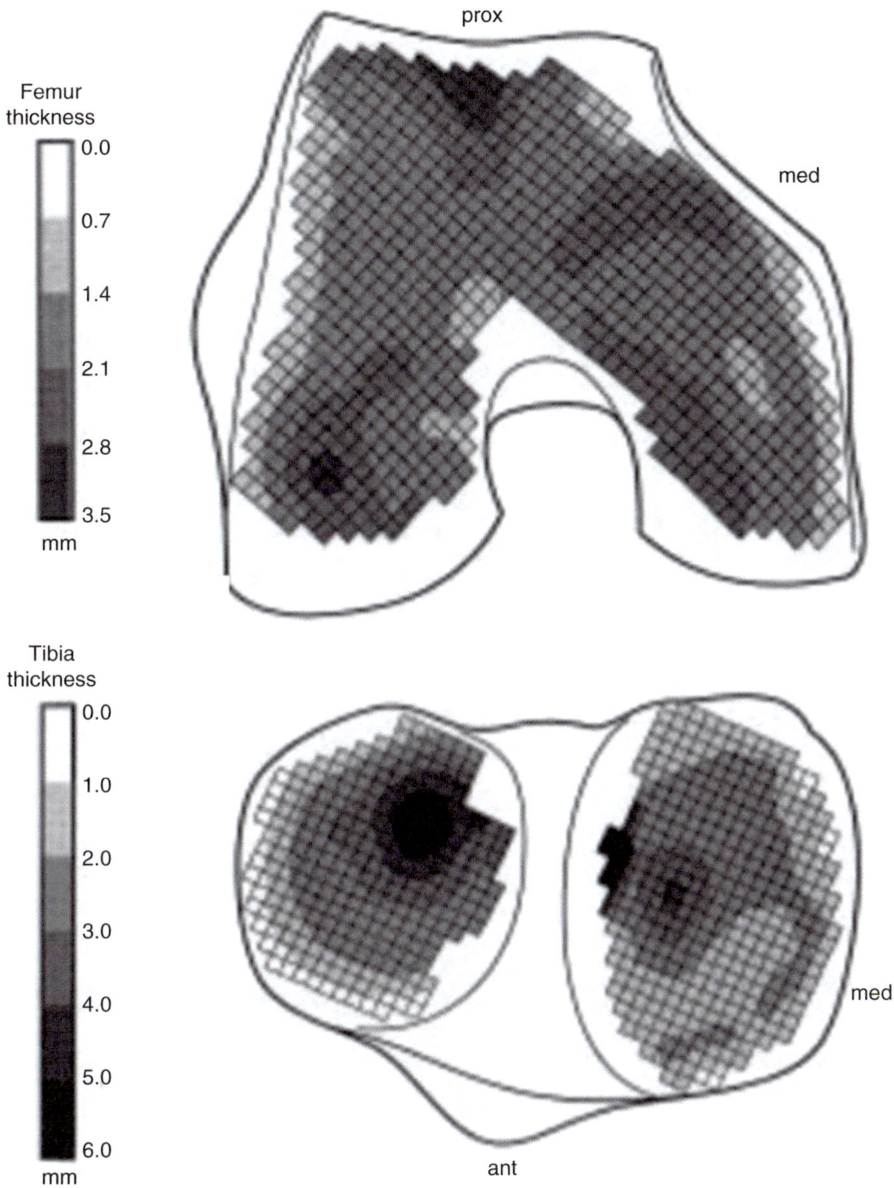

Fig. 4.10 The cartilage thickness over the femoral and tibial surfaces was mapped using a stereophotogrammetry technique accurate to 0.1 mm. There was considerable variation in thickness with some indication that the thickest cartilage occurred over areas of most frequent weight-bearing (Cohen et al. 1999). This data has implications to the deformations which occur during weight-bearing and hence to the changing lengths of the major ligaments around the knee. Such length changes will have significant effects on the laxity during weight-bearing phases of activity (Cohen et al. 1999). (Reprinted with permission from *Osteoarthritis & Cartilage*)

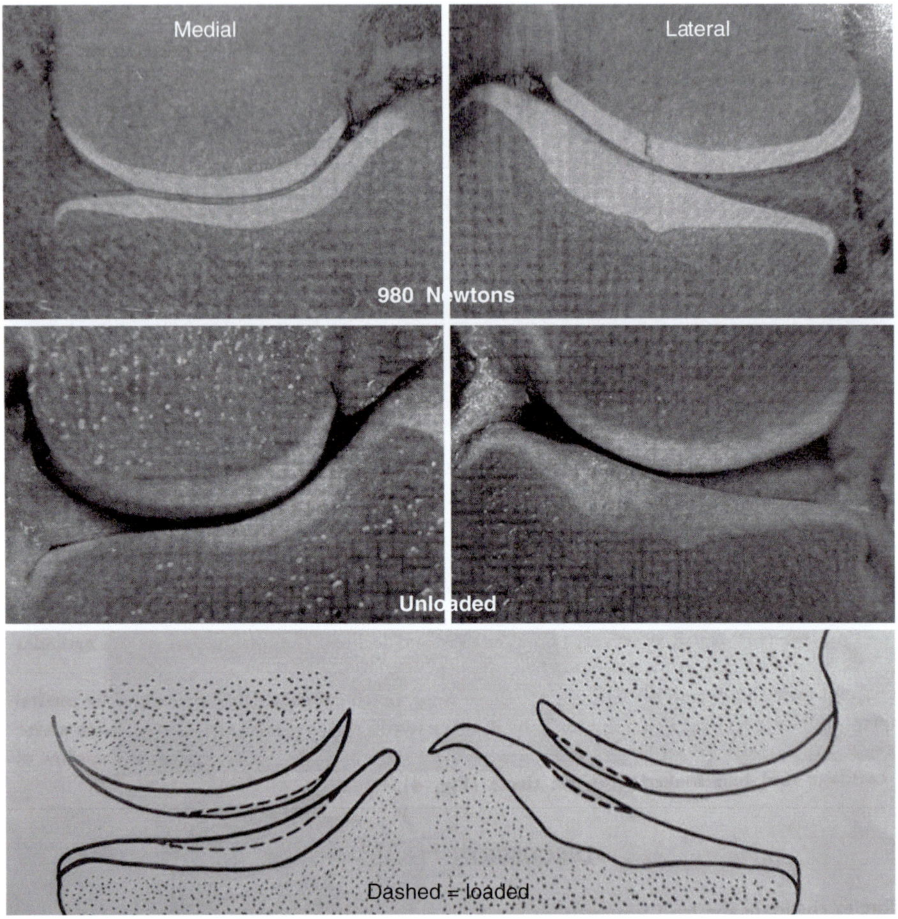

Fig. 4.11 Knees were loaded, frozen, sectioned, and photographed. After thawing, another photograph was taken. This figure shows the regions of cartilage deformation and the magnitude. Deformation of each cartilage layer was approximately 1 mm. The variation in cartilage thickness can be seen, especially on the tibia. Peter Walker observed this work in progress, on a visit to Tsunenori Takei's lab at Shinshu University in about 1978 (Takei 1979). (Reprinted with permission from *Journal of the Japanese Orthopaedic Association*)

artificial knee need to substitute for the function of the articular surfaces and the menisci. The medial side of the knee does provide anterior-posterior stability, particularly if there is a compressive force acting. Hence in a conventional condylar knee, there should be some sagittal tibial dishing medially, even if the lateral side is flat. If one or both cruciate ligaments are resected, the dishing will need to be increased accordingly. Again, if the medial-lateral asymmetry is to be replicated, the medial dishing should be greater than the medial. Based on the above criteria, some ACL + PCL preserving designs may be under-constrained, while in cruciate resecting designs, most are symmetric, although they will in general still provide adequate stability. Considering that the muscles in many arthritic patients are weaker than normal, more than anatomic constraint seems advisable. The constraint in any particular design can be determined by the ASTM constraint test or by software simulating that test.

How Has Laxity and Stability Been Incorporated into the Designs?

A combination of laxity and stability has been incorporated into artificial knee designs by the radii of the femoral condyles in the frontal and sagittal view being smaller than the radii of the tibial surfaces. The closer the radii between the femur and tibia, the higher the stability and the lower the laxity, and vice versa. For designs which preserve the cruciate ligaments, there should be relatively large differences in the radii, to the point where the tibial surfaces are shallow. When the cruciates are resected, there needs to be smaller differences in the radii, so that the bearing surfaces provide the stability which was normally carried by the cruciate ligaments.

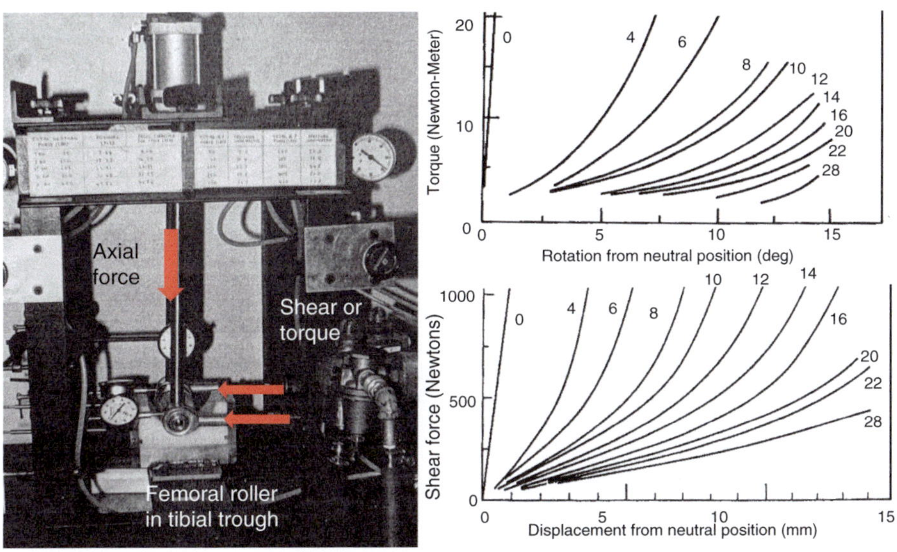

Fig. 4.12 Equipment for measuring the laxity of total knees, designed by Walker. Knee geometry was represented by rollers in troughs with different combinations of sagittal radii. The laxity was determined by the difference between the femoral and tibial sagittal radii (numbers next to each curve). A difference of 0 mm indicates complete conformity, for which displacement and rotation were small. As the shear force or torque were increased, or as the difference in radii increased, the laxity increased. The values shown in the graphs are for an axial force of 1000 N, about one half the maximum force in activity. To maintain the laxities to normal levels in the absence of the cruciate ligaments, moderate to high conformity is needed

References

Aglietti P, Insall JN, Walker PS, Trent P. A new patella prosthesis. Design and application. Clin Orthop Relat Res. 1975;107:175–87.

Bingham JT, Papannagari R, Van der Velde SK, Gross C, Felson DT, Rubash HE, Li G. In vivo cartilage contact deformation in the healthy tibiofemoral joint. Rheumatology. 2008;47(11):1622–7.

Brantigan OC, Voshell AF. The mechanics of the ligaments and menisci of the knee joint. J Bone Joint Surg (Br). 1941;23(1):44–66.

Cohen ZA, McCarthy DM, Kwak SD, Legrand P, Fogarisi F, Ciacchio EJ, Ateshian GA. Knee cartilage topography, thickness, and contact areas from MRI; in-vitro calibration and in vivo measurements. Osteoarthritis & Cartilage. 1999;7:96–109.

Frankel VH, Burstein AH, Brooks DB. Biomechanics of internal derangement of the knee. Pathomechanics as determined by analysis of the instant centers of motion. J Bone Joint Surg Am. 1971;53(5):945–62.

Freeman MA, Swanson SA, Zahir A. Total replacement of knee using metal polyethylene two-part prosthesis. Proc R Soc Med. 1972;65(4):374–5.

Freeman MA, Swanson SA, Todd RC. Total replacement of the knee using the Freeman-Swanson knee prosthesis. Clin Orthop Relat Res. 1973;(94):153–70.

Gunston FH. Polycentric knee arthroplasty. Prosthetic simulation of normal knee movement. The J Bone Joint Surg (Br). 1971;53(2):272–7.

Hallen LG, Lindahl O. The “screw-home” movement in the knee-joint. Acta Orthop Scand. 1966;37(1):97–106.

Hsieh HH, Walker PS. Stabilizing mechanisms of the loaded and unloaded knee joint. J Bone Joint Surg Am. 1976;58(1):87–93.

Kahn H, Walker PS, Zuckerman JD, Slover J, Jaffe F, Karia RJ, Kim JH. The potential of accelerometers in the evaluation of stability of total knee arthroplasty. J Arthroplast. 2013 Mar;28(3):459–62.

Krause WR, Johnson RJ, Wilder DG. Mechanical changes in the knee after meniscectomy. J Bone Joint Surg Am. 1976;58(5):599–604.

Liu F, Kozanek M, Hosseini A, Van der Velde SK, Gill TJ, Rubash HE, Li G. In vivo tibiofemoral cartilage deformation during the stance phase of gait. J Biomech. 2010;43:658–65.

Luger E, Sathasivam S, Walker PS. Inherent differences in the laxity and stability between the intact knee and total knee replacements. Knee. 1997;4(1):7–14.

Markolf KL, Mensch JS, Amstutz HC. Stiffness and laxity in the knee – the contribution of the supporting structures. J Bone Joint Surg Am. 1976;58(A)(5):583–94.

Markolf KL, Graff-Radford A, Amstutz HC. In vivo knee stability. A quantitative assessment using an instrumented clinical testing apparatus. J Bone Joint Surg Am. 1978;60(5):664–74.

Pinskerova V, Maquet P, Freeman MA. The anatomic literature relating to the knee from 1836 to 1917: an historic note. Clin Orthop Relat Res. 2003;410:13–8.

Piziali RL, Rastegar JC. Measurement of the non-linear, coupled stiffness characteristics of the human knee. J Biomech. 1977;10(1):45–51.

Shepherd DET, Seedhom BB. Thickness of human articular cartilage in joints of the lower limb. Ann Rheum Dis. 1999;58:27–34.

Takei T. Deformation of the articular cartilage and joint space of the human knee joint under static load. J Japan Orthop Ass. 1979;53:577–93.

Tuke MA, Freeman MAR. ‘Knee Prosthesis’ US Patent No. 5, 219, 362. Filed Feb. 1992, issued June 15, 1993.

Walker PS, Shoji H. Development of a stabilizing knee prosthesis employing physiological principles. Clin Orthop Relat Res. 1973;(94):222–33.

Walker PS, Wang CJ, Masse Y. Joint laxity as a criterion for the design of condylar knee prostheses. Conference on Total Knee Replacement, Institution of Mechanical Engineers, London, UK, 16–18 September 1974.

Wang CJ, Walker PS. Rotatory laxity of the human knee joint. J Bone Joint Surg Am. 1974;56(1):161–70.

5 Fixation Using Acrylic Cement

What Are the Basic Principles of Cemented Fixation, and How Durable Is It?

Before the artificial hip and knee were introduced, metal components for resurfacing one side of the joint were being used to treat arthritis. However for resurfacing both sides of the joint, there were two major challenges: how to fix the components rigidly to the bones such that the fixation would be durable and identifying materials with sufficiently low friction and wear. This chapter will describe why acrylic cement was chosen for fixation and the way in which it should be used at surgery. Initially the mechanics of the fixation of uncemented components will be discussed as this led to the recognition of why some type of cementing was considered to be necessary.

Implants Without Fixation

Hip prostheses such as the Austin Moore stem for replacing an arthritic femoral head or for treating a femoral neck fracture were widely used in the 1950s and 1960s. Fixation of the component to the femur was by an intramedullary stem press fit into the canal, sometimes augmented by bone graft. In many cases however, the stem loosened in the canal due to the axial and torsional forces, causing subsidence and pain. In the knee, uncemented metal tibial plateaus of the McKeever or MacIntosh types were frequently used (McKeever 1960; Macintosh and Hunter 1972). Their design rationale was different. McKeever focused on biomechanical design criteria: "There must be an optimal relation between surface area and the range of functional stress to be borne by the prosthesis and transmittal to the bone." "An endoprosthesis must be self-retaining…..so that the normal forces in the joint hold it in place." "The direction of stress transfer between the prosthesis and the bone must be constant." "The stress transfer from prosthesis to bone must take place at a single level." This referred to a situation where a stem could transfer loads directly to cortical bone, bypassing trabecular bone which would then experience "stress protection" and become porotic.

P. S. Walker, *The Artificial Knee*, https://doi.org/10.1007/978-3-030-38171-4_5

The emphasis of MacIntosh was: "The aims are to correct the varus or valgus deformity and restore normal stability by taking up the slack in the collateral ligaments." However these metal tibial plateaus, while finding a useful application for certain indications, experienced an incidence of sinkage, bone resorption, and loosening with some pain (Scott et al. 1985). Even the addition of anterior screws used in Townley's tibial plateau design (Townley 1988, originally published 1964) could not prevent bone resorption and loosening over time. The likely reason was the mechanics at the interface between the rigid metal component and the exposed ends of the trabecular bone across the resected proximal tibial surface. Firstly, there would not be a precise fit, so that the patches of contact would be overstressed; secondly, there would be interface micromotions due to the changing compressive and shear stresses during activities. It was clear that rigidly fixing the implant component to the bone where the forces were uniformly distributed was essential. A possible solution would be to use a grouting material between the implant and the bone, where the grout would penetrate into the interstices of the trabecular bone. The criteria for the material were biocompatibility, sufficient mechanical strength, and practical to use at surgery.

Origin and Use of Acrylic Cement

A solution applied to a surface replacement hip was first used by Edward Haboush (1953). Haboush was an orthopedic surgeon at the Hospital for Joint Diseases in New York (now NYU Langone Orthopedic Hospital). Haboush was regarded as being extrovert and inventive by his colleagues. In his paper, it is clear that he was familiar with basic engineering principles: "I have also found it highly desirable to secure the head or ball in position on the femur by means of a quick-setting resinous material, such as a quick-hardening acrylic resin and also to secure the socket in position in the pelvic arch, by means of a similar quick-setting resin which serves not only to bond the elements together but to afford a cushioning action which absorbs and distributes the shock throughout a greater area of the bone structure and this minimizes wear, erosion and pain." At surgery, a powder (polymer) and a liquid (monomer) were mixed together, and after a few minutes, a doughy stage was reached allowing the cement to be applied in the joint. After a few more minutes, the cement hardened, fixing the component to the bone. This setting property of the acrylic cement allowed the surgeon enough time to apply the cement and position the components before the cement hardened. Although Haboush used photoelasticity to demonstrate how cement produced uniform force transfer, mechanical problems with the hip components limited further advancement of his work to only a few cases.

It is likely that Charnley obtained the idea of using acrylic cement from a conference in Copenhagen in 1951 or from Edward Haboush soon after (Waugh 1990). However, Charnley subsequently carried out a great deal of experimental work and materials development in conjunction with a manufacturing company, so that the acrylic could be used practically for hip surgery. One important characteristic of the acrylic was its biocompatibility in solid form. Charnley explained the role of the

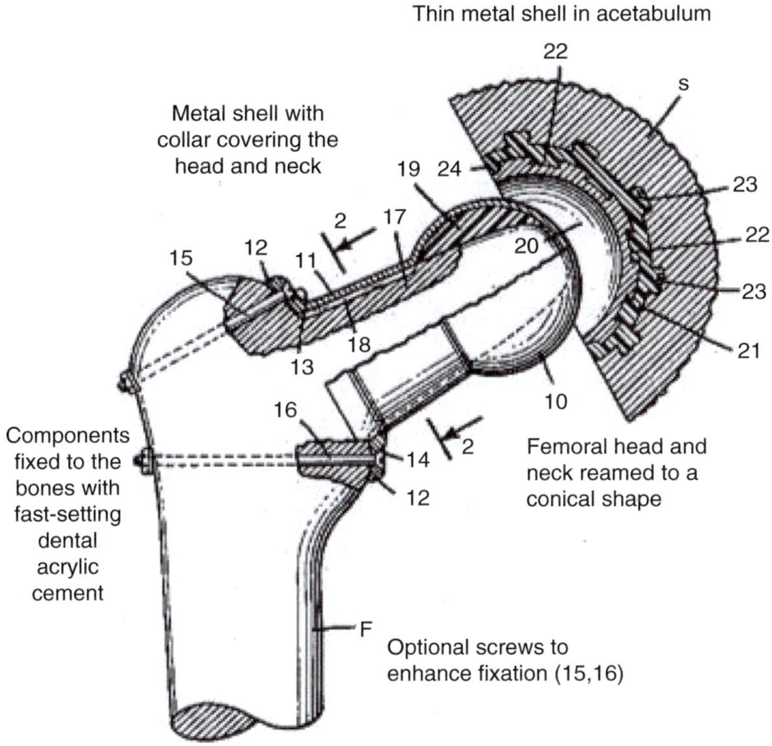

Fig. 5.1 Edward Haboush from the Hospital for Joint Diseases in New York (now NYU Langone Orthopedic Hospital) was first to use fast-setting dental acrylic cement for anchoring components to the bone, applied to a surface replacement type of artificial hip joint. He designed several versions of the device and implanted them in patients from 1951. The figure shows his US patent filed in February 1952 (Haboush 1953). (Reprinted with permission from Bulletin of the Hospital for Joint Diseases)

cement in providing an accurate cast of the surface of the bone whether in the femoral canal or in the acetabulum. This would transmit stress evenly over all parts of the interface between the acrylic and cancellous bone. The cement was then used in the total hip.

Over the next few years, Charnley studied the use of acrylic cement in the hip and reported his findings in 1970 in a book entitled *Acrylic Cement in Orthopaedic Surgery* (Charnley 1970). He prepared histological sections from the hips of deceased patients, showing the minimal tissue reaction and durability of the interface. He also emphasized the surgical technique and an understanding of the mechanical principles: "Failures after using acrylic cement are basically the same as the failures of all forms of orthopaedic surgery: namely, mechanical failures from an inadequate understanding of mechanical detail. These failures…. result from fundamental errors in biomechanical theory underlying these procedures, errors which the concept of cement eliminates." An important aspect was reduction of the interface motion to

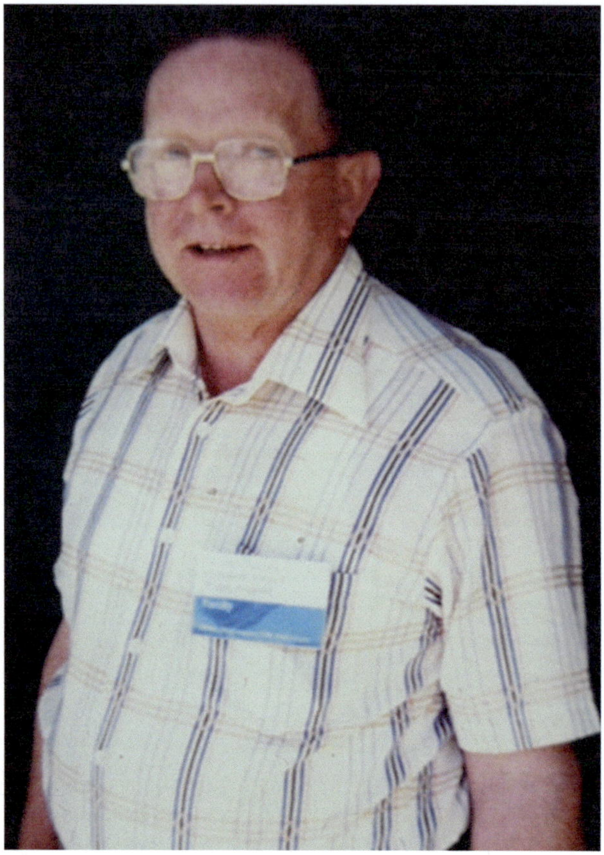

Fig. 5.2 John Charnley's extensive experience and research on the use of acrylic cement in the hip joint set the stage for the use of cement in the artificial knee, by demonstrating that it was both safe and effective. One disadvantage of using cement in the hip was the high pressures generated in the femoral canal during stem insertion, forcing monomer and fat into the circulation. However this did not apply to the knee where the problem was often obtaining enough pressure at the tibial bone interface to achieve sufficient cement penetration. (Photo taken c 1980) (© Peter S Walker)

insignificant values by the interposition of cement between the implant and the trabecular bone, the cement interlocking with the trabeculae: "The superficial layer of the cancellous bone in contact with the cement will move as one with the cement surface when load is applied. The deflection of the cancellous structure under load will take place inside the bulk of the cancellous bone. In this way we can explain the paradox of the transmission of load from a hard to soft substance without relative motion taking place between the surfaces in contact." Charnley explained the mechanism of cement intrusion into the cancellous bone of the walls of the femoral canal: "The insertion of the tapered stem of the prosthesis expands the stiff dough (cement) and injects it into the cancellous lining." After the mid-1960s, there were an increasing number of US surgeons who had spent the requisite training time at Charnley's hip center and were using the Charnley hip. It was not long before US companies started to make their own artificial hip designs, and in the early 1970s, knees were to follow. However, considering the importance of fixation to the success of the devices, there was a surprising delay in scientific studies on the mechanics of fixation, especially for the knee. This can largely be explained by the higher priority given to the study of the systemic effects caused by the monomer of the cement, as well as on the effects of the heating of the cement during polymerization on the trabecular bone.

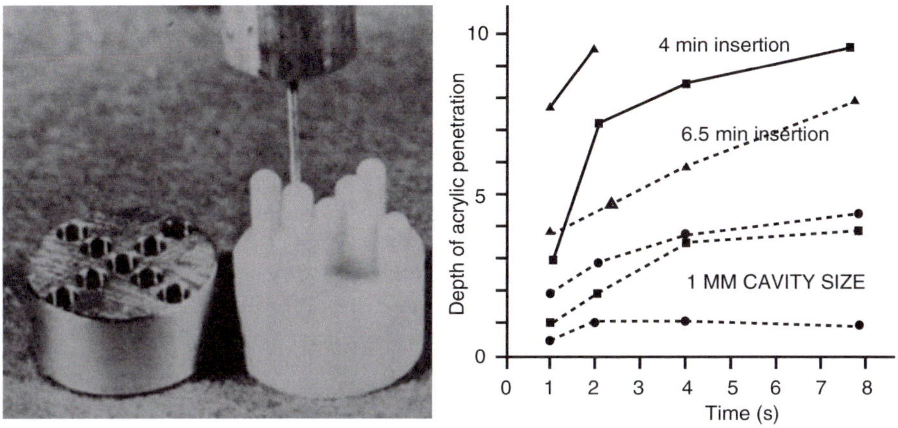

Fig. 5.3 Early fundamental experiments on the depth of penetration of acrylic cement under different conditions. The smaller the time after mixing and the less viscous, the greater the depth of penetration. The higher the applied pressure, the greater the depth. The smaller the holes, the less the depth (Markolf and Amstutz 1976). (Reprinted with permission from Clinical Orthopaedics & Related Research)

At surgery, it was necessary to account for the rheological behavior of the cement, including the variations in properties due to time, ambient temperature, and handling. The initial liquidy state changed during only a few minutes from low viscosity to high viscosity with rubberlike viscoelasticity. Consequently the timing of the introduction onto the bone surface and the mechanical pressures applied greatly affected the degree of interdigitation. In controlled experiments using holes drilled in blocks, the depth of penetration was higher for an earlier time of introduction, for larger hole diameters, and for larger applied pressure, as expected (Markolf and Amstutz 1976). But after only 1–2 seconds after pressure application, the rate of penetration slowed down significantly. This led to the conclusion that no matter what the introduction time of the cement and placing the component, the greatest penetration would be obtained by only a few episodes of vigorous finger packing. These experiments provided general guidelines for the use of acrylic cement in surgical conditions, although if a specific depth of penetration was required for a particular component, whether hip or knee, and for cancellous bone of low or high density, more detailed experimentation would be needed.

Cement-Bone Interface

While the above work was applied to hip replacement, in the case of the artificial knee, although their usage expanded in the early 1970s, similar experiments were not carried out until the late 1970s. By then, it was evident that loosening of the tibial component was a major problem in many designs even after only 1–2 years. Loosening was evidenced by radiolucent lines (RLLs) at the interface between the cement and the bone on the radiographic images. In many of these cases, the RLLs were restricted to about 1 cm width on the lateral and medial sides and did not progress in extent or thickness. This was termed a nonprogressive RLL which was not considered to be a problem. However, in many cases, the RLLs became more extensive over time, even involving the entire interface. This was called a progressive RLL, a serious problem in that it represented a complete dissociation of the component and cement from the underlying bone. Histological examinations indicated that there had been a lack of cement penetration into the cancellous bone with bone resorption beneath the cement, replaced by fibrous tissue. Beneath that was a thin layer of new cortical bone, a subchondral layer.

Part of the explanation for the radiolucent lines was evident from biomechanical experiments carried out at the Hospital for Special Surgery in the early 1970s although the significance was not fully recognized at the time. The first piece of evidence was that the load between the femur and the tibia in the normal knee was transmitted over elliptical-shaped contact areas which were anteriorly located in early flexion and posteriorly located in high flexion (Walker and Hajek 1972). This would exert a rocking effect on an artificial tibial component, transmitting both tensile and compressive stresses to the underlying trabecular bone. The density and strength of this bone were found to be highly variable, especially in arthritic knees where deformity resulted in areas of very low density on the relatively unloaded side of the knee (Behrens et al. 1974): "The natural trabecular pattern may have been altered to such an extent that the bone is not suited to support the forces from insertion of a prosthetic implant the significance of this work related....to the design and surgical technique....of condylar replacement knee prosthesis".

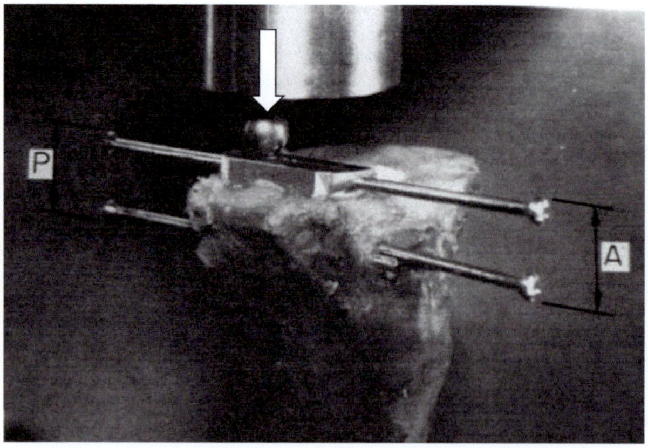

Fig. 5.4 Experiments to determine the micromotion of a tibial component relative to the tibial surface. Loads were applied (white arrow) to a ball bearing at different AP locations along the top of the component. Anterior A and posterior P distances were measured to indicate the relative component-bone motions. For anterior or posterior loading, distraction of the component occurred at the opposite end to the load, detrimental to fixation (Walker et al. 1976). (Reprinted with permission from Journal of Biomechanics)

The fixation was investigated experimentally on unicompartmental components cemented to tibias and loaded in different ways (Walker et al. 1976). Such components were currently part of the Unicondylar and Duo-condylar knee systems which were being used clinically at the time. In the experiments, as an indicator of fixation, the relative micromotions between the components and the surface of the bone were measured. For central loading, all-plastic components deflected in a U-shape, deforming the underlying bone as well as the component. When a metallic component representing metal-backing was loaded centrally, there was uniform deflection into the trabecular bone but of smaller magnitude. For off-center loading, lift-off between the component and the bone occurred on the end opposite to the loading for both plastic and metal components. The lift-off was even more pronounced when the trabecular density varied across the surface. For example, on the medial condyle, the central area of trabecular bone is frequently stiffer than that at the anterior and posterior. That situation produced a "seesaw" effect on a tibial component loaded off-center. It was recommended that the surgeon drill cement keyholes in the bone at the anterior and posterior of the tibial surface to counteract the tilting. It was also noted that the small surface area of unicompartmental components would also cause higher stresses on the bone surface with potential compressive failure of trabeculae. These negative factors eventually led to the abandonment of separate tibial components in favor of one-piece components which had a much larger surface area. The obvious exception was for unicompartmental knees.

Other possible causes were investigated for the development of the RLL seen on the radiographs of clinical cases. With components of small surface area such as in the Polycentric knee, and in the early condylar replacements with separate medial and lateral components, the contact stresses could be abnormally high, causing mechanical failure of the trabecular bone immediately below the cement. The effect would be exacerbated if the components were made from polyethylene, because deflections beneath the loading points would cause stress concentrations beneath. The reason for this is that for a convex femoral component loaded against a flat polyethylene component, the contact area is small, only about 10 mm in diameter. Due to the low modulus of elasticity of the polyethylene and the thickness of the component, typically 8 mm or even less, the high surface stress transmits to the underlying trabecular bone with little attenuation. Even if the component had a metal-backing to increase rigidity, if the loading occurred near the anterior or posterior edges, tilting of the component would occur with high compressive stresses under the load and tensile stresses at the opposite edge. The tension could cause separation of the cement from the trabecular bone, especially if the cement was not well interdigitated.

Another factor which could cause interface failure was the amount of constraint between the femoral and tibial components. For example, in two of the earliest designs, the Freeman-Swanson and the Geometric, the tibial bearing surface was in close conformity with the femoral surface. The rationale was to minimize the contact stresses on the polyethylene surface, thereby reducing the wear. In addition, it would provide both rotational and anterior-posterior stabilities, an important factor when most of the knees treated at that time were very unstable. However, a negative effect was that transmission of the shear and torque forces would cause high stresses at the cement-bone interface. Even if the patients were not very active, there would likely be sufficient episodes of twisting and sudden stops and starts, to disrupt the interface.

Yet a further factor was the varus and valgus moments which could occur in everyday activities. Even in normal individuals, due to the adduction moment acting on the knee, the forces on the medial condyle are higher than on the lateral condyle by a ratio of about 3:2. If the artificial knee components were misaligned by only a few degrees, the ratio would be higher. In some activities, all of the load could pass through the medial side, with lift-off occurring on the lateral side. Such uneven loading would overstress the trabecular bone and cause compressive failure at the interface on the medial side. This uneven varus or valgus loading condition would affect certain designs of tibial component more than others. However the worst effect was thought to be with all-plastic components with relatively thin plastic.

Joe Miller MD, an orthopedic surgeon, and Bill Krause PhD, a biomechanical engineer, from McGill University in Montreal, Canada, realized that a lack of understanding of the principles of cement fixation was having a negative effect on the clinical results of artificial knee replacement (Krause et al. 1982a, b). According to them there was limited appreciation of the need for cement penetration and of the methods for achieving that: "acrylic cement applied manually in the usual fashion to cancellous surfaces results in virtually no penetration of the cement into the interfaces between the boney trabeculae, and as a result, no interlock is achieved." Such an interface would allow micromotion to occur between the cement and the trabecular bone. In addition, the load would not be transmitted across sufficient surface area of trabeculae. In combination, this condition would lead to bone resorption and radiolucent lines. The solution proposed (Miller et al. 1992) was: "an improved interlock can be produced by using acrylic cement in a liquid stage, applying it to the boney surfaces using a pressurization system which induces an actual penetration of the cement into the interstices of the cancellous bone….This would resist movement as a result of compression, shear and tensile loading and would result in a more even transfer of stress from prosthesis to cement to bone".

Krause prepared multiple specimens where metal plates of constant area were cemented onto trabecular bone from the proximal tibia. The lower surface of the plate was grooved to rigidly bond to the cement. Different preparation methods were used including cleaning and drying the bone, pressurizing the cement as it was applied, and using the cement in a more liquid or doughy form. The strength of fixation was defined by the tensile force needed to distract the metal plate with the cement adherent from the trabecular bone. The failure was characterized by where the failure occurred, in the cement or in the trabecular bone either directly below the cement or some distance below. Finger-packing doughy cement on an untreated tibia resulted in minimal depth of penetration which increased to 2–3 mm if the bone surface was first water lavaged. The lavage removed not only blood and fat from the bone surface, but also trabecular fragments produced during the resection of the tibial surface. There was a further increase in cement penetration to 5–10 mm when more liquidy cement was pressurized with a

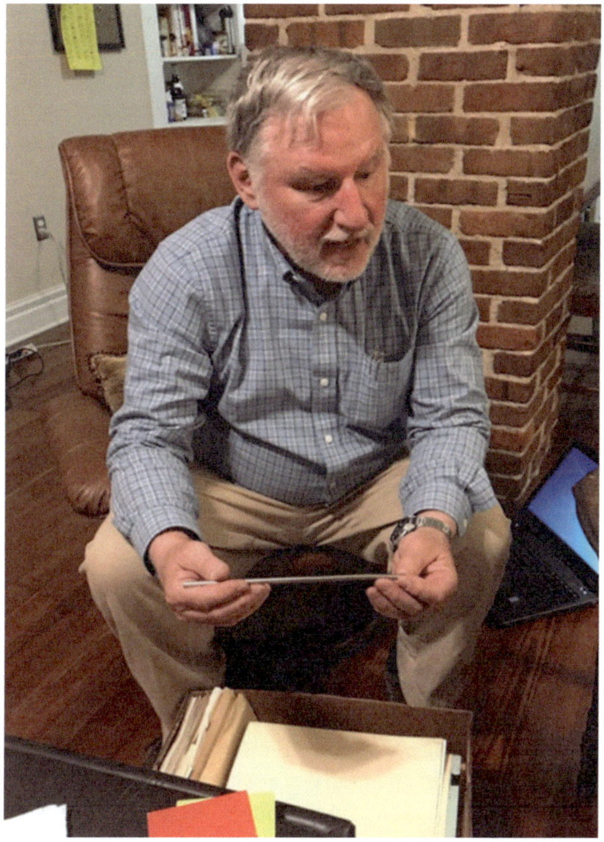

Fig. 5.5 In the late 1970s and early 1980s, Bill Krause PhD worked with Joe Miller MD at McGill University, Montreal, on cementing technique for artificial knees. They carried out the first systematic experimentation on the importance of cement penetration to achieve adequate interface tensile strength and developed methods for achieving the required cement penetration. (Photo taken on interview at the ORS/AAOS meeting, New Orleans, 2018) (© Peter S Walker)

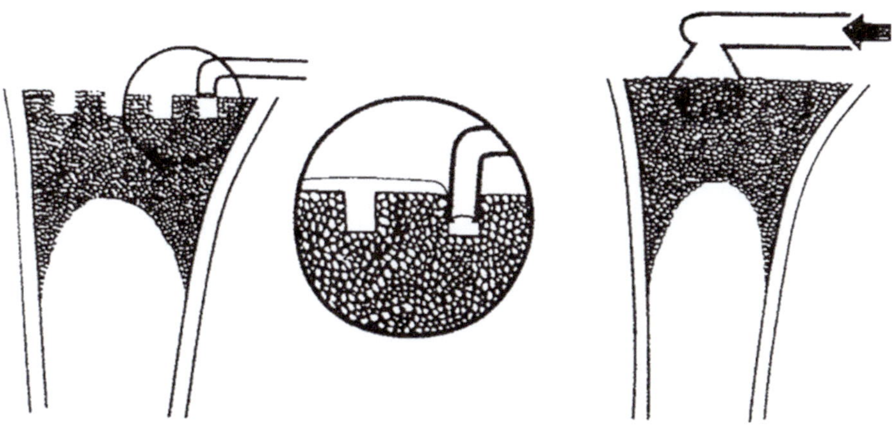

Fig. 5.6 Different methods for achieving cement penetration into the cancellous bone, using nozzles to inject cement into the surface and into small holes drilled into the surface. This resulted in a mechanically superior interface (Miller et al. 1979). (Reprinted with permission from William R Krause PhD)

cement gun into a lavaged surface. The tensile strength to pull the cement out of the trabeculae paralleled the depth of penetration, with the pressurized samples giving at least twice the strength of the finger-pressed. However "….there was a great deal of scatter in the results for each series of tests. This scatter resulted from possible differences in porosity from sample to sample, as well as the location of each sample." The two most important variables affecting fixation strength were the depth of penetration and the density of the trabecular bone. Both of these had upper limits however. Beyond 2–3 mm of penetration, the strength did not increase further. This was explained by observing that cement engagement of about two levels of transversely oriented trabeculae was sufficient. With very dense bone, the cement filaments between adjacent trabeculae had only a small tensile strength. The opposite effect occurred with porotic bone where in this case it was the thin trabeculae that failed in tension.

In practice there is a disadvantage to cement penetration of more than a few millimeters. Firstly, there would be thermal effects on the encased trabecular bone as the cement hardened. Secondly, if a revision was needed in the future, extra tibial resection depth would be needed to reach new trabecular bone. However, trabecular strength reduces steadily with depth below the surface. In addition, cement which is liquidy enough to be applied with a syringe would spread over the edges of the bone during application, which is difficult to remove. Probably for these reasons, application of cement using a syringe was not generally practiced. On the other hand, the importance of achieving several millimeters of cement penetration across the entire tibial surface has now been recognized by most surgeons. This is usually achieved by surface lavage, applying the doughy cement in as soft a condition as possible, and pressurizing manually across the surface. Even so, there is often inadequate cement penetration at the periphery because of the loss of pressure. This deficiency is still in need of a practical solution.

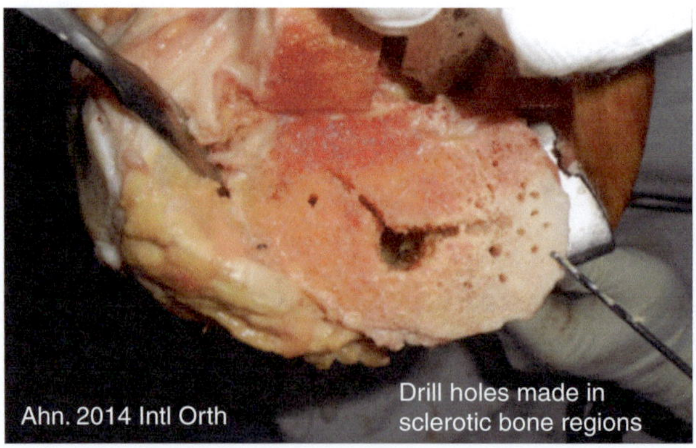

Fig. 5.7 For durable fixation of the tibial component, Krause, Krug, and Miller (1982) emphasized that 2–3 mm of cement penetration must be achieved across the entire tibial surface. Brushing and water lavage were the first step. In cases where there was sclerotic bone, such as on the medial side, small drill holes were made. On application of the cement, pressurization was applied

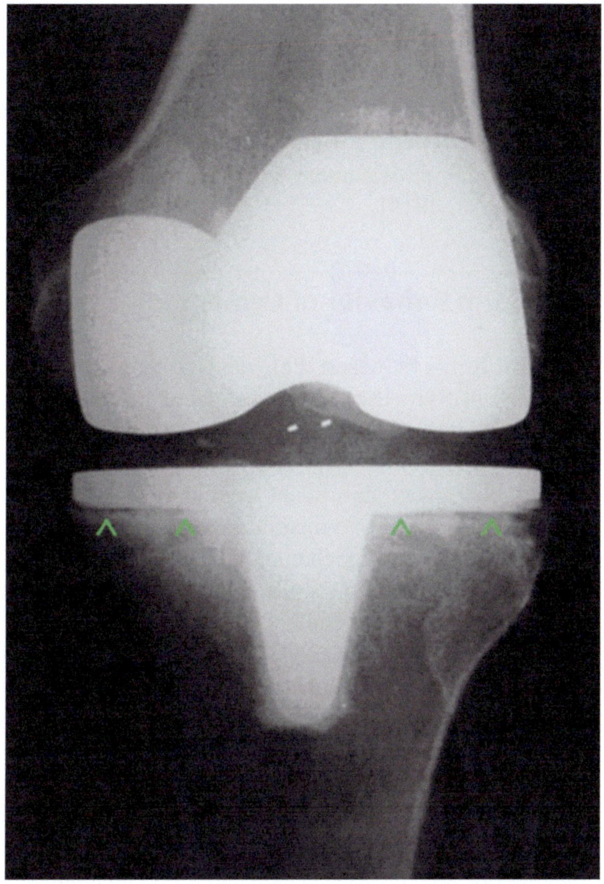

Fig. 5.8 An anterior radiograph of an artificial knee. Radiolucent lines at the interface indicating bone resorption and replacement with fibrous tissue. This is likely the result of low cement penetration at the sides (green arrows), allowing cement-bone micromotion to occur

Back to the 1970s, it was evident that even though interface loosening was a recognized problem with many designs, more attention was given to femoral-tibial conformity, and enhancing fixation with large pegs, rather than focusing on cement penetration and tensile strength of the interface. Nevertheless, for certain designs of total knee replacement, cement fixation turned out to be adequate, with long-lasting results even up to 20 years and more. For example, for the AGC knee, using a non-modular tibial component with molded polyethylene, the survivorship for aseptic loosening was 95% at a 25-year follow-up (Ritter et al. 2016). For a PS total knee at a mean of 12 years, there had been no revisions for loosening out of 89 young (< 60 years) active patients (Meftah et al. 2016). A 20-year follow-up of the PFC knee, designed in the 1980s, showed a survivorship for loosening of 98% (Patil et al. 2015). A mean 15-year follow-up of a wide range of implant designs and surgeons showed 98.8% survivorship for loosening (Vessely et al. 2006). Even a knee that was designed in 1973, the Total Condylar, for 45 knees in 30 surviving patients at 20-year follow-up, only 4 had been revised. Radiolucencies were prevalent, which could be attributed to an inadequate cement technique in that era of the surgeries, but this had not resulted in any cause for revision (Rodriguez et al. 2001). With such results, it might be concluded that cemented fixation, even with imperfect techniques in many cases, was an effective method of fixation for the long term, for tibial components with central pegs. For the femoral component, loosening has seldom been a problem, attributed to the wraparound shape of the component, yet the penetration depth of cement at follow-up has been found to be surprisingly small (Howard et al. 2014).

Long-Term Behavior of Cement

Recently, Kenneth Mann PhD and colleagues from the Biomaterials Institute, University of Syracuse, NY, investigated whether the cement-bone interface maintained its integrity in long-term follow-up. The basis for the work was to determine whether cemented fixation could be considered to be satisfactory in the long term or whether there was significant degradation over time. Autopsy specimens were obtained, and innovative methods were developed for studying the interfaces both morphologically and mechanically. The specimens ranged from 3- to 22-year follow-up, in patients aged 54–90 years. Rectangular prisms 8 mm × 8 mm in section were cut down into the cement below the metal tibial tray and into the underlying trabecular bone. Micro-CT was used to make three-dimensional computer models of the specimens. Different colors showed the trabecular bone, the cement, and the bone cavities in the cement where the bone has once been located. A major finding was: "Resorption of the trabecular bone below the tibial tray starts at the cement border (at the extent of cement penetration into the bone bed) and progresses into the cement layer. The amount of resorption increases with time in service, and may be more prevalent in older donors, although the age effect was not statistically significant here" (Goodheart et al. 2017). The mechanism for reduced interlock of the cement in the bone appeared to be resorption of the bone at the boundary with the cement, with the resorption gradually spreading into the cement over time. In the early stages, the process would seem not to have a serious effect on the fixation. However, the more the resorption at the interface, the weaker the resistance to shear and tension. The resorption process was time related, but the age of the patient had much less effect. The authors pointed to strain shielding and biological effects as reasons for the resorption.

Since the interfaces would transmit load from the implant to the trabecular bone beneath, it would be interesting to determine the deformations of the bone and how much micromotion there was between the cement and the bone (Miller et al. 2016). Specimens were placed in fixtures, and a charge-coupled device (CCD) camera attached to a microscope was used to obtain images during the loading. Apart from the autopsy specimens, fresh cadaver tibias were used to obtain "time of surgery" lab specimens. The findings were as follows: "When loaded, there is a small amount of micromotion between the trabeculae and cement, with a greater degree of micromotion near the cement border compared to deep within the cement layer. With in vivo service, local trabecular resorption causes gaps between the trabeculae and cement

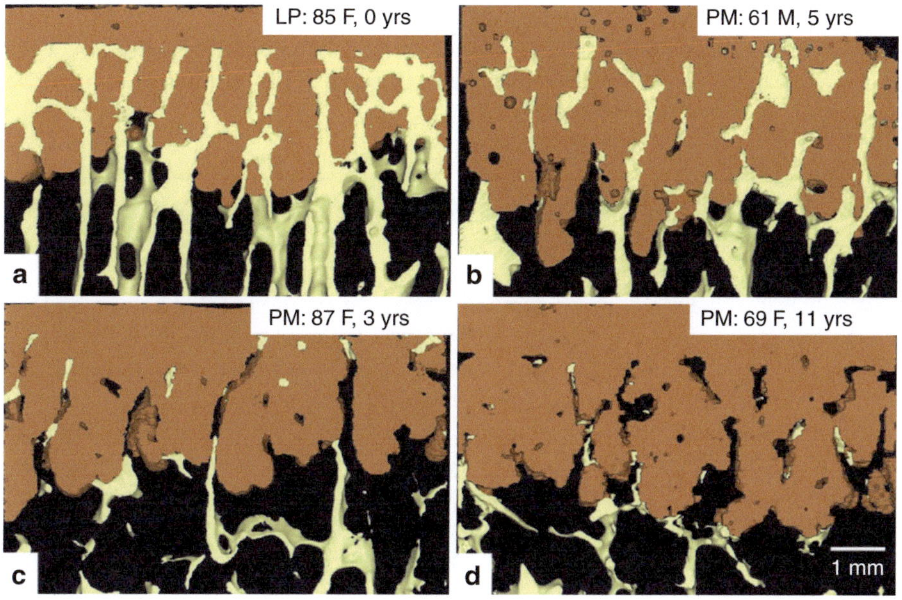

Fig. 5.9 New sectioning methods were devised for showing the penetration of the cement (brown) within the trabecular bone (yellow) and the changes over time, on autopsy specimens. Top left **a**, prepared in lab. **b**, **c**, and **d** show progressive loss of the embedded trabecular bone in specimens. More initial interlock at surgery resulted in better interfaces at follow-up with less resorption and micromotion (Miller et al. 2016). (Reproduced with permission from Journal of Orthopaedic Research)

surface to become much larger. The larger gaps allow for more micromotion near the cement border." The gaps were an average of 14 and 40 microns in the lab and autopsy specimens, respectively. Under loaded conditions the relative average micromotions were 1 and 10 microns. These are small values but could still contribute to some resorption of the bone and fibrous tissue formation. To obtain further insights, a finite element model was formulated to determine the bone strains under the different interface conditions (Srinivasana et al. 2017). This work was carried out by a collaboration with Nico Verdonschot PhD, Director of the Orthopaedic Research Lab at Nijmegen University in the Netherlands. The calculated micromotions were similar to the experimental data, validating the model. It was found that the trabecular bone at the interface with the cement was strain-shielded by as much as 35–61%. This alone could be responsible for the gradual loss of the bone over time.

This research has produced a fascinating description and analysis of the cement-bone interface of tibial components over an extended time period. Fixation of the tibial component in early artificial knees was problematic. This situation was gradually improved by more robust component designs and by better cement technique. The implant designs from the autopsy samples in the Syracuse study are very similar to, or the same as, the designs used today. Hence the results of the study can be taken to represent today's artificial knees. To what extent the degraded interfaces affected the function of the donors of the samples is not evident from the papers referenced. It is conceivable that a degraded interface could eventually affect the function of an active patient after many years of service, but further research will be needed to investigate that in detail.

What Are the Basic Principles of Cemented Fixation, and How Durable Is It?

The goal is to achieve a uniform depth of cement penetration of 2–3 mm around the entire interface, in order to provide sufficient bonding to minimize micromotions due to compressive, shear, and distraction forces. To achieve this, the trabecular bone must be cleaned of fat, blood, and bone debris, prior to applying the cement at sufficiently low viscosity under pressure. There is evidence of gradual degradation of the interface in long-term follow-up, but so far there has been no sign of accelerated late loosening. However further evidence is still needed of the integrity of cemented interfaces in the long term in younger and more active patients.

References

Behrens JC, Walker PS, Shoji H. Variations in strength and structure of cancellous bone at the knee. J Biomech. 1974;7(3):201–7.

Charnley J. Acrylic cement in orthopaedic surgery. Edinburgh: S. Livingstone Ltd.; 1970.

Goodheart JR, Miller MA, Oest ME, Mann KA. Trabecular resorption patterns of cement-bone interlock regions in total knee replacements. J Orthop Res. 2017;35(12):2773–80.

Haboush EJ. A new operation for arthroplasty of the hip based on biomechanics, photoelasticity, fast-setting dental acrylic, and other considerations. Bull Hosp Joint Dis. 1953;14(2):242–77.

Howard KI, Miller MA, Damron TA, Mann KA. The distribution of implant fixation for femoral components of TKA: a postmortem retrieval study. J Arthroplast. 2014;29(9):1863–70.

Krause WR, Krug W, Miller J. Strength of the cement-bone interface. Clin Orthop Relat Res. 1982a;163:290–9.

Krause WR, Miller J, Ng P. The viscosity of acrylic bone cements. J Biomed Mater Res. 1982b;16(3):219–43.

Macintosh DL, Hunter GA. The use of the hemiarthroplasty prosthesis for advanced osteoarthritis and rheumatoid arthritis of the knee. J Bone Joint Surg. 1972;54B(2):244–55.

Markolf KL, Amstutz HC. Penetration and flow of acrylic bone cement. Clin Orthop Relat Res. 1976;(121):99–102.

McKeever D. Clin Orthop Rel Res. 1960;18:86–95.

Meftah M, White PB, Ranawat AS, Ranawat CS. Long-term results of total knee arthroplasty in young and active patients with posterior stabilized design. Knee. 2016;23(2):318–21.

Miller J, Krause WR, Krug WH, Kelebay LC. Low viscosity cement. Clin Orthop Rel Res. 1992;276:4–6.

Miller MA, Goodheart JR, Khechen B, Janssen D, Mann KA. Changes in micro-gaps, micromotion, and trabecular strain from interlocked cement-trabecular bone interfaces in total knee replacements with in vivo service. J Orthop Res. 2016;34:1019–25.

Patil S, McCauley JC, Pulido P, Colwell CW Jr. How do knee implants perform past the second decade? Nineteen- to 25-year followup of the press-fit condylar design TKA. Clin Orthop Relat Res. 2015;473(1):135–40.

Ritter MA, Keating EM, Sueyoshi T, Davis KE, Barrington JW, Emerson RH. Twenty-five-years and greater, results after nonmodular cemented total knee arthroplasty. J Arthroplast. 2016;31(10):2199–202.
Rodriguez JA, Bhende H, Ranawat CS. Total condylar knee replacement: a 20-year followup study. Clin Orthop Relat Res. 2001;388:10–7.
Scott RD, Joyce MJ, Ewald FC, Thomas WH. McKeever metallic hemiarthroplasty of the knee in unicompartmental degenerative arthritis. Long-term clinical follow-up and current indications. J Bone Joint Surg Am. 1985;67(2):203–7.
Srinivasana P, Miller MA, Verdonschot N, Mann KA, Dennis Janssen D. Strain shielding in trabecular bone at the tibial cement-bone interface. J Mech Behav Biomed Mater. 2017;66:181–6.
Townley CO. Articular-plate replacement arthroplasty for the knee joint. Clin Orthop Relat Res. 1964;1988(236):3–7.
Vessely MB, Whaley AL, Harmsen WS, Schleck CD, Berry DJ. The Chitranjan Ranawat award: long-term survivorship and failure modes of 1000 cemented condylar total knee arthroplasties. Clin Orthop Relat Res. 2006;452:28–34.
Walker PS, Hajek JV. The load-bearing area in the knee joint. J Biomech. 1972;5(6):581–9.
Walker PS, Ranawat C, Insall J. Fixation of the tibial components of condylar replacement knee prostheses. J Biomech. 1976;9(4):269–75.
Waugh W. John Charnley the man and the hip. Chapter 11: Springer; 1990.

6 Uncemented Fixation

Is Uncemented Fixation Reliable Enough to Replace Cemented?

In the early development of the artificial knee, fixation of the components to the bone using acrylic cement was generally considered to be the way forward. Its success with total hips had already been demonstrated, and it was assumed that it would be equally successful in the knee. Furthermore, press-fit components for the knee were not seen to be viable based on the previous experience, while cement was becoming available. Nevertheless, a number of drawbacks of cement were being recognized. There were thermal effects on the adjacent bone due to the heat generated during polymerization. Systemic effects, due to fat and monomer entering the bloodstream caused by cement pressurization during component placement, were considered a serious risk. In many cases, the bonding of the cement to the trabecular bone was weak due to inadequate cement penetration. Localized areas of interface failure were frequently observed on radiographs. Despite these factors, in some of the early designs the fixation seemed to be satisfactory, at least in the short term. At the same time, there were negative signs which indicated that fixation might not be as durable as for the hip. The main reason was considered to be the complex forces on the tibial component which could result in cement-bone micromotion or failure of the underlying trabecular bone. As a result, an alternative method of fixation was proposed. The idea was that the components would have a porous surface into which the bone would grow, providing a rigid and long-lasting bond.

Early Experience with Porous Ingrowth

At Clemson University, South Carolina, during the 1960s, Sam Hulbert PhD founded a Bioengineering Department and in 1969 started an annual conference in biomaterials which eventually led to the formation of the International Society for Biomaterials. Hulbert and his research associates started a program on porous ceramics (Klawitter and Hulbert 1971): "Using present day techniques (including cementing) it is usually impossible to achieve a method of permanent mechanical fixation which will have more than a small amount of the strength of

P. S. Walker, *The Artificial Knee*, https://doi.org/10.1007/978-3-030-38171-4_6

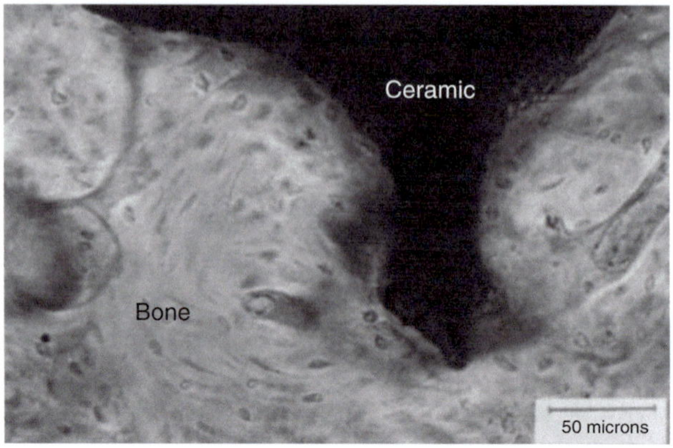

Fig. 6.1 Bone ingrowth into the porous surface of aluminum oxide material. A cylinder had been implanted into the cortex of a canine femur for 4 months (Klawitter and Hulbert 1971). (Reprinted with permission from Journal of Biomedical Materials Research)

the intact bone." "One possible solution to the problem of skeletal attachment is to provide a porous material into which bone can grow and thus create a material capable of direct tissue attachment". For that purpose they focused on new methodologies for obtaining bone ingrowth for orthopedic implants. They chose a calcium aluminate ceramic material and fabricated small cylindrical pellets with different pore sizes ranging from 50 to 200 microns. For comparison, the diameter of a human hair is about 180 microns, only a fifth of a millimeter. The ceramic pellets were pressed into holes which were drilled into the mid-shafts of canine femora, for up to 22 weeks. Elaborate methods were developed for studying the tissue which infiltrated the pores in the ceramic. Using a diamond saw, sections of only 75 microns in thickness were cut and ground. The sections were studied using microradiography, electron microprobe analysis, and light microscopy. The skill and originality in developing these techniques at that time cannot be underestimated. It was found that: "Under the conditions of the experiment, pore interactions greater than one hundred microns (0.1 mm) were necessary to obtain mineralized bone ingrowth." For the ceramic samples with the highest porosity, depths of bone ingrowth up to 1.5 mm were obtained.

This work was featured at annual conferences held at Clemson University in the early 1970s. The meetings were presided over by the charismatic Sam Hulbert, supported by the scientific faculty including Jerome Klawitter, Barry Sauer, and Alan Weinstein. Considerable excitement was generated during these meetings, porous ceramic materials being predicted to be on the verge of revolutionizing the fixation of joint replacements. For practical application, Klawitter patented an idea for a unicondylar tibial plateau consisting of an aluminum oxide ceramic component with dense material at the upper part and porous material at the base for bone ingrowth (Klawitter and Bhatti 1977). The idea could have been applied to a complete tibial component covering the entire upper tibia. However, it was not feasible to manufacture the femoral component in the same way because there was no experience with ceramic-on-ceramic as a bearing material in the knee with partially conforming bearing surfaces. The alternate was to bond a thin coating of porous ceramic to a metallic femoral component

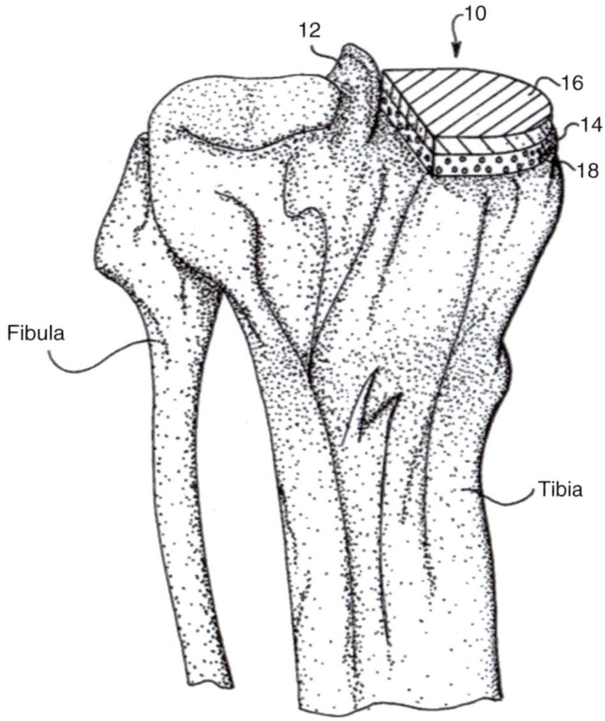

Fig. 6.2 The idea of a tibial plateau composed of a solid alumina ceramic bearing surface integral with a porous ceramic base, which interfaced with trabecular bone, was patented in 1977 by Klawitter and Bhatti. (US Patent number 4000525A. Filed 1975, issued 1977)

and a tibial tray component. This presented the technical difficulty of producing a bond which would not dissociate over time. In addition, a thin layer could fragment due to the high cyclic loads during activities. Due to these intractable difficulties, the research group shifted their attention to dental implants where solid implants with selected areas of porous coating could be fabricated. Also, Sam Hulbert left Clemson University in 1973 to be Dean of Engineering at Tulane University, while other members of the group also took up new positions shortly after Sam Hulbert left. But the pioneering work of this group set the scientific standards for other laboratories investigating porous coatings for the fixation of knee joint replacements.

At the same time as the Clemson University work began, Jorge Galante MD, an orthopedic surgeon at Rush Presbyterian Hospital in Chicago, and Bill Rostoker PhD, a Professor of Metallurgy at the University of Illinois, formed a collaboration to develop the idea of using pads made from thin titanium fibers compressed together and sintered. The surface of the pads consisted of irregular and elongated openings into which bone could readily grow (Galante et al. 1971). If a pad was pressed into a cavity in a solid implant component made from either titanium alloy or cobalt-chrome alloy, it could be rigidly attached to the component by sintering. An important advantage of this porous material was that it had sufficient compliance and strength to withstand cyclic loading while maintaining mechanical integrity: "The material could not fail by crack propagation and exhibited a compliance in the same range as that of trabecular bone" (Lembert

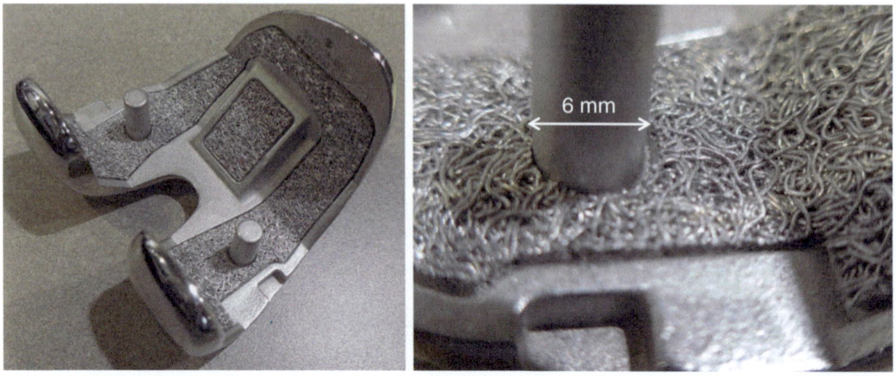

Fig. 6.3 The Miller-Galante knee, designed by Joe Miller, Jorge Galante, and Tom Andriacchi. The fiber-metal porous pads were made from kinked thin titanium wires sintered together and then sintered to the femoral and tibial surfaces. In animal experiments and in the application to bone tumor prostheses, bone readily invaded the porous structure. The fiber diameter was approximately 0.2 mm, and the pore sizes 0.2–0.4 mm. The fiber-metal pads were then applied to a modified IB knee and the Miller-Galante MG knee (shown here). The tibial component (not shown) had three pegs to provide initial stability for bone ingrowth to occur

et al. 1972). In animal experiments using a femoral stem prosthesis coated with the porous material, mean pore sizes up to 390 microns were investigated. In most areas of the stem, bone ingrowth occurred without an interposed layer of fibrous tissue between the bone and the fibers. The shear strength of the interface was similar to that when the stems were fixed using acrylic cement. During subsequent years, further research on the fiber-metal material was carried out, including application to segmental replacements such as distal femurs and proximal tibias, where extensive bone ingrowth occurred. In the late 1970s, a total hip stem with fiber-metal pads showed extensive bone ingrowth in patients (Landon et al. 1986).

Meanwhile, in London, England, Michael Freeman FRCS had decided that press-fit fixation where the components were directly interfaced to the bone was viable after all, so long as there were fixation pegs to resist shear and torque forces. Freeman designed an all-plastic tibial component with grooved pegs laterally and medially which provided strong resistance to pull-out, as reported to the Orthopaedic Research Society in 1981. In 1983, Freeman reported on a series of cases performed since 1977, although not all components were uncemented and there were also design changes during that time (Freeman et al. 1983). Comparisons between cemented and uncemented showed similar results, but in many of the cases, there was a postoperative range of flexion of less than 90 degrees, partially explained by the preoperative condition of the patients. But despite the ingenuity of the design, the overall results did not generate sufficient enthusiasm for either the design or the fixation method, possibly because much of the interest in uncemented fixation had already switched to porous coatings.

Returning to Chicago, based on over 10 years of laboratory research including animal trials and experience with a total hip, Jorge Galante, in collaboration with

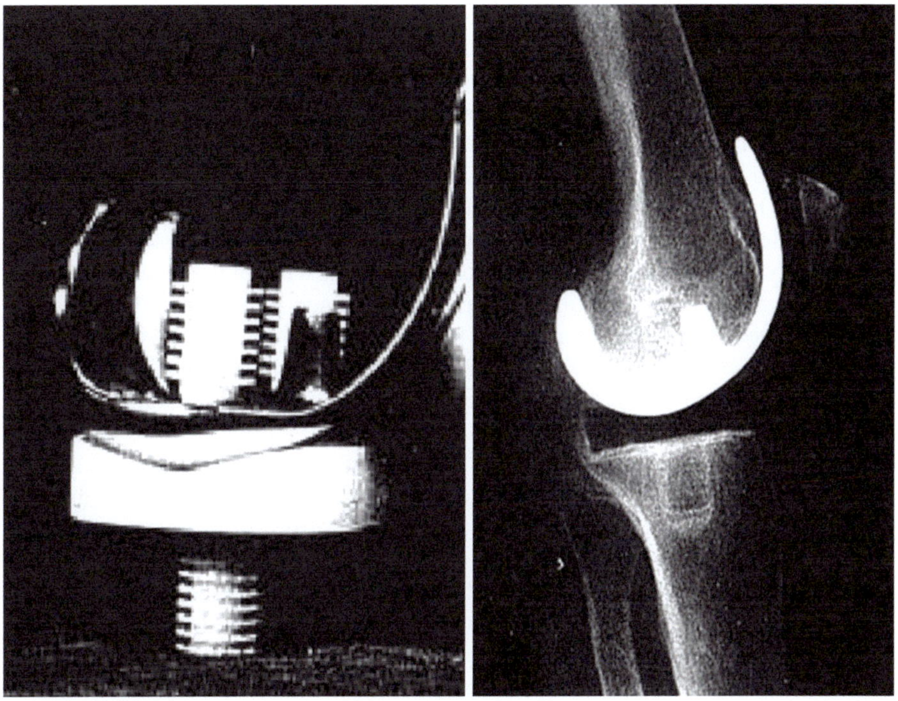

Fig. 6.4 An uncemented version of the Freeman-Samuelson was used from 1977. Polyethylene pegs with circumferential groves (known as "magic pegs") were an interference fit in holes drilled into the trabecular surfaces. Radiographically, a layer of dense cortical bone formed around the pegs. No gross loosening was observed. The clinical results were similar to those using cement (Freeman et al. 1983). (Reprinted with permission Clinical Orthopaedics & Related Research)

Tom Andriacchi PhD and Joe Miller MD from Montreal, designed the Miller-Galante knee in 1984. Andriacchi's contribution, backed up by gait analysis studies, was to produce a tibial surface of low constraint while preserving the cruciate ligaments so as to minimize the shear stresses transmitted to the interface between the tibial component and the bone. By that time it was known that micromotion at the interface could seriously inhibit the ingrowth of bone and lead to a fibrous tissue interface, quite the opposite of what was intended. The mechanical fixation of the tibial component to the resected surface of the tibia was by four porous-coated pegs approximately 10 mm in diameter and length. However to provide a more rigid connection, four long cancellous screws were passed through the center of each peg into the underlying cancellous bone. This use of screws was evidently intuitive because there were no recorded mechanical tests that would provide quantitative data of reducing micromotion at the interface. It does however indicate they were aware that in order for ingrowth to occur, a process which could take several weeks, the porous surface had to interface with the trabecular bone without any relative motion, whether shear or distraction. Later lab studies did show the substantial increase in rigidity of the initial fixation provided by the screws (Volz et al. 1988).

While the Miller-Galante (MG) porous-coated knee was used extensively in the late 1980s and into the 1990s as one of Zimmer's premier knees, most of the usage was in a hybrid form, where the femoral component was uncemented and the tibial component cemented. The rationale was explained in several articles, a notable one by Kraay et al. in 1991: "Retrieval studies of uncemented tibial components have demonstrated that very little bone ingrowth actually occur into these implants, challenging the long-term durability of this method of fixation with both uncemented and cemented femoral components, however, aseptic loosening has occurred only infrequently. Recently the hybrid method of fixation, with an uncemented femoral component and a cemented tibial component has been introduced." However the success of the MG knee was dampened because problems emerged with the metal-backed patella component (Joseph and Kaufman 1990). This was a mechanical failure resulting in loosening and even fragmentation of the fiber-metal, with fibers entering the joint itself. This problem adversely affected the follow-up results and prompted Joseph and Kaufman to state: "This should stimulate research and analysis in the laboratory so that future mistakes in design can be avoided." While this was a sound suggestion, artificial knee development was still a new endeavor, and laboratory methods had not been devised for every facet of the design process. Certain aspects, in this case the patella design, were perceived as obvious, not requiring any elaborate testing. The main emphasis was on designing long-lasting implants, porous coatings being seen as the way to provide that.

Another influential application of porous coating to a total knee was based on the work of Bob Pilliar PhD and others in the late 1970s and early 1980s (Pilliar 1983). Pilliar's idea was to start with a femoral component and a tibial tray made from cast Co-Cr alloy, the most common material used for total knee components at the time, and then to apply porous coatings to the surfaces which interfaced with bone. To produce the porous coating, powdered Co-Cr alloy was used in the form of tiny spherical beads layered on to the surface of the implant and coated with a liquid binder to maintain the beads in close proximity. After sintering, small neck regions of fusion occurred between adjacent beads and between the beads and the solid substrate. Tests on round beams with and without porous coating showed that the process and structure of the coating did not affect the fatigue strength of the Co-Cr specimen, an important consideration in the highly stressed regions of knee components. Durability was attributed to the smooth connections between the beads and the solid structure, avoiding sharp corners which would cause stress concentrations and weaken the structure. Animal tests using plugs of porous Co-Cr implanted into the femoral cortex showed excellent bone ingrowth for average pore sizes of 50–400 microns. The higher end of this range was chosen for application to total knees to allow for the inevitable small micromotions at the bone-implant interface before bone ingrowth occurred.

By 1983, there had been several years of successful experience of the Co-Cr porous coating applied to artificial hip stems. Now it was considered the time to apply the same technology to total knees, but a suitable artificial knee design was needed. Pilliar had been working on the porous technology with a Canadian branch of the British Oxygen Company, with a technically oriented sales representative,

Bob Kenna. They connected with David Hungerford MD and Ken Krackow MD, surgeons at Johns Hopkins University, with the proposition of applying their porous coating technology to a new knee design. In a very short time, they formulated original ideas not only for an artificial knee design but also for the instrumentation. The femoral component was based on the shape of the anatomic femur. The tibial component had a metal-backing, while the plastic insert was of low conformity to allow freedom of motion, similar to that of the Miller-Galante knee. The beaded Co-Cr porous coating was applied to both the femoral and tibial components, as well as to the patella component. For the instrumentation, Hungerford and Krackow developed the Universal Instruments which were based on achieving anatomic alignment of the components. The group met with David Fitzgerald, the CEO of Howmedica in New Jersey, to discuss his interest in developing this new knee system using the porous coating technology. At the time, the company's main total knee was the Kinematic Knee system using cemented fixation, designed by Peter Walker, Director of Product Development, in collaboration with surgeons at the Robert Breck Brigham Hospital in Boston: Clem Sledge, Fred Ewald, Bob Poss, and Bill Thomas. Moreover the Kinemax Knee, an advancement of the Kinematic, was already well under development. However, Howmedica lacked porous coating technology which was by now being promoted by Zimmer on the Miller-Galante knee, while other companies were also developing porous coatings. This was the ideal opportunity for Howmedica.

Even though much preparatory work had already been carried out, production of a new total knee system was still a formidable task. Time was of the essence because of the gaining popularity of the Miller-Galante knee. However, David Fitzgerald sensed that this dynamic and enthusiastic group, with an innovative approach to total knee design and surgical technique, could make a major impact and even elevate

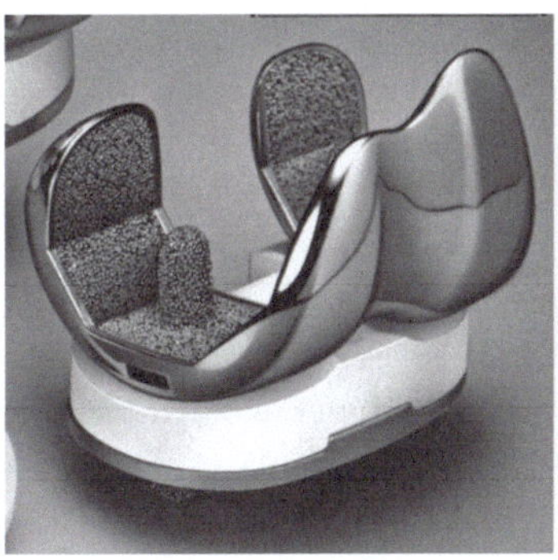

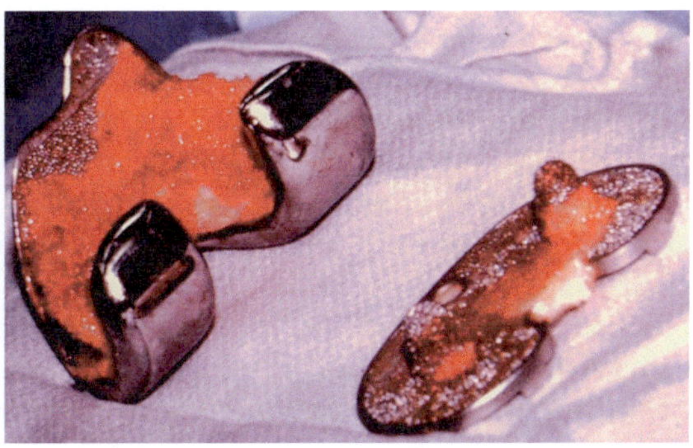

Fig. 6.5 The PCA knee (left) designed by David Hungerford MD, Ken Krackow MD, and Bob Kenna. The bone-facing surfaces were coated with sintered cobalt-chrome beads for bone ingrowth. The polyethylene insert surface was hot-pressed for a precisely contoured smooth surface. The Universal Instruments were designed for anatomic placement of the components. In the retrieval specimen (right), bone is seen adherent to most of the femoral surfaces, due to bone ingrowth into the pores. In the tibia, only about 25% of the surface and the pegs have adherent bone. Fibrous tissue is invading the pores over the remaining surface

Howmedica above Zimmer in the knee area. An entire mezzanine floor was constructed in the Howmedica plant, and prime staff were assigned to accomplish the knee project in the shortest possible time. Internally, Bob Kenna single-mindedly pushed forward the work at a rapid pace, dealing with every aspect and using the technical knowledge he had acquired in his previous work. As well as the porous coating technology, Kenna developed a new way of forming a smooth contoured bearing surface on the tibial insert, a process called "hot-pressing." The idea was to machine the surface to an approximate shape and then to place the component into a metal die which was heated up to mold the final surface. The surface was smooth and shiny, giving the component a hi-tech appearance compared with the usual machined surfaces of artificial knees at that time. The Universal Instruments was another innovative aspect of the knee system, by now called the PCA knee, the porous-coated anatomic. Hungerford and Krackow were accomplished surgeons, and mainly due to Krackow's mathematical background, they recognized the importance of component alignments in relation to the applied forces during activity. For example, they pointed out the anatomic alignment of the joint line in the frontal plane, which meant cutting the tibia at 2–3 degrees of varus, with the distal femur cut appropriately to maintain the correct mechanical axis of the leg. This was depicted in a colorful slide showing that in a normal individual, the joint line was parallel to the ground during activity.

After about a year of clinical trials by Hungerford and Krackow, the use of the PCA knee was extended to an early user group in the USA and then progressively expanded. This was achieved by well-organized lectures, starting off in the USA, but soon including many other countries, facilitated by Hungerford and Krackow's fluency in several languages. On his office wall, David Hungerford had a map of the world with pins indicating the countries where they had given instructional lectures. Their aim was to leave no country unvisited, a goal that was almost realized! Many of the lecturing events were supported by other surgeons, who were early users of the PCA knee. There was also a special group of leading surgeons in Europe, Jean-Louis Briard being a prominent member. The quality of the presentations was of the highest level, projecting a new way forward for artificial knee replacement, surpassing the rather traditional designs and surgical techniques.

After introduction of the PCA knee, there were several follow-up studies by the originators and by independent users in the ensuing years. One article raised an alarm about loose beads and radiolucent lines mainly around the patella and tibial components (Cheng and Gross 1988). In another article there was a much higher incidence of radiolucent lines around the tibial component for an uncemented PCA compared with the same designs used in cemented mode (Collins et al. 1991). Subsidence anteriorly or antero-medially was also noted, possibly due to the large amount of anterior bone resection as a consequence of a horizontal resection plane rather than with the usual 5 degrees of posterior slope. Fibrous tissue ingrowth rather than bone ingrowth was noted in revised tibial components, indicative of inadequate stability of the interface especially in the time period after surgery. A number of corrective modifications were made to the PCA knee, and a stabilized type was added. The resulting new system, the Duracon, produced good long-term results whether used in cemented or uncemented modes.

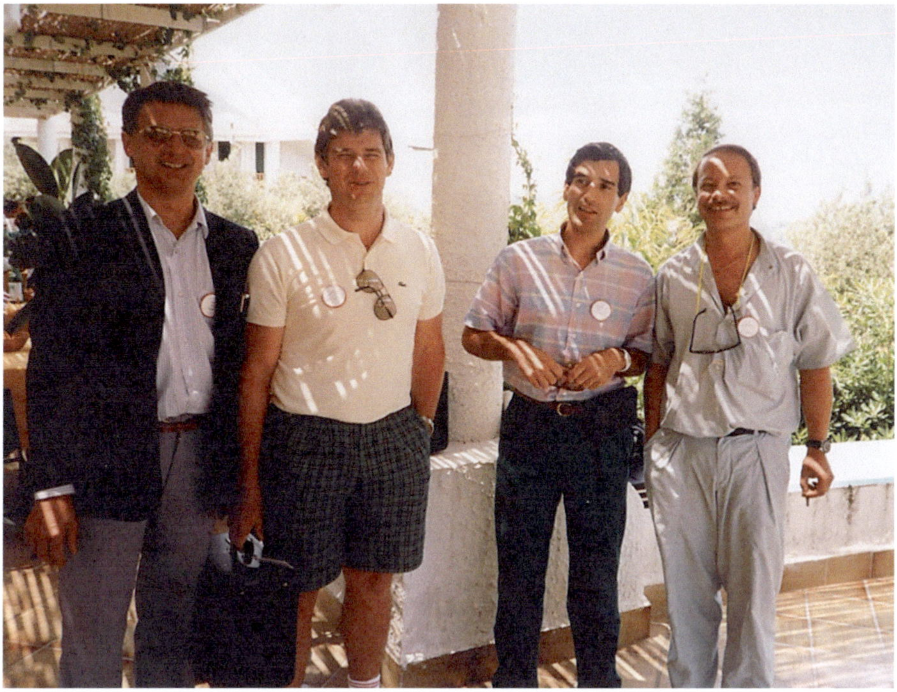

Fig. 6.6 At the many workshops on the PCA knee around the world, Dave Hungerford and Ken Krackow involved local surgeons who were early users. This photo (left to right: Jean-Louis Briard, Marc Raguet, Jean-Louis Prudhon, Gerard Deschamps) was taken in Sicilia in 1982. (© Peter S Walker)

In 1984, Bob Volz MD, a surgeon from Tucson, Arizona, in collaboration with Gerald Engh MD and John Moreland MD, introduced the Anatomic Modular Knee (AMK) with porous coating. Along with several other porous-coated designs at that time, there were reported cases with inadequate bone ingrowth on the tibial component. To address this, Bob Volz devised a new biomechanical testing method to investigate the initial stability of uncemented tibial components (Volz et al. 1988). Volz had a strong interest in biomechanics and was particularly interested in improving tibial fixation which had hitherto been a problem with some uncemented components. While porous-coated components were a possible advancement, Volz recognized that the components must maintain initial rigid fixation before bone ingrowth took place. The interface micromotions were compared between several porous-coated designs: his own AMK, the Miller-Galante, the Ortholoc, and the PCA. The experiments consisted of eccentrically loading the components cyclically for 300,000 cycles and measuring the subsidence as well as the distraction between the component and the bone. Volz found that uncemented component stability was greatly enhanced by peripheral cancellous screws, an important element being prevention of interface distraction on the side of the component opposite to the applied load. "The ability of a noncemented tibial component to resist micromotion….

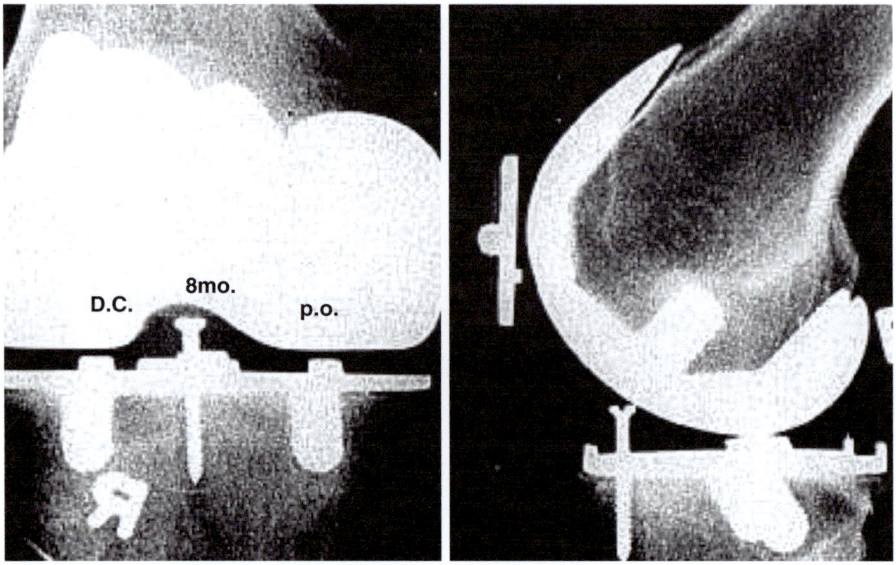

Fig. 6.7 Frontal and sagittal plane radiographs of an 8-month follow-up of a porous-coated anatomic (PCA) artificial knee. Efforts have been made to take the radiograph exactly along the plane of the base of the tibial component, such that the interface is not obscured. Close proximity of the trabecular bone to the porous surface can be visualized (Hungerford and Kenna 1983). (Reprinted with permission from Clinical Orthopaedics & Related Research)

would appear to be a critical determinant of the success bone might have in invading a porous surface. The shape of the surgically prepared proximal tibia (flat) leads little intrinsic stability to a flat metal plate placed on its surface.…Tibial designs secured with four screws provided the best stability." This was a vitally important guideline for other porous-coated designs, as well as the AMK. Shortly after this work, Walker et al. (1990) developed a method for studying the interface in response to offset compression, shear and torque loading, using Tekscan to show the interface micromotions which occurred. The purpose of the study was to determine which combinations of pegs and keels would provide the least overall micromotion. A central peg augmented with short pegs laterally and medially, or augmented with keels, was the most effective. Screws would likely have further reduced the micromotions.

After there had been a few years of clinical experience of the early uncemented designs, Myron Spector wrote a considered appraisal of the status of component fixation using porous coatings (Spector 1987). While recognizing that there were early problems with cement, he emphasized that successful bone ingrowth would need certain conditions for it to succeed, such as initial mechanical stabilization, not easily achieved. Also if porous-coated pegs or stems were used, they could cause extensive stress-shielding, a very important consideration at that time when such factors had not been considered. To avoid this, Spector proposed the use of porous polymeric coatings such as polysulfone or polyethylene, and although he showed promising results with a hip stem, he never applied

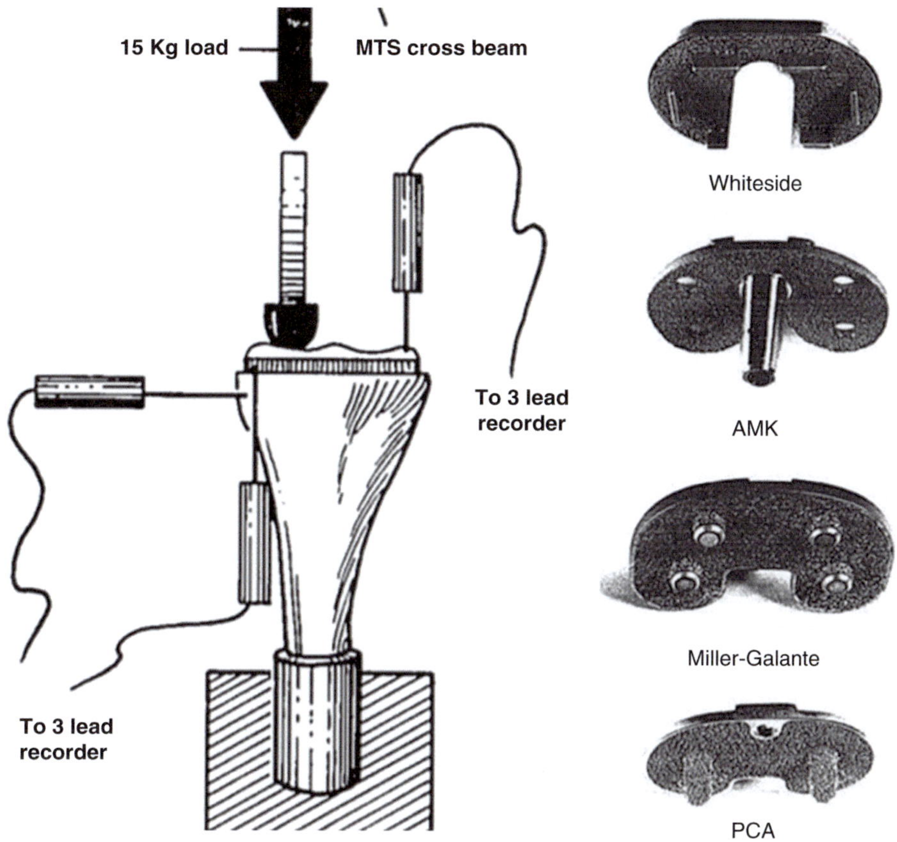

Fig. 6.8 Experimental determination of the stability of fixation of uncemented tibial baseplates. A cyclic load from 5 to 115 Kg was applied for 300,000 cycles. Subsidence and lift-off were measured with transducers. All components gradually subsided over time. The maximum lift-off was only 100 microns with the AMK due to 4 cancellous screws (see holes in baseplate) and central stem. The other designs showed subsidence and lift-off from 200 to 500 microns. This explained the variability in bone ingrowth, where above 100 microns micromotion could prevent ingrowth from occurring (Volz et al. 1988). (Reprinted with permission from Clinical Orthopaedics & Related Research)

the material to the knee. In any case, there was evidence that polymeric coatings did not have sufficient mechanical strength, while bonding to a metal substrate was problematic.

A number of new designs subsequently emerged which were definite improvements to the first uncemented designs. These included the Natural Knee designed by Aaron Hofmann MD and Roy Bloebaum PhD, the LCS by Fred Buechel and Michael Pappas, the AGC by Merrill Ritter, and the Ortholoc by Leo Whiteside. All of these designs were later reported to have 94–100% survivorship at 10 years follow-up (Meneghini and Hanssen 2008). The natural knee had a superior porous coating made from cancellous-like titanium (Bloebaum et al. 1992). The LCS may have benefited from low interface stresses due to the freedom of rotation of the tibial insert (Buechel and Pappas 1989). In the AGC, the molded polyethylene and the monoblock construction of the metal-reinforced tibial component would produce less wear particles, which likely avoided bone lysis at the interfaces after up to 20 years follow-up time (Small et al. 2013). For the Ortholoc, the resected bone surface was coated with bone slurry from the patient's trabecular bone generated during the surgical procedure, and the tibial component was initially stabilized with lag screws (Whiteside 2001). The use of bone slurry was adopted for other porous-coated designs. It is interesting that all the uncemented designs except the AMK used several short fixation pegs on the tibial component. This is in contrast to the design of cemented components which in most cases used the successful large central peg. For the uncemented components, the screws essentially substituted for the central peg which may not have been as effective in uncemented application.

In the designs where screws were used, radiographically, there was an incidence of bone lysis around the screws. This was attributed to the accumulation of small polyethylene particles which had migrated down the holes in the tibial tray. The wear particles themselves were caused by backside wear between the polyethylene insert and the base of the metal tray. This led to improvements of the insert-tray locking mechanism and to polishing of the base of the trays. Looking at the overall situation, Meneghini and Hanssen concluded that "cementless fixation is probably the future of knee arthroplasty, particularly in young patients with an active lifestyle." While the main reason for their prediction was that cementless fixation would be more durable in that group of patients, another motivation for moving in that direction was the reduced operating time.

Scientific Evaluations

In parallel with the development of uncemented artificial knees, studies were being conducted on the scientific aspects. The requirement for the close proximity of the porous surface and the absence of relative motion had been shown to be essential for bone ingrowth to occur (Martens et al. 1980). Experiments where porous surfaces were implanted without being subjected to physiological loads, such as porous plugs inserted into transverse holes in the femoral cortex, would give optimistic data of the bone ingrowth which occurred, which might not apply to dynamic conditions: "Consistent bone ingrowth was observed for implants in nonfunctional conditions if the pore size exceeded 70 microns. Ingrowth in functional loading conditions requires rigid initial stability of the implant and intimate contact of implant coating and surrounding bone tissue." This proposition was supported in later experiments (Goodman and Aspenberg 1992) where the greater the interface motion, the more the surrounding tissue became fibrous tissue rather than bone. This work showed why interfaces developed in different ways, either with bone ingrowth or with fibrous tissue, depending on the local mechanical conditions.

The above experimental methods can be regarded as preclinical evaluations, where the intention was to reproduce the mechanical conditions believed to occur in vivo in order to predict the relative performance of different component designs, surgical techniques, and bone properties. Ideally, methods such as these should have been an integral part of the design process for every new uncemented artificial knee design. However this was not always the case in the early designs of uncemented knees, mainly because the equipment for carrying out such experiments was not generally available and the methods had not been developed until after clinical trials had been initiated. The main method for evaluation of the porous-bone interface was radiography, which could readily be applied to every case postoperatively. Zonal analysis methods were defined where the status of the interface regions in frontal and sagittal views was characterized. Bone ingrowth, a fibrous interface, a sclerotic bone line, and local cysts were features which could be discerned. Bone completely adjacent to the implant surface was regarded as indicating bone ingrowth. However frequently there were areas of radiolucency indicating a fibrous tissue interface, with only smaller areas indicating bone ingrowth. The interface of the medial and lateral edges of the component, areas with the greatest micromotion, most often showed radiolucency. Progressive radiolucency over time was considered to be indicative of loosening. This method of interface evaluation became standard and was easy to perform routinely. It was however subject to some underestimation of radiolucent lines if the x-ray beam was not exactly in line with the surface of a component, such that radiolucency could be obscured by metal.

A totally new method for evaluating the fixation of artificial knee components was devised in Lund, Sweden, in the early 1970s by Goran Selvik PhD, a mathematician, working with Leif Ryd MD and Lars Lidgen MD (Ryd 1986). Selvik's thesis

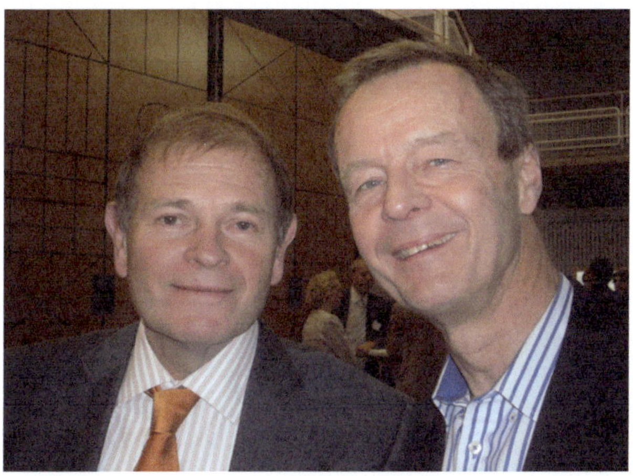

Fig. 6.9 Rik Huiskes PhD (left) directed a laboratory in Nijmegen, Netherlands, which developed advanced iterative finite element computer modelling to predict the bone remodeling around implants and the effect on fixation. He was Editor of the Journal of Biomechanics from 1979 to 2009, tripling the journal in size. He was considered the most influential orthopedic biomechanics researcher in Europe. Leif Ryd MD from Lund in Sweden, starting from the theoretical work of Goran Selvik, developed the application of RSA to measuring the subsidence of artificial knee components over time, thus predicting their longevity. The method was applied extensively to determining the efficacy of uncemented components. RSA is still in use today (Photo c 1995). (© Peter S Walker)

was published in 1974, entitled "Roentgen stereophotogrammetry: a method for the study of the kinematics of the skeletal system." The generalized method, called RSA for short, was lucidly described by Selvik as follows: "If two adjacent objects each have at least 3 identifiable points which can be identified in any direction of view, and two radiographs are taken from different directions, it is then possible to use the coordinates of the 6 points to calculate the position of an axis system defined in one of the objects relative to an axis system defined in the other object: the position being defined by a translation between the origins of the axis systems, and an ordered rotation of 3 angles to bring one axis system in line with the other. Because of the divergence of the x-ray beam from a single point and the unknown location of the points in a global axis system, a calibration process is also necessary where additional points are included in the field of view as the x-rays are taken of the objects. In the application of the method to studying the fixation of tibial components, usually four (for redundancy and enhanced accuracy) tantalum beads are embedded in the tibial component itself, while four beads are injected into the trabecular bone beneath the component. If biplanar radiographs are taken immediately after surgery and then at various times of follow-up, it can be determined if the component has moved relative to the bone, and by how much."

The movement, or subsidence, of the component into the bone over a time period could be expressed by the three displacements and three rotations or, in a simpler way, by the maximum displacement of any of the beads in the component, called "maximum total point motion" (MTPM). Another metric was "inducible displacement," the motion which occurred between unloaded and loaded conditions, the patient at rest and then standing on the knee. During the 1980s many RSA studies were carried out of cemented, press-fit, and porous-coated artificial knees at different follow-up times. For cemented tibial components: "A smaller number of prostheses....showed continuous migration, and had migrated significantly more than others after 6 months. An indication can thus be obtained as early as half a year....as to whether the prosthesis will migrate continuously or not." This last sentence highlights the value of the RSA method, in that new designs, such as with porous coatings, can be compared with a reference cemented design, as to whether it had more or less migrating cases. At the time of Ryd's articles (1986), the conclusion for currently used porous-coated knees was: ".... biologic ingrowth type of fixation displayed micromotion, both as migration and inducible displacement. Stable bony ingrowth was ruled out in most cases." "The inducible displacement occurred within the soft tissue of the....interface." "Radiolucent zones may be of both tensile and compressive origin." This painted a pessimistic picture of porous ingrowth, at least of the component designs and types of porous surfaces which were investigated.

A revolutionary change from cement to porous ingrowth was not yet ready to occur. The main reason appeared to be the inability to prevent micromotion at the component-bone interface in the weeks after surgery, which would prevent bone ingrowth from occurring. Instead, fibrous tissue ingrowth and not bone ingrowth was too prevalent. Nevertheless, this referred mainly to the tibial component, whereas in contrast, porous-coated femoral components, although less studied, were well fixed with few reports of loosening. For that reason, from the late 1980s, hybrid fixation was commonly adopted, although even then, there were still many more cemented than uncemented femoral components being used (Volz and Benjamin 1990; Kraay et al. 1991). Not surprisingly, the quest to design a successful uncemented knee continued, but this time with the mechanical testing methods that had been developed and the clinical follow-up capabilities of RSA.

Since about the year 2000, there have been further advances in porous coating technologies (Harwin et al. 2017). One example called "trabecular metal" is a tantalum structure that looks exactly like trabecular bone. Using this material, tibial components were fabricated as "monoblocks" where the polyethylene insert was fused into the porous surfaces of the metal backing. The component had substantial pegs at the lateral and medial sides to minimize the interface micromotion caused by varus and valgus moments. Clinical follow-ups showed interfaces with positive signs of bone ingrowth and the absence of radiolucencies. Some companies are experimenting with 3D printed metal backings for tibial components. Advantages of this approach are that almost any structure can be manufactured and the coating becomes integral with the solid metal substrate. The EOS company is the main driving force behind this method, with its advanced technology in 3D printing metals such as cobalt-chrome and titanium. Polyetheretherketone (PEEK), a rigid plastic, which is already used for the femoral components of a particular total knee design, is also amenable to 3D printing manufacture and has a modulus nearer to the bone than either metal or polyethylene.

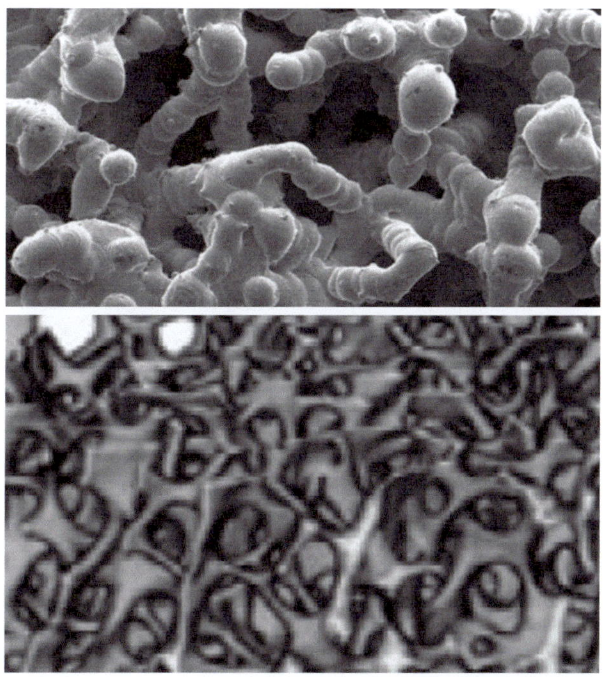

Fig. 6.10 A porous structure made by 3D printing titanium on the surface of knee components (Stryker) compared with trabecular structure at the proximal tibia (Saers et al. 2016). Bone growing in to the irregular 3D printed structure is expected to provide a bond with minimal micromotion due to the irregularities of the structure. The relative scale of the figures is approximate. (Reprinted with permission from Stryker and from Journal of Human Evolution)

Despite impressive clinical results and demonstrable ingrowth of the more recent designs, Bill Barger MD took a conservative approach, based on the successful and reliable long-term results of cemented knees: “Until mid-to-long-term data is available that shows significant benefit in appropriate candidates, widespread adoption of cementless total knees cannot be scientifically or economically justified” (Bargar 2015). This is a surprising viewpoint taken by the person who first introduced a robotic system for preparing the bone for implant components. In 1986, Bill Barger, together with “Hap” Paul, developed Robodoc for accurately shaping the femoral canal for uncemented hip stems. Recently a new company, Think Surgical, was formed, which has initiated clinical trials of artificial knee robot surgery in the USA. Several companies have recently introduced robotic solutions for more accurate knee surgery, applicable to both cemented and porous-coated components. It might be thought that preparing accurate bone surfaces for porous-coated implants would result in enhanced ingrowth. This view is supported in the conclusions of Newman et al. (2018) who stated that: “The newer cementless TKA designs have shown excellent survivorship, functional outcomes and satisfaction rates in not only young but elderly populations.” But change may come about slowly due to confidence and familiarity with cement, the higher implant cost of uncemented artificial knees, and the requirement of a more exacting surgical technique.

Is Uncemented Fixation Reliable Enough to Replace Cemented?

The two advantages of an uncemented knee are that the surgery would be quicker, and it will potentially not be subject to the long-term degradation of a cemented interface. At this time, there is evidence that some uncemented interfaces have overcome the short-term loosening problems of the earlier interfaces. However before uncemented can be confidently used on a more routine basis, further conditions are required: the design of the component and the initial fixation method fixation must be such that there will be no migration over the first 2 years, as shown by RSA; the bone ingrowth must be substantial that it is likely to maintain sufficient strength in the long-term; retrieval data is needed to determine if long-term degradation would apply in a similar way to cemented interfaces.

References

Bargar WL. CORR Insights(R): the Mark Coventry Award: trabecular metal tibial components were durable and reliable in primary total knee arthroplasty: a randomized clinical trial. Clin Orthop Relat Res. 2015;473(1):43–4.

Bloebaum RD, Rubman MH, Hofmann AA. Bone ingrowth into porous-coated tibial components implanted with autograft bone chips. J Arthroplast. 1992;7(4):483–93.

Buechel FF, Pappas MJ. New Jersey low contact stress knee replacement system. Ten-year evaluation of meniscal bearings. Orthop Clin North Am. 1989;20(2):147–77.

Cheng CL, Gross AE. Loosening of the porous coating in total knee replacement. J Bone Joint Surg. 1988;70(3):377–81.

Collins DN, Heim SA, Nelson CL, Smith P, 3rd. Porous-coated anatomic total knee arthroplasty. A prospective analysis comparing cemented and cementless fixation. Clin Orthop Relat Res 1991(267):128-136.

Freeman MA, McLeod HC, Levai JP. Cementless fixation of prosthetic components in total arthroplasty of the knee and hip. Clin Orthop Relat Res. 1983;(176):88–94.

Galante J, Rostoker W, Lueck R, Ray RD. Sintered fiber metal composites as a basis for attachment of implants to bone. J Bone Joint Surg Am. 1971;53(1):101–14.

Goodman S, Aspenberg P. Effect of amplitude of micromotion on bone ingrowth into titanium chambers implanted in the rabbit tibia. Biomaterials. 1992;13(13):944–8.

Harwin SF, Patel NK, Chughtai M, et al. Outcomes of newer generation cementless total knee arthroplasty: beaded periapatite-coated vs highly porous titanium-coated implants. J Arthroplast. 2017;32(7):2156–60.

Hungerford DS, Kenna RV. Preliminary experience with a total knee prosthesis with porous coating used without cement. Clin Orthop Rel Res. 1983(176):95–107.

Joseph J, Kaufman EE. Preliminary results of Miller-Galante uncemented total knee arthroplasty. Orthopedics. 1990;13(5):511–6.

Klawitter JJ, Bhatti NA. Ceramic prosthetic implant suitable for a knee joint plateau. US patent 4,000,525. Filed Aug. 21, 1975, Issued Jan 4, 1977.

Klawitter J, Hulbert S. Application of porous ceramics for the attachment of load bearing internal orthopedic applications. J Biomed Mater Res. 1971;5(6):161–229.

Kraay MJ, Meyers SA, Goldberg VM, Figgie HE 3rd, Conroy PA. "Hybrid" total knee arthroplasty with the Miller-Galante prosthesis. A prospective clinical and roentgenographic evaluation. Clin Orthop Relat Res. 1991;(273):32–41.

Landon GC, Galante JO, Maley MM. Noncemented total knee arthroplasty. Clin Orthop Relat Res. 1986;(205):49–57.

Lembert E, Galante J, Rostoker W. Fixation of skeletal replacement by fiber metal composites. Clin Orthop Relat Res. 1972;87:303–10.

Meneghini RM, Hanssen AD. Cementless fixation in total knee arthroplasty: past, present, and future. J Knee Surg. 2008;21(4):307–14.

Martens M, Ducheyne P, De Meester P, Mulier JC. Skeletal fixation of implants by bone ingrowth into surface pores. Arch Orthop Trauma Surg. 1980;97(2):111–6.

Newman JM, Sodhi N, Khlopas A, et al. Cementless total knee arthroplasty: a comprehensive review of the literature. Orthopedics. 2018;41(5):263–73.

Pilliar RM. Powder metal-made orthopedic implants with porous surface for fixation by tissue ingrowth. Clin Orthop Relat Res. 1983;(176):42–51.

Ryd L. Micromotion in knee arthroplasty. A roentgen stereophotogrammetric analysis of tibial component fixation. Acta Orthop Scand Suppl. 1986;220:1–80.

Saers JPP, Cazorla-Bak Y, Shaw CN, Stock JT, Ryan TM. Trabecular bone structure variation throughout the lower limb. J Human Evol. 2016;97:97–108.

Selvik G. Roentgen stereophotogrammetry: a method for the study of the kinematics of the skeletal system. Reprint from the original 1974 thesis. Acta Orthopaedica Scandinavica Supplementum no. 232, Vol. 60.1989

Small SR, Ritter MA, Merchun JG, Davis KE, Rogge RD. Changes in tibial bone density measured from standard radiographs in cemented and uncemented total knee replacements after ten years' follow-up. Bone Joint J. 2013;95-b(7):911–6.

Spector M. Historical review of porous-coated implants. J Arthroplast. 1987;2(2):163–77.

Volz RG, Nisbet JK, Lee RW, McMurtry MG. The mechanical stability of various noncemented tibial components. Clin Orthop Relat Res. 1988;(226):38–42.

Volz RG, Benjamin JB. The current status of total joint replacement. Investig Radiol. 1990;25(1):86–92.

Walker PS, Hsu HP, Zimmerman RA. A comparative study of uncemented tibial components. J Arthroplast. 1990;5(3):245–53.

Whiteside LA. Long-term followup of the bone-ingrowth Ortholoc knee system without a metal-backed patella. Clin Orthop Relat Res. 2001;388:77–84.

7 Femoral Component and Patella

To What Extent Do Femoral Component Shapes Mimic Normal Anatomy?

The forerunner of an anatomically shaped femoral component for the knee was the mold arthroplasty for the hip, described by Smith-Petersen and Aufranc (1947). The word "arthroplasty" was defined as "an operative procedure undertaken for the purpose of creating a joint mechanically suited for lasting function." The hip mold was a thin hemispherical shell made from cobalt-chrome alloy (Vitallium) that was interposed between the reamed surfaces of the femoral head and the acetabulum. It was expected that due to the close conformity of the surfaces, the sliding action, and the cyclic loads, hyaline articular cartridge would form on the cancellous bone surfaces. Even though the results in the hip were not uniformly successful, the concept was applied to the distal femur in 1958 (Hodge 1991). From molds of cadaveric femurs, thin-walled Vitallium shells were made, with the outer surface being an anatomic replica. Both the internal and external surfaces were polished so that new cartilage could form on the femoral and tibial condyles. At surgery, while the distal femur was shaped to fit the implant, there was no shaping of the proximal tibia. To provide rigid fixation of the shell, a long intramedullary stem was attached. It was notable that the shell included the patella surface, an advantageous feature that was not included on some of the artificial knees designed more than 10 years later. But because there was only one size of the right and left components, it is likely that there would be a kinematic mismatch in many cases, explaining the poor ranges of flexion obtained, while the hard convex surfaces would inevitably overstress and erode the cartilage and bone on the tibia. Even so, Andrew Hodge MD was justified in saying in 1991 that "Vitallium-mold arthroplasty of the knee was the foundation for the current condylar-design femoral components of the modern total knee arthroplasties." The component was called the MGH femoral condyle, referring to the Massachusetts General Hospital in Boston where it was designed.

P. S. Walker, *The Artificial Knee*, https://doi.org/10.1007/978-3-030-38171-4_7

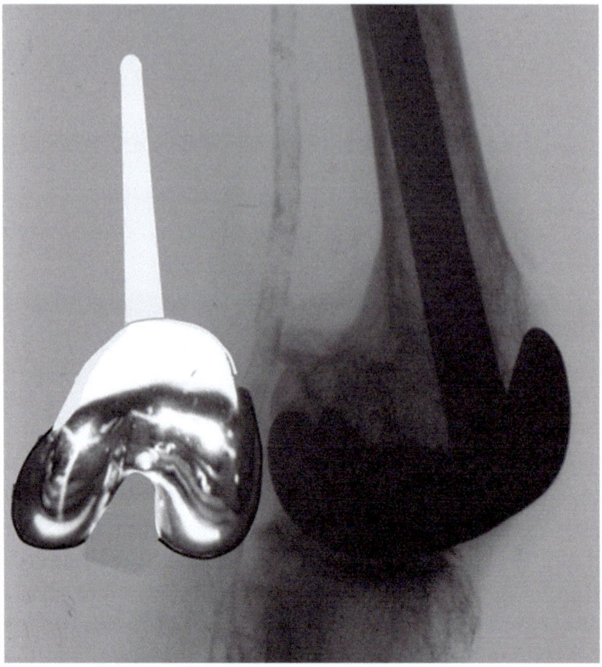

Fig. 7.1 Vitallium mold arthroplasty, known as the MGH femoral condyle. The left picture shows the anatomic shape of the condyles and the intramedullary stem for fixation and alignment. The implant was used from about 1958. The sagittal view radiograph shows a long-term follow-up from the Brigham and Women's Hospital in Boston. The tibial surface has gradually molded to the shape of the femoral condyles. (Reprinted with permission from Journal of Arthroplasty)

Early Femoral Component Designs

By the time of the landmark conference on total knee replacement, held in London UK in 1974 and organized by the Institution of Mechanical Engineers and the British Orthopaedic Association, numerous designs of artificial knee replacement were already in use. Most originated in Europe and the USA but also in Japan and other countries. At one extreme there were fixed axis metallic hinges with long intramedullary stems for fixation. The rationale of one of these hinges, the Shiers, was expressed by the designer as follows: "The object of the exercise is to produce a painless knee that will bend. The simplest and strongest method of achieving this object is by replacing the worn or damaged joint surfaces with a hinge." At the other extreme were the compartmental designs consisting of a metallic component which resurfaced the femoral condyles and a plastic component resurfacing the tibial plateau. Such designs could be compartmental or could resurface both the lateral and medial sides of the knee with one-piece components. The cruciate ligaments could be preserved or resected.

An intermediate design between the hinge and the compartmental was the Freeman-Swanson which had been used in patients since 1970. The femoral component was characterized by simplicity of design, strength of construction, and ease of implantation. The straight cut across the distal end of the femur, perpendicular to the femoral axis, highlighted the requirement that femoral components needed to be aligned in a specified way relative to the femur. The large surface area of the femoral

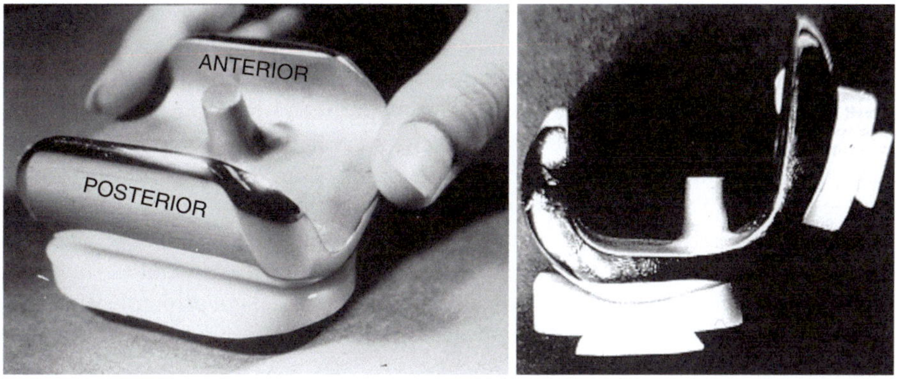

Fig. 7.2 The original Freeman-Swanson artificial knee design, first implanted in 1970 in London, England. The bearing was a cylindrical surface in a trough to maximize the contact area and minimize the wear. There was no patella flange. The designers introduced the concepts of resecting both cruciate ligaments to facilitate correct alignment and balancing, make a square cut across the distal end of the femur to define frontal alignment, and make fitting of the femoral component much easier. A few years later, a patella flange was added, together with a patella component with close conformity to the anterior flange. (Reprinted with permission from Institution of Mechanical Engineers, London UK)

component was intended to minimize the stresses between the component and the femoral bone and between the femoral and tibial bearing surfaces. The design may have been initially too simplified in that it did not have a patella groove nor an extended trochlea for the patella to articulate against in early flexion. This initial configuration was based on the premise that freedom of patella motion was preferable to constraining the patella in a medial-lateral direction. Medial-lateral displacement was similarly unconstrained between the femoral and tibial components, which led to instability in some patients.

The first of the compartmental resurfacing knees was designed by Frank Gunston while he was working as a fellow with John Charnley in Wrightington, England (Gunston 1971; Gunston and MacKenzie 1976). Gunston graduated in engineering before becoming a surgeon, thus having the ideal background to produce an innovative knee replacement. Although Gunston intended to replace only the femoral and tibial bearing surfaces, the configuration of the femoral component was by no means intuitive. Rather than replacing the femoral condyles with metal runners covering the entire bearing surfaces, Gunston made a narrow half disc which fitted into a slot cut into the center of each femoral condyle in the sagittal plane. This had several practical advantages. Firstly, it was difficult to shape a worn femoral condyle by cutting away a uniform layer of bone. It was much easier to cut a slot in the condyle using a handsaw. Secondly, when the component was inserted into the slot in a bed of doughy cement, it could be positioned so that the bearing surface projected 1–2 mm from the original bearing surface which was still preserved on either side of the slot. However, there would inevitably be some mismatch because in the sagittal plane, the distal radius of the condyle is larger than the posterior radius on both the lateral and medial condyles. Since the component was matched more to the smaller posterior radius, the anterior part of the component would be recessed. This would actually be an advantage in that the patella would then not impinge on the inner edges of the component. The constant radius also made the component easy to manufacture, important because the implants were made in Charnley's Biomechanical Workshop which was equipped with only basic machine tools. The hemi-disc-shaped components would be strongly fixed to the condyle because the large surface area at the sides of the component would efficiently transfer axial forces in shear. For consistency, a similar design principle was used for the tibia, where slots were cut into the tibia in an anterior-posterior direction, although in this case the slot was v-shaped.

A limited number of Polycentric knees were carried out by Gunston at Wrightington Hospital due to time constraints. In most of the knees, both the lateral and medial sides were replaced, due to the cases being primarily rheumatoid arthritis. When Gunston returned to Winnipeg in 1969, he chose not to pursue his design commercially, continuing to make the components locally, but only carrying out a small number of cases. However Lowell Peterson and Richard Bryan from the Mayo Clinic in Rochester, Minnesota, met with Gunston and were interested in using the design. Initially they produced Gunston's design in the Mayo Clinic workshops but soon started working with companies including Howmedica. Peterson and Bryan modified the femoral and tibial components by making them "wide-track." The part of the femoral component which entered the slot on the femoral condyle was the same, but the bearing surface was widened, thinking that this would provide better load transfer onto the femoral condyles. In follow-up studies of the original design (Gunston and MacKenzie 1976; Lewallen et al. 1984) and the wide-track design (Bloom and Bryan 1977), there were no fixation or bone fracture problems with the femoral component. It is likely however that the bone strength of the femur would have been better preserved with the wide-track version, but this was not studied.

Because of the preservation of the normal joint geometry and the cruciate ligaments, it might be expected that the postoperative function of the Polycentric knee would be close to normal. This was investigated by Ed Chao PhD, director of the Biomechanics Laboratory at the Mayo Clinic, using an elaborate gait analysis system (Chao and Stauffer 1974). He used electrogoniometers to measure the rotations at the knee and force plates to measure ground reaction forces. Among Chao's goals were to identify the most significant gait parameters on which functional performance of the total knees can be compared and provide objective criteria for evaluating function. Chao found that the motion curves for a Polycentric knee were close to those of the normal opposite side, though he noted that the maximum flexion was less than normal, which even applies to artificial knees today. Ed Chao was undoubtedly a pioneer in the development of the measurement of objective biomechanical functional parameters in the study of artificial knees and comparison with normal knees.

In parallel with Gunston's work in the late 1960s, a more conventional compartmental design was being produced in Hamburg, called the St. Georg Sledge (Englebrecht and Zippel 1973). "Under the guidance of the collateral ligaments the sledge (femoral component) finds a suitable gliding area on the block (tibial component) keeping full range of movement of the knee joint….the surgeon….is not forced to consider the exact placement of two equally adjusted implants. The prosthesis can be inserted medially, laterally or bilaterally." Comparing the metal hinges with the condylar resurfacing types, as well as being at opposite extremes in size, bone removal, and canal invasion, the motions provided were completely different. The hinge allowed only flexion-extension, while the resurfacing knees allowed anterior-posterior and medial-lateral displacements as well as internal-external rotation. Surgical placement of a hinge was relatively straightforward with stability guaranteed, whereas for resurfacing, accurate component placement and balancing of ligaments were essential. This was particularly the case for the sledge knee because the surface of the tibial component was completely flat offering no constraint in any direction. The purpose of this was so that the femoral component can find a suitable sliding area and the surgeon will not be forced to consider the exact placement. Even with this much freedom of motion, the average range of flexion was only about 100 degrees in a 4-year follow-up, the same as for the St. Georg intercondylar hinge. An important element of the St. Georg design was that the sagittal and frontal radii of the femoral component were closely matched to the anatomic shapes, based on measurements from 50 knees. The femoral runners themselves were a constant 2–3 mm thickness, with two pegs for fixation, but the authors did not explain their technique for preparing the femoral condyles. A 3–10-year follow-up of 53 cases of the sledge knee used as bicondylars gave additional insights into the performance of the femoral component (Stockley et al. 1990). There was one case of impingement of the femoral runner against the medial tibial eminence due to lateral subluxation, and there was one case where the posterior part of a femoral runner fractured due to overhang with no cement support. While small in numbers, there are certain requirements for unicompartmental femoral components used on one or both condyles. The different lateral and medial geometries require different shapes for each. Sufficient sizes are necessary. The bearing geometry between the femoral and tibial components needs to restrict medial-lateral displacement, for which accurate instrumentation is required. There must be sufficient bending strength based on the thickness of the runners or reinforcement fins, to carry the functional forces without failure.

As well as the hinges and compartmental knees, at the 1974 London meeting, numerous other designs were presented, some with ingenious mechanisms. Most of the designs had similar goals: minimize the amount of bone resection needed yet still provide sufficient stability and fixation; utilize the collateral ligaments to provide varus-valgus stability; allow for sufficient laxity for normal function; reduce the fixation stresses on the components; and provide more inherent stability than afforded by simple condylar resurfacing types.

The Link arthroplasty invented by Michael Devas (Devas 1974) was a narrow all-metal hinge where a flat "finger" projecting from the tibia was housed in a circular cavity embedded in the distal femur: "While requiring no resection of the distal femoral and proximal tibial condyles, this device still functioned mechanically as a uniaxial hinge." It was considered that "an old person when walking neither rotates the knee nor locks it into full extension….therefore it has not been considered necessary to build in rotation…".

Another intercondylar design, the Attenborough stabilized gliding prosthesis (Attenborough 1974), took an opposite approach: "Flexion and extension should approximate to the normal knee and some rotation and lateral flexion should be possible….full extension should be completely stable....but these movements should increase gradually with increasing flexion….there should be anterior-posterior stability." Hence Attenborough was advocating a restoration of the laxity and stability characteristics of the normal knee. The femoral component was a complete resurfacing of the condyles and patella trochlea while the tibial component was a one-piece resurfacing with dished lateral and medial bearing surfaces, partially conforming with the femoral condyles. Each component had a short but bulky stem for fixation. In the center there was a loose hinged element which controlled the motions described above. The design was a middle ground between a hinge and a condylar replacement in that the laxity did not require long stems, but the intercondylar stability substituted for the resected cruciate ligaments and to some extent supplemented the collaterals. The design possessed many elements of future successful total knees.

The Deane knee (Deane 1974) was another design which reproduced normal knee laxity, stability in extension, and progressive laxity with flexion. The lack of varus-valgus constraint allowed for components where intramedullary fixation was not necessary. This knee actually reversed the materials, the femoral component being plastic and the tibial being metal, which minimized the total bone resection. An intercondylar cam produced an instant center of rotation path which changed with flexion, a concept which was demonstrated by Frankel and Burstein in 1971. The shape of the cam was to a large extent reproduced in the posterior stabilized or PS designs produced in the mid- to late 1970s.

A number of condylar replacement designs had also been produced. The femoral bearing surfaces were similar to the anatomic femur, while the tibial surfaces were generally dished both laterally and medially. This was in contrast to the anatomic tibia where the lateral condyle is convex in the sagittal plane and where the medial surface is raised anteriorly but has only shallow concavity centrally. However the medial concavity can be considered to be augmented by the meniscus, which is not the case laterally due to the mobility of the meniscus. Condylar replacement designs at that time included the Kodama-Yamamoto, the Townley, the Leeds (Seedhom), the Geometric, the Duo-condylar and Duo-patella, and the Total Condylar.

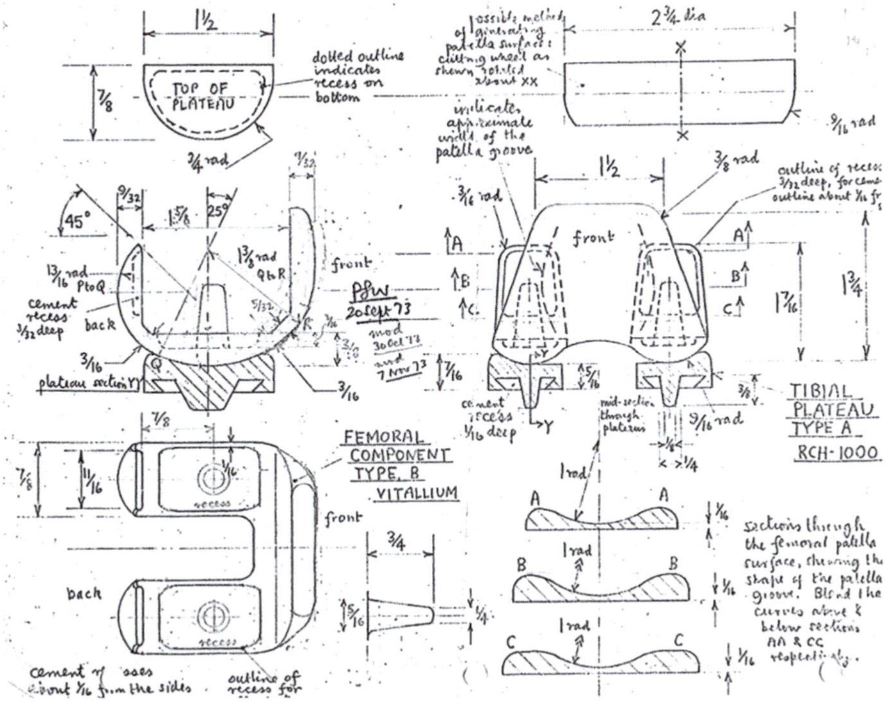

Fig. 7.3 The design drawing for the first Total Condylar knee dated 1973. The component fitted both right and left knees. Pockets for cement were provided distally and posteriorly. This version had separate tibial plateaus. The one-piece component with a central peg was designed separately. It is noted that computer-assisted design software did not exist at that time. The design was an equal group effort between Chit Ranawat, John Insall, and Peter Walker

Anatomically Shaped Femoral Components

In all cases, the femoral component shape was based to a large extent on normal anatomy. For some of the designs, the sagittal profile was obtained from radiographs or from slicing knee specimens. One exception was the Geometric knee (Coventry et al. 1972) where the surfaces were spherical, with the same radii in the frontal and sagittal planes. The reasons were that it would present a uniform geometry to the dished tibial surfaces throughout flexion and that it would be relatively easy to machine and polish accurately. In Bahaa Seedhom's Leeds knee design (Seedhom 1972) however, he replicated anatomic shapes: "....because there is a close relation between the geometry, ligamentous attachments and the joint movements, it follows that the prosthesis geometry must not depart too far from that of the natural knee if we are to preserve the ligaments and cause as little distortion of

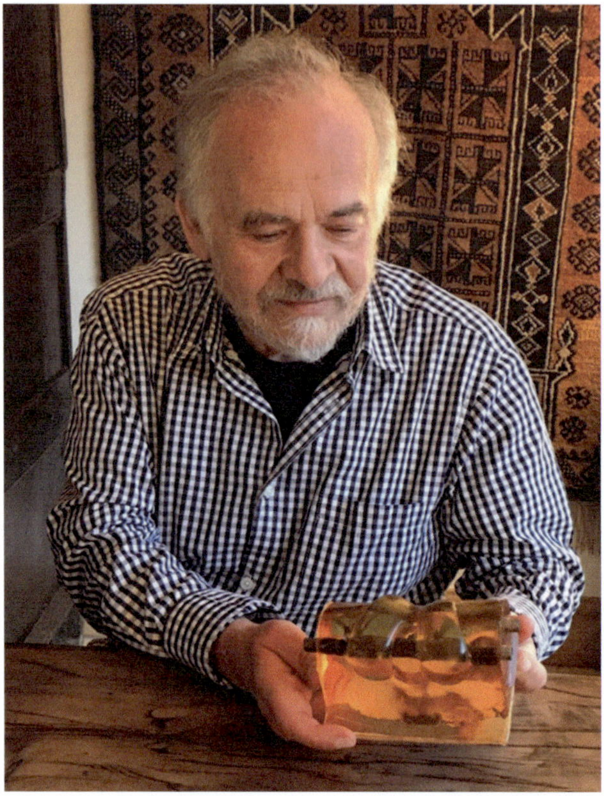

Fig. 7.4 Bahaa Seedhom PhD with a casting of a femoral component of the anatomically shaped Leeds knee which he designed in the early 1970s. In his position at University of Leeds, England, he hosted numerous Japanese fellows, who carried out a succession of innovative biomechanical studies on the knee. Seedhom founded a company making artificial ligaments, and he continues as general manager. He lives in a farmhouse on the Yorkshire Moors near Harrogate (Photo taken at interview in 2018). (© Peter S Walker)

the natural movement as possible. Furthermore, it was necessary to have a large range of flexion which meant less conformity of the bearing surfaces." Seedhom appreciated just how sensitive the laxity and stability were to small changes in the lengths of the ligaments which in turn was controlled by the shape of the bearing surfaces, especially on the femoral side. To be consistent with this, a sufficient number of femoral sizes were required. From a large number of knee specimens, Seedhom selected representative specimens of different sizes and made exact molds of the surfaces. From each mold, a metal femoral component was produced as a shell of uniform thickness. The divergence of the lateral and medial condyles from each other of 15 to 20 degrees, clearly visualized on a distal view of the femur, was reproduced in order to provide anterior-posterior stability. An intercondylar notch in the femoral component allowed for cruciate ligament preservation. The shape of the femoral component was not unlike that of the MGH femoral condyle, but Seedhom incorporated it within a full artificial knee system with multiple sizes.

Frederick Ewald MD, an orthopedic surgeon from the Robert Breck Brigham Hospital in Boston, also invented an innovative total knee with an anatomically shaped femoral component (Ewald 1975). He filed a US patent in 1971 which was issued in 1974. The femoral component was in the form of a shell, on which he added a short intramedullary stem for stabilization, but this was not intended to be cemented. The femoral component design overall was based on the MGH femoral condyle, described at the beginning of this chapter. In both Seedhom and Ewald's designs, the surface of the femoral component that interfaced with the femoral condyles was anatomic in shape, and consequently the component was very difficult to fit accurately at surgery, even though cement was used for fixation. Another difficulty at surgery was balancing of all four ligaments: even though the femoral component was anatomic in shape, the variation in shape between individual knees could result in mismatches in ligament length and tension patterns. The difficulties in fitting and the ligament balancing, as well as the cost of manufacturing the anatomic shapes, were the main reasons why these two designs, though elegant in form, were withdrawn only a few years after introduction. In retrospect, with moderate tibial dishing, the designs would likely have functioned well without the cruciates and hence would have been easier to insert surgically.

Patella Flanged Components

All of the above femoral component designs, with the exception of the Geometric and the Duo-condylar, had a patella flange. Although there is little documentation in the early literature of the advantages of the patella flange, it was generally recognized that there would be better fixation of the femoral component to the distal femur due to the larger surface area. It also avoided the surgical difficulty in non-flanged designs of providing a smooth transition at the anterior edge of the component and the anatomic trochlea above. Most importantly, it provided a smooth continuous track for the natural or artificial patella. A cartoon of the patellofemoral "distress" in non-flanged femoral components was drawn by Seedhom in the proceedings of the 1974 Conference on Total Knee Replacement.

For early resurfacing femoral components without patella flanges, additional fixation was needed other than relying simply on the flat or curved surfaces of the femoral component. The solutions used were either a central peg to be cemented a short distance into the intramedullary canal or two short pegs cemented into the lateral and medial condyles where the cancellous bone is sufficiently strong. Designs which used such means were the Geometric and the Duo-condylar. Femoral components with a patella flange may have been thought to have sufficient fixation due to the wraparound shape from posterior to anterior, but this is not the case for two reasons. Firstly, as the component is placed on to the distal femur at surgery, it is difficult to pressurize the cement on the anterior and posterior surfaces. Even if there are a few degrees of divergence of these surfaces, on insertion at surgery, the metal component tends to scrape the cement ahead of it, rather than pressurizing it into the cancellous bone surfaces. Secondly, when the knee is flexed past 90 degrees, the compressive forces on the posterior condyles have a force component which tries to push the femoral component off the end of the femur. The consequence of these factors is that the fixation, as for the non-patella flanged components, needs to be augmented by a central peg or two side pegs.

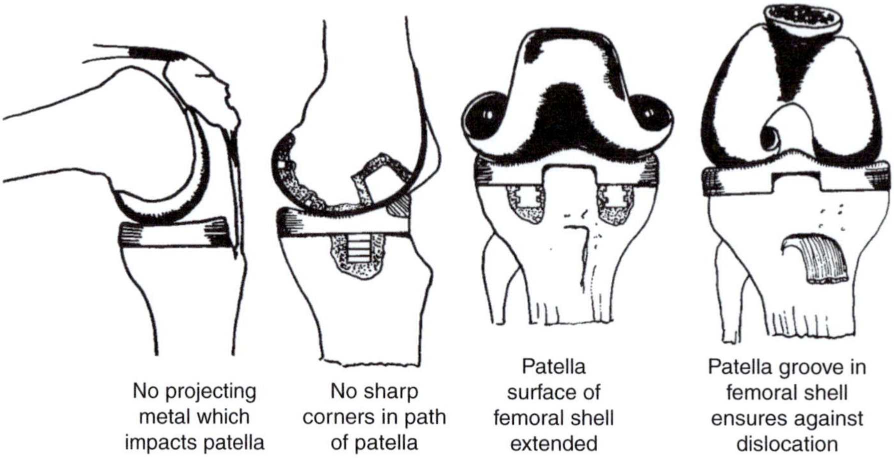

Fig. 7.5 Guidelines for designing the trochlea of the femoral component to ensure smooth continuous sliding, low contact stresses, and stability. This was presented at the 1974 conference in London, at a time when several implants still did not have an anatomical type of design as in the Leeds knee (Seedhom 1974). (Reprinted with permission from Institution of Mechanical Engineers, London UK)

This was well appreciated by Townley who designed one of the first flanged femoral components (Townley 1988). An important feature of Townley's femoral component was that there were five separate facets facing the bone: the distal surface, the anterior and posterior surfaces, and 45 degree chamfers at the anterior and posterior. These surfaces were straight-line approximations to the sagittal curve of the distal femur. Such facets are now standard on almost all femoral components, because it is easier to cut straight surfaces than curved surfaces, given the practicalities of the equipment used for joint replacement surgery. Even now with robot-assisted cutting tools, straight lines are still quicker than curves though not as bone preserving. Another feature which Townley included was pockets in the femur-facing facets of the femoral component, for containment of cement. This would give the cement mantle some integrity and avoid thin layers which could fragment under load. Other early designs, such as the Total Condylar, adopted the pocket feature.

Multiple Sizes

Most of the condylar designs were only made in a few sizes, mainly for economic reasons. However, it was not sufficiently recognized that accurately reproducing the original femoral sagittal profile was necessary for maintaining taut ligaments throughout flexion to achieve anatomic laxity and stability in every case. Seedhom did however provide a rationale for the number of sizes necessary based on a radiographic study of 131 knees (Seedhom 1972). He found close correlations between

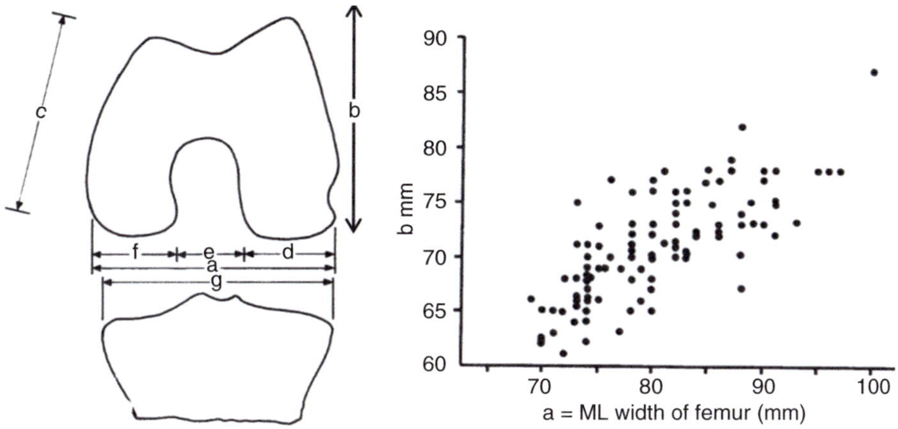

Fig. 7.6 Bahaa Seedhom carried out a systematic dimensional analysis of the femur and tibia to determine key dimensional parameters of the components for his anatomic knee design. From 101 radiographs and 20 cadaveric knees, he determined the relations between the parameters, illustrating the deviations from an exact correlation. One example is shown for the AP width to the ML width. To limit the AP or ML error between the component and a given knee to 3 mm, he calculated that five sizes would be needed of the femoral component (Seedhom et al. 1972). (Reprinted with permission from Wear)

many of the dimensional parameters and chose the medial-lateral width as the reference parameter with which to scale the other dimensions. With a 6 mm spacing in the medial-lateral dimension between sizes, he determined that only four sizes were needed to cover the population. While 6 mm seems large by today's standards, the largest error in a given knee would only be 3 mm or 1.5 mm per side. It has been noted that Seedhom used actual cadaveric specimens to make molds for the four sizes, so the radii of the condyles and the patella groove in the anterior-posterior (AP) and medial-lateral (ML) views would be automatically scaled. In a separate study however, Seedhom took sagittal and frontal slices through the condyles so that he could calculate the contact stresses on the polyethylene surfaces for the tibia, as the basis for wear experiments.

Today, artificial knee systems have as many as 12 sizes of femoral components, right and left, and, in some systems, additional sizes to include different medial-lateral widths. The dilemma in defining dimensions, notably the AP and ML, is the variations in their ratio, which is increased when different genders and ethnicities are included. The AP dimension is the main factor controlling kinematics, whereas there is a condition on the ML dimension that there should be less than 2–3 mm of overhang on any side. While the ML dimension could simply be made narrow enough to avoid overhang, this would result in too much exposed cancellous bone, as well as reduced varus-valgus stability. The conclusion from different studies based on fitting of large femoral databases of femurs in the computer concluded that the more sizes, the better but with little further gains after the 12 sizes mentioned above (Dai et al. 2014; Morris et al. 2016).

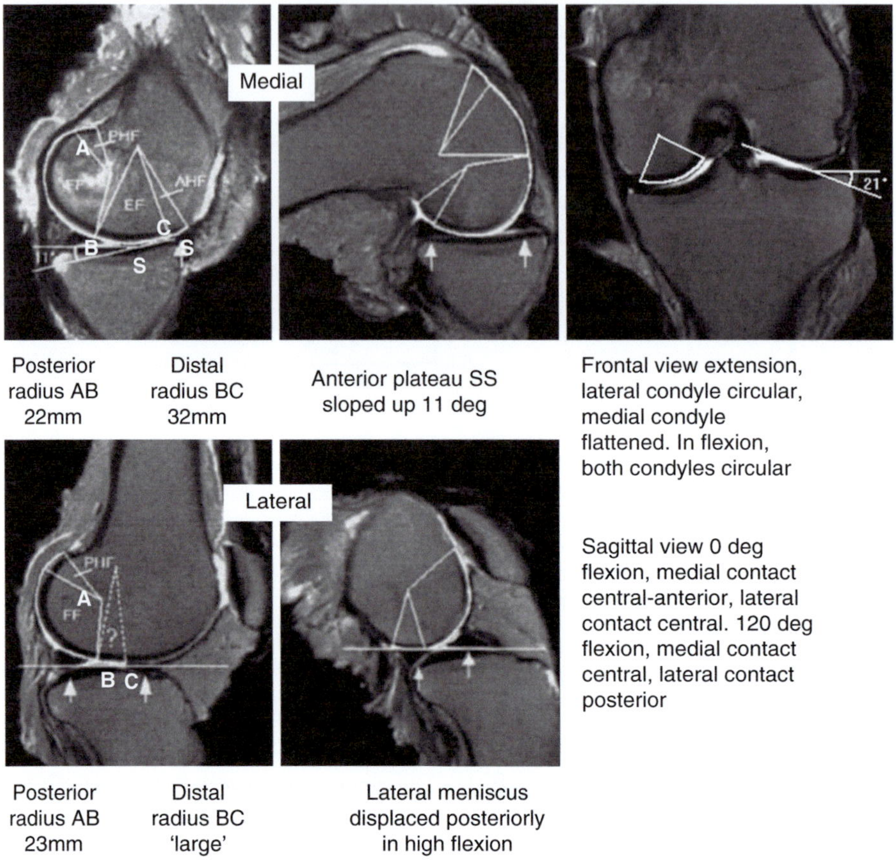

Fig. 7.7 MRI studies of knee specimens were used to characterize the shapes of the femoral and tibial bearing surfaces, the contact point locations, and the positions of the menisci. Describing the condylar profiles as connecting arcs is useful for practical purposes such as artificial knee design and modelling. The tibial slope on the medial side is seen as a result of the anterior region being sloped upwards. Some anterior-posterior restraint is provided on the medial side due to the tibial surface shape and the relatively immobile meniscus. Medial-lateral restraint is provided by the upward slopes on the inner tibial plateaus (Martelli and Pinskerova 2002). (Reprinted with permission from *Journal of Bone & Joint Surgery B*)

The sagittal profiles of the femoral condyles are likely to affect the kinematics, as well as the contact areas. In the anatomic knee, there are differences between the lateral and medial profiles (Martelli and Pinskerova 2002). Laterally, the profile which contacts the tibia during the flexion range was of a constant radius, with only a few millimeters distally where the radius is large. On the medial side, the distal region up to about 30 degree flexion had an average radius of 32 mm, while from 30 degrees to maximum flexion, the radius averaged 22 mm. Martelli and Pinskerova also pointed out that the medial profile could be represented by a radius which gradually reduced from distal to posterior. These authors also described the interaction of the femoral

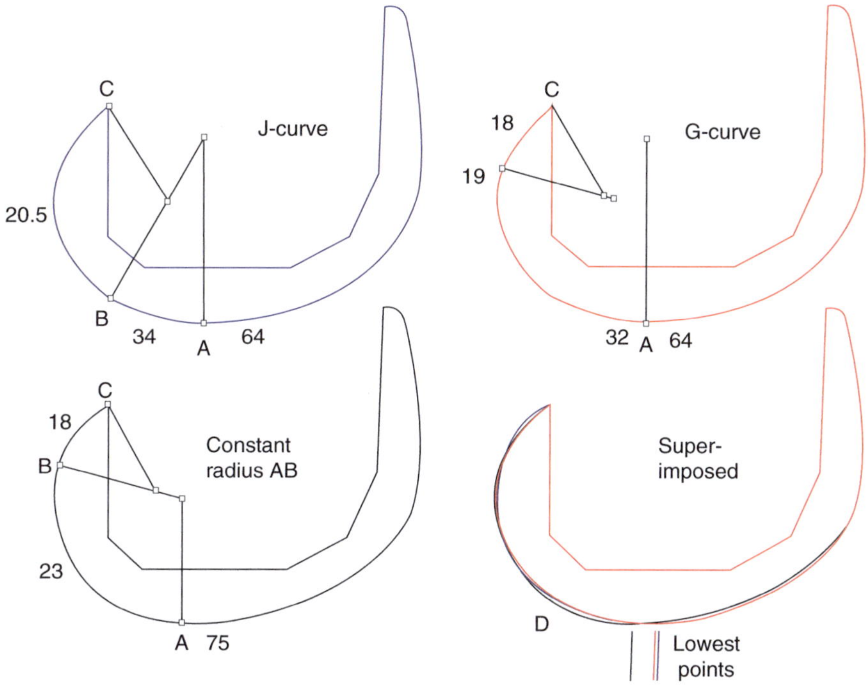

Fig. 7.8 Different schemes for constructing the sagittal profile of the femoral component. J-curve = two radii, A to B and B to C. G-curve = gradually decreasing radius from distal A to posterior C. Constant radius = constant from distal A to posterior B. The radii in millimeters are marked adjacent to the curve segments. When the curves are superimposed, the maximum deviation at D is 1 mm. The lowest point is 4 mm more posterior for the constant radius

condyles with the menisci and with the very different shapes of the lateral and medial tibial plateaus. The complex interactions are generally not reproduced by the articulating surfaces of an artificial knee, and certainly, the femoral condyles alone will not determine the kinematics. Artificial knees use three main schemes for the sagittal profiles from distal to posterior. Firstly, a constant radius resembles the anatomic lateral condyle. Secondly, a larger distal radius and a smaller posterior radius resembles the anatomic medial condyle; this is called a J-curve. Thirdly, a gradually reducing radius from distal to posterior again resembles the medial condyle; this is called a G-curve (Pfitzner et al. 2018). There are an infinite number of ways to construct these curves. However when they are superimposed, there appears to be only small differences in the profiles. One difference however is that the lowest point on the profile which will contact the tibial surface in early flexion may be more anterior for the J-curve and the G-curve than for the constant radius. A final point about the profiles is that if the goal is to mimic anatomy, the lateral condyle should be of constant radius, while the medial condyle should be a G-curve or J-curve. But again, this would need to be matched with asymmetric tibial surfaces.

Patellofemoral Joint

One aspect of femoral component design, the patellofemoral joint, received relatively little attention in early studies. This is remarkable considering that the quadriceps action is the driver of function for which a smooth-acting and stable patella is essential. It is likely that designers carried out basic measurements of the femoral groove on radiographs or on specimens, without making that aspect into a major study for publication. There was one exception to this, the work of Paolo Aglietti MD and associates in the Biomechanics Laboratory of the Hospital for Special Surgery (Aglietti et al. 1975). Aglietti, from Florence in Italy, was a surgical fellow of John Insall, chief of the knee service. Aglietti questioned whether a patella resurfacing component should be anatomic in shape or possibly some other shape which would be more suitable for an artificial knee. Working with John Insall, Peter Trent, a masters of mechanical engineering from Columbia University, and Peter Walker, Paolo designed a resurfacing component for the patella (Aglietti et al. 1975). The idea was that the artificial patella could be used as an independent implant or used

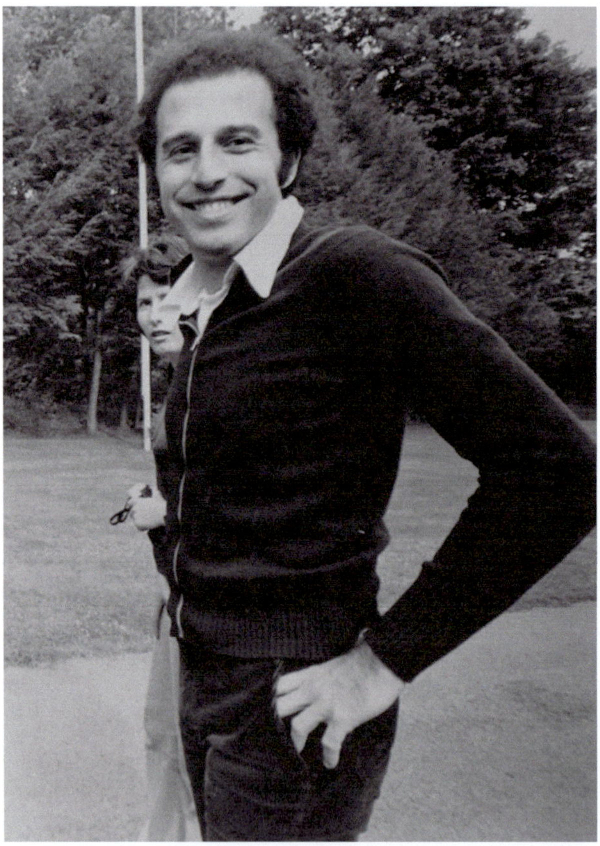

Fig. 7.9 Paolo Aglietti MD was a fellow in John Insall's Knee Service at the Hospital for Special Surgery (HSS) in the early 1970s, when this picture was taken. He participated in the design of the early HSS knees including the instrumentation. He carried out lab studies for the design of the dome patella, widely used today. He was coeditor with John Insall on the first edition of *Surgery of the Knee*. Paolo later returned to Florence to be Professor of Orthopedics, where he became a founding member of the Italian Knee Society. He maintained a strong relation with John Insall and HSS throughout his career. (© Peter S Walker)

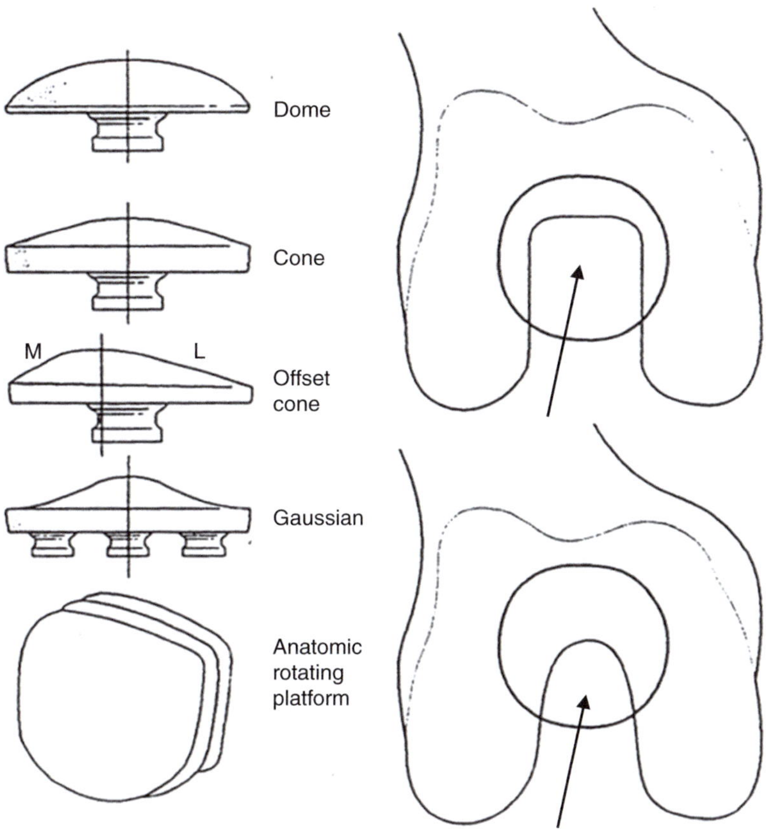

Fig. 7.10 Different possible configurations for the shape of an artificial patella. The offset cone is the closest resemblance to anatomic, but the most widely used design is the simple dome due to its simplicity and its ability to tilt in different directions without edge loading. The shape of the intercondylar region (arrows) affects contact area and stability

with the Total Condylar knee which was by then being used clinically. Dimensional parameters were measured from 80 resected patellae from surgical cases, ranging from "normal" to severely arthritic with grossly abnormal shape. Using this data, a dome-shaped patella was designed made from metal for use with an anatomic femur and from polyethylene to be used with the Total Condylar. Contact locations of normal intact knee specimens and those with a dome inserted were determined using an acrylic casting technique. Similar contact patterns were observed. Stability tests using a test rig were also carried out on specimens, where the Q-angle was varied. The dome was equal in medial-lateral stability to an anatomic patella. The conclusion was "The dome-shaped prosthesis conformed reasonably to all the femurs we have tested so far and located well into the groove, allowing some inherent stability. The symmetrical shape eliminates any ambiguity in insertion, and also accepts twisting and tilting with no change in contact area and with little stress on the fixation." So even though the anatomic patella has two distinct facets, the lateral longer than the medial, the dome was considered to be the best solution because of its adaptability to any shape of groove in any alignment. Even though there might be tilting or rotation, the dome will still provide coherent lateral and medial contact areas without any edge loading. In clinical application, in artificial knees the plastic dome patella did develop two patches of wear and deformation, indicative of exceeding the yield stress. However at that stage, the stresses would be reduced and would be tolerated by the plastic over a long time period without severe wear. This was largely due to the fact that in walking, the most frequent activity, the patello-femoral forces are less than the body weight, whereas in high flexion, even though the forces are higher, the frequency of loading is much less. At the same time, the intercondylar cutout, between the femoral condyles as in the femoral component of most of today's artificial knees, has shown disadvantages. Soft tissue distal to the resurfaced patella has become trapped between the condyles causing a snapping or popping as it releases, a phenomenon that has been more frequent with the posterior stabilized (PS) designs where the intercondylar housing has been more extensive and not sufficiently rounded.

Comparing today's femoral component designs of standard condylar replacements with those of the 1970s, the shapes have not in general evolved from being symmetric and geometric to being asymmetric and anatomic, as might be expected. While most designs have asymmetry in the overall peripheral shape especially in the patella flange area, only a few designs have differences in the sagittal profiles between the lateral and medial sides. Those designs that do have condylar asymmetry are mostly those where one or both cruciate ligaments are preserved, whereas for the PS designs, medial-lateral asymmetry is not considered necessary. In one study, the differences in geometry between the femoral component and its host

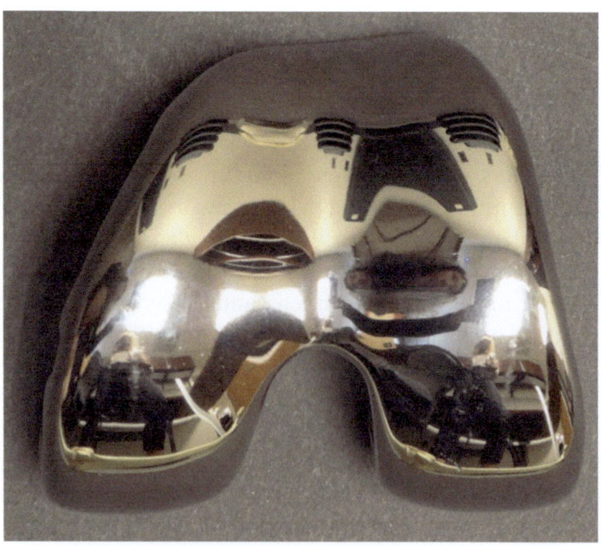

Fig. 7.11 A typical condylar femoral component with convex bearing surfaces to control medial-lateral sliding, with an anatomically shaped trochlea for retention of the patient's patella or for a plastic resurfacing, with a right-left flange shape to better fit the bone surface, and with a rounded intercondylar space for retention of the posterior cruciate

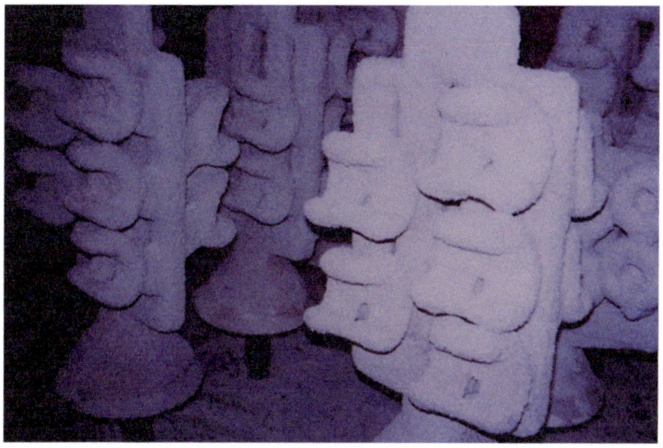

Fig. 7.12 The process for manufacturing femoral components from cobalt-chrome alloy, using the "lost wax" process. Ceramic coats the original wax models. The wax is melted out, after which molten metal is poured into the cavity. The components are mounted on a "tree," and connecting holes are made between components, so the molten metal will fill many components at the same time. After the metal hardens, the ceramic is removed, leaving individual femoral components. (Photo taken in manufacturing plant of Howmedica, now Stryker)

femur, combined with variations in surgical placement, were shown to result in dimensional discrepancies up to 6 mm (Akbari et al. 2018). This would make it difficult to balance the knee, while kinematic abnormalities might occur. Remarkably, the patella is symmetric in the majority of knee systems, despite the obvious asymmetry of the anatomic patella with a longer lateral facet than medial. The likely reason for this situation is that there have not been any compelling clinical advantages in asymmetry, nor disadvantages of symmetry, to cause a widespread movement to asymmetry.

To What Extent Do Femoral Component Shapes Mimic Normal Anatomy?

Most of the earliest designs were simplified shapes, not resembling normal anatomy either in the sagittal radii or in the overall contours. The exceptions to this were the MGH femoral condyle, designed to be used without a tibial component, the Ewald artificial knee which was based on the MGH, and the Leeds knee which was made from actual molds of anatomic specimens. Today, cruciate sacrificing designs usually have the same sagittal profiles laterally and medially, in contrast with normal anatomy; cruciate preserving knees usually have different lateral and medial condyle shapes. While the key dimensions and multiple sizes can provide a reasonably close match to any knee, the overall surface shapes of the femoral components are not anatomical and can deviate by several millimeters from a host femur. The discrepancies may cause some deficiencies of kinematics and function.

References

Aglietti P, Insall JN, Walker PS, Trent P. A new patella prosthesis. Design and application. Clin Orthop Relat Res. 1975;107:175–87.

Akbari S, Boulos P, Saavarsson SK, Ramm H, Fu CKJ, Miller S, Zachow S, Anglin P. Changes in knee shape and geometry resulting from total knee arthroplasty. Proc Inst Mech Eng H. 2018;232(1):67–79.

Attenborough GG. Total knee replacement using a stabilized gliding prosthesis. Conference on Total Knee Replacement, Institution of Mechanical Engineers, London UK, 16-18 September 1974.

Bloom JD, Bryan RS. Wide-track polycentric total knee arthroplasty. Clin Orth Rel Res. 1977;128:210–3.

Chao EY, Stauffer RN. 1974 Biomechanical evaluation of geometric and polycentric knee arthroplasty. Conference on Total Knee Replacement, Institution of Mechanical Engineers, London UK, 16-18 Sept 1974.

Coventry MB, Finerman GA, Riley LH, Turner RH, Upshaw JE. A new geometric knee for total knee arthroplasty. Clin Orthop Relat Res. 1972;83:157–62.

Dai Y, Scuderi GR, Penninger C, Bischoff JE, Rosenberg A. Increased shape and size offerings of femoral components improve fit during total knee arthroplasty. Knee Surg Sports Traumatol Arthrosc. 2014;22(12):2931–40.

Deane G. The Deane Knee: a new concept in knee joint design. Conference on Total Knee Replacement, Institution of Mechanical Engineers, London UK, 16-18 September 1974.

Devas M. Link arthroplasty of the knee. Conference on Total Knee Replacement, Institution of Mechanical Engineers, London UK, 16-18 September 1974.

Englebrecht E, Zippel J. The sledge prosthesis model St. Georg. Acta Orthrop Belg. 1973;39(1):203–9.

Ewald FC. Metal to plastic total knee replacement. Orthop Clin North Am. 1975;6(3):811–21.

Frankel VH, Burstein AH, Brooks DB. Biomechanics of internal derangement of the knee. Pathomechanics as determined by analysis of the instant centers of motion. J Bone Joint Surg Am. 1971;53(5):945–62.

Gunston FH. Polycentric knee arthroplasty. Prosthetic simulation of normal knee movement. J Bone Joint Surg (Br). 1971;53(2):272–7.

Gunston FH, MacKenzie RI. Complications of polycentric knee arthroplasty. Clin Orthop Relat Res. 1976;(120):11–7.

Hodge WA. Vitallium-mold arthroplasty of the knee. A case report with 30-year follow-up study. J Arthroplast. 1991;6(3):195–7.

Lewallen DG, Bryan RS, Peterson LF. Polycentric total knee arthroplasty. A ten-year follow-up study. J Bone Joint Surg Am. 1984;66(8):1211–8.

Martelli S, Pinskerova V. The shapes of the tibial and femoral articular surfaces in relation to tibiofemoral movement. J Bone Joint Surg (Br). 2002;84-B:607–13.

Morris WZ, Gebhart JJ, Goldberg VM, Wera GD. Implant size availability affects reproduction of distal femoral anatomy. J Knee Surg. 2016;29(5):409–13.

Pfitzner T, Moewis P, Stein P, Boeth H, Trepczynski A, von Roth P, Duda GN. Modifications of femoral component design in multi-radius total knee arthroplasty lead to higher lateral posterior femoro-tibial translation. Knee Surg Sports Traumatol Arthrosc. 2018;26:1645–55.

Seedhom B. A technique for the study of geometry and contact in normal and artificial knee joints. Wear. 1972;20:189–99.

Seedhom BB, Longton EB, Dowson D, Wright V. The Leeds Knee. Conference on Total Knee Replacement, Institution of Mechanical Engineers, London UK, 16-18 September 1974.

Smith-Petersen MN, Aufranc OE, Larson CB. Principle of mold arthroplasty as applied to the hip. Surg Clin North Am. 1947;27:1303–6.

Stockley I, Douglas DL, Elson AA. Bicondylar St. Georg sledge knee arthroplasty. Clin Orth Rel Res. 1990;(255):228–34.

Townley CO. Total knee arthroplasty: a personal retrospective and prospective review. Clin Ortho Rel Res. 1988;236:8–22.

Tibial Component

8

What Are the Best Configurations for Durability?

The tibial component provides a low-friction and wear-resistant bearing surface for the femoral component, as well as constraints to displacements and rotations. In order to avoid loosening over time, the component must have the means for rigid fixation to the resected tibial surface.

Opposite Extremes of Tibial Component Design

The earliest tibial component designs had strikingly different configurations. The Freeman-Swanson consisted of a plate of polyethylene covering the entire resected tibial surface without provision for retaining the cruciate ligaments. This was based on the knee pathology for which the design was intended: "the theoretical advantage of retaining the cruciate ligaments was not realized in those severely disabled knees in which these ligaments are often damaged" and "hence the largest possible area in one plane is presented to the tibia…thus minimizing the chances of compressive failure of the bone" (Freeman et al. 1973). On the other hand, Gunston's Polycentric tibial components were small polyethylene runners to be embedded in V-shaped slots in the proximal tibia. This design resulted from an entirely different set of design criteria to Freeman and Swanson's: "Separate replacement of the diseased joint surfaces using cement…permits adjustment of the relative levels of the prosthetic surfaces. Collateral ligament laxity may be reduced and varus or valgus deformity decreased" (Gunston 1971). Freeman and Swanson placed a higher priority on minimizing the stresses on the trabecular bone of the proximal tibia, over retaining the cruciates; whereas Gunston's criteria were the opposite.

The Freeman-Swanson can be thought of as a mechanistic approach, where the joint stability was provided by the component geometry, while the alignment was based on making the bone cuts relative to defined axes in the femur and tibia. It was assumed that "when the prosthesis has been correctly implanted the soft tissues will be tight in extension but a little lax in flexion." In the clinical follow-ups, some patients reported varus-valgus instability which could be attributed to the initial surgical technique where "the bone ends were resected at right angles to their long

P. S. Walker, *The Artificial Knee*, https://doi.org/10.1007/978-3-030-38171-4_8

axis." This would leave the limb in some varus compared with normal alignment where the distal femoral condyles are aligned an average of 5–6° to the anatomic axis. The Gunston design was an anatomic approach where the goal was restoration of the levels and contours of the original bearing surfaces and correct tensing of the ligaments to perform their normal functions. Separate components for each condyle were important to enable individual adjustment, difficult to achieve with a single one-piece component. At the same time, alignment of four different components both in height, rotation, and medial-lateral position would not be easy for the surgeon, and there was a limited surface area of the tibial components for fixation.

Application of Anatomic Experiments

Subsequently, several tibial components intermediate to the Freeman-Swanson and Gunston were designed, preserving a complete bridge of tibial bone in the center. At the Hospital for Special Surgery in 1970, Peter Walker and Joe Hajek, an orthopedic resident, determined the location of the contact areas in knee specimens throughout flexion (Walker and Hajek 1972). Their method was to remove the menisci, fill the cavity with soft acrylic cement, load the knee in an Instron machine, and then remove the hardened acrylic casting. The holes in the casting on the lateral and medial sides signified the contact areas. From a composite of the contact areas over a full range of flexion, they made a model of a tibial component with an anterior bridge. The tibial spines were replicated to provide medial-lateral constraint and limit internal-external rotation: "The weight-bearing surface curves upward toward the intercondylar area to provide medial-lateral and rotary stability, but provides no stability in the anterior-posterior plane." Anterior-posterior stability was to be provided by the preserved cruciate ligaments and "allow normal patterns of motion as characterized by the variable instant centers."

When the Duo-condylar knee was designed, however, based on the above study, the crossbridge was abandoned to allow for individual component placement as with the Gunston (Ranawat and Shine 1973). The provision of several thicknesses allowed for individual tightening of each compartment. The correct medial-lateral spacing of the two separate components at surgery was obtained by an insertion instrument locating in holes on the front of the components. Nevertheless, the use of separate components was discontinued after a few years due to fixation problems, even though the components covered the full extent of the normal contact areas.

Metal Tibial Tray and Modularity

In the late 1960s, a completely new approach to tibial component design was being developed by Nas Eftekhar, a surgeon from Columbia Presbyterian Hospital in New York (Eftekhar 1978). Eftekhar had spent 18 months at Wrightington Hospital in England with John Charnley. There he learned the technique of low-friction hip arthroplasty. He overlapped with Frank Gunston and was interested in his knee design, but considered that the small components designed by Gunston would not provide sufficient strength of fixation. On his return to the USA, Eftekhar was appointed at Columbia Presbyterian Hospital where he established programs for artificial hips and knees. Working in his own lab and with some involvement from Howmedica (now Stryker), he designed the Intramedullary Adjustable knee, which was an adaptation of Gunston's knee. Eftekhar's femoral component consisted of two Gunston components without the full half-disc shape, joined by a crossbridge on which there was an intramedullary stem. The tibial component was a metal plate covering the entire proximal tibia where Gunston plastic components were pressed into recesses. The metal plate had a central intramedullary stem for fixation and two small side pegs to resist rotary forces. The design rationale was stated as: "The principle fixation mechanism was achieved by intramedullary elements of the prosthesis (metal stems) and the differential plastic heights were press-fitted into the metallic component of the tibia to prevent cold flow of the plastic with the hope of preventing loosening." Eftekhar had decided that the cruciate ligaments were not necessary for an artificial knee, which made it easier to achieve balancing. The plastic

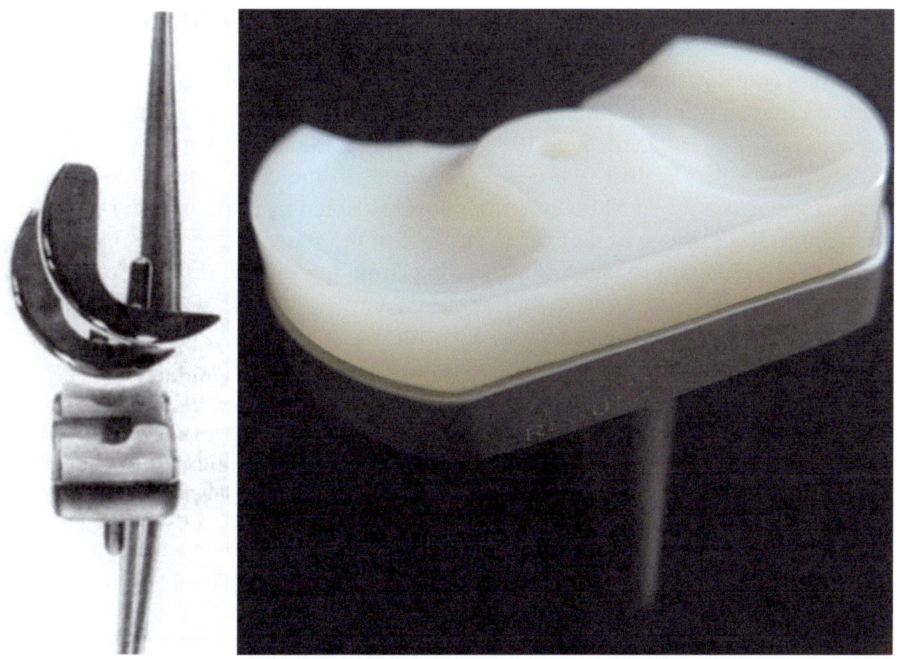

Fig. 8.1 While on a Fellowship at Charnley's Hip Center in the late 1960s, Nas Eftekhar MD became familiar with Gunston's Polycentric design. On returning to New York, he worked with Howmedica in adapting the components for stronger fixation (left). The plastic inserts could be adjusted individually for height. The metal tray was intended to enhance fixation. Later, Eftekhar used the same idea but this time modified the Total Condylar design, providing a metal-backed tibial component with a one-piece plastic. It provided more rotational laxity than the Total Condylar. This was the first metal-backed component to be designed for an artificial knee (Eftekhar 1978). (Left, Reprinted with permission from Clinical Orthopaedics and Related Research. Right, photo of sample courtesy of William Macaulay MD)

thicknesses of 6, 10, 14, and 20 mm seem to be too widely spaced by today's standards. This design was used in patients from 1970 till 1974. When the Total Condylar knee was being produced by Howmedica in 1973, Eftekhar utilized the Total Condylar femoral component with the addition of a stem and a one-piece plastic insert which seated into a tibial tray. But by now, Howmedica was in full production of the Geometric knee, while the Total Condylar became an even higher priority. Consequently, the Eftekhar knee was not widely adopted and faded out after a few years. Another major reason was that surgeons were not ready to revert to long cemented intramedullary stems, going back to the days of all-metal hinges. Nevertheless Eftekhar‘s tibial components were the first metal-backed designs, with the advantages of rigidity of fixation and interchangeability of the plastic inserts.

While Eftekhar's tibial tray design had sufficient strength, this was not the case for some subsequently designed metal trays. For example the Kinematic knee showed an incidence of tray fracture of an estimated 1–2% (Abernethy et al. 1996). Cracks initiated at the corners of a posterior rectangular-shaped notch which provided clearance for the posterior cruciate. Associated factors were lack of bone support under the metal tray and undercorrected varus deformity. Other contributing factors were that the tray itself was too thin, in order to minimize the amount of bone resection, and a pyramidal pattern on the base to grip the cement which acted as a stress concentration. A finite element analysis showed that the development of a fibrous tissue layer beneath the tray increased the stresses to the point where fracture was possible (Paganelli et al. 1988). As a result of this failure mode, a study was initiated by Peter Walker who was Director of the Biomedical Engineering Department at the Royal National Orthopaedic Hospital in Stanmore, UK, affiliated with University College London. The purpose of the study was to develop a testing method for predicting whether a metal tibial tray design would fail in service. In collaboration with surgeons, radiographic data was obtained from clinical cases where fractures had occurred. Consistent with the above study by Paganelli, it was found that all of the failures occurred when there had been a fibrous tissue interface beneath the tray medially. This led to a test scenario where half of the tray was clamped rigidly, while a cyclic load was applied to the overhanging part of the component (Ahir et al. 1999). The result of this work was a standard adopted by the ASTM entitled: "Cyclic fatigue testing of metal tibial tray components of total knee replacements."

Conformity and Cruciate Preservation

The scheme of an anterior bridge to preserve the cruciate ligaments was used in the early 1970s in the Leeds, the Ewald, and the Geometric knee designs. The rationale was to maintain a one-piece component, which was easier for surgery, to retain both cruciate ligaments, and to provide extra-fixation from the bridge. Even so, comparing separate components to a single component with an anterior bridge, the utility of the bridge can be questioned, especially with an all-plastic component. The increase in surface area for fixation is small in relation to the areas of the lateral and

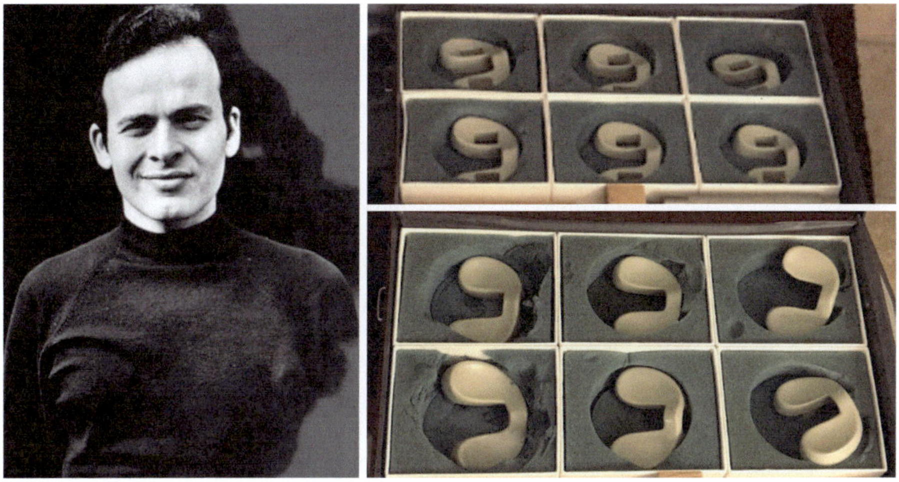

Fig. 8.2 Bahaa Seedhom Ph.D. designed the Leeds knee with all-plastic tibial components where the polyethylene was compression molded for enhanced wear resistance. There were three sizes right and left. The peripheral shape was based on anatomic specimens. The holes in the trial components (top right) were for drilling holes in the tibia, which lined up with fixation pegs on the base of the components. (© Peter S Walker)

medial condyles themselves, while the removal of the anterior tibial bone weakens the attachment of the anterior cruciate ligament, in some cases causing the ligament to avulse. Nevertheless the advantage of joining the lateral and medial plateaus with the consequent ease of surgery was the main priority. In the case of the Geometric, the tibial bearing surfaces were in close conformity with the femoral surfaces with only a small amount of mismatch to allow for some rotational laxity. It transpired that the close conformity had two disadvantages. The average flexion angle in an early series was only 87°, but in addition, there was an average of seven degrees of extension lag (Skolnick et al. 1976). The likely reason for this was that in preserving the cruciate ligaments, there needed to be provision for up to 10 mm of anterior-posterior displacement of the femur on the tibia during the flexion range, which would not be possible due to the high femoral-tibial conformity. The close conformity between the bearing surfaces under loaded conditions would allow almost no displacement or laxity. On the contrary, the intention was to provide a stable knee joint by adjusting the tibial thickness: "laxity of capsular and ligamentous structures is taken up by the so-called spacer effect of the components."

Another effect of the high conformity was on the fixation of the components. Even at 2 years follow-up, there was 12% of loosening while "lucent lines were noted at the tibial cement-bone interface in all cases of loosening and in about 80% of the remaining knees." The authors considered that "uncorrected varus alignment of the knee was thought to be the primary cause of loosening" with other factors being inadequate medial bone support and incorrect component seating. In addition, the component conformity would have caused high shear and tensile stresses at the cement-bone interface, but the fixation pegs were relatively small. Also at that time, there was little recognition of the need for adequate cement penetration into the trabecular bone. After several years of widespread clinical use, the Geometric knee was replaced by other designs. Nevertheless, the Geometric was the first total knee in the USA to have been designed initially by an engineer, Bob Averill, followed by bringing together a number of prominent surgeons from different institutions. Over the first 2 years, the group refined the design and developed the surgical instrumentation. There were many iterations involving cadaveric trials and mechanical testing. When the knee was first introduced at the AAOS Annual Meeting in 1972, there was an impressive exhibit with demonstrations by the developers, generating enormous interest among the surgeon community.

At about the same time that the Geometric knee was introduced, Charles Townley started using a cruciate-preserving design he had been refining for many years. The Townley Anatomic knee was however only used by Townley in the first few years due to the delay in finding a manufacturer who would widely promote it. Townley's efforts on a knee replacement design began in the early 1960s when he introduced the articular-plate replacement, consisting of a thin metal shell for tibial resurfacing, fixed to the bone with two screws through anterior metal lugs. At the same time, Townley had designed an anatomically shaped femoral component, but this was not implemented because it would need to have been made in metal and there was a reluctance to use metal-on-metal in a non-conforming bearing. However once metal and polyethylene knees fixed with acrylic cement had been introduced by Freeman and Swanson in England in the late 1960s, Townley saw this as the solution. Townley's goal in reconstructing the knee had always been to restore normal anatomy and function: "optimal results require proper implant design and surgical technique that restore the normal joint anatomy mechanics and kinematics" (Townley 1985). Not surprisingly, the bearing surfaces were a close reproduction of the anatomic shapes, the components were made as thin as possible, and the cruciates were preserved. The tibial component was all-plastic with a central cutout for the cruciates and an anterior bridge to join the lateral and medial sides. The tibial bearing surfaces were shallow to allow sliding and rotations to occur between the femur and the tibia: "For optimal postoperative motion, the normal synchronized relation between the ligaments and the articular outlines of the femoral condyles must be retained. This requires anatomic design contouring and accurate size selection and technical positioning of the implants."

The results of the Townley were better than those of the Geometric knee both in durability and range of flexion. Townley claimed only 2% revision for loosening in over 500 cases followed for 2–11 years. "The postoperative motion was at least 90° in 91%, between 110–120 in 21%, and in excess of 120° in 12%." Both the favorable motion and fixation results can be attributed largely to the low conformity between the femoral and tibial components such that there would be relatively low shear forces transmitted to the tibial component. Nevertheless the low loosening rate is not easy to understand considering that thin plastic components are known to deform under weight-bearing, while the stresses on the surface are transmitted directly to the surface of the trabecular bone with little attenuation. The answer may

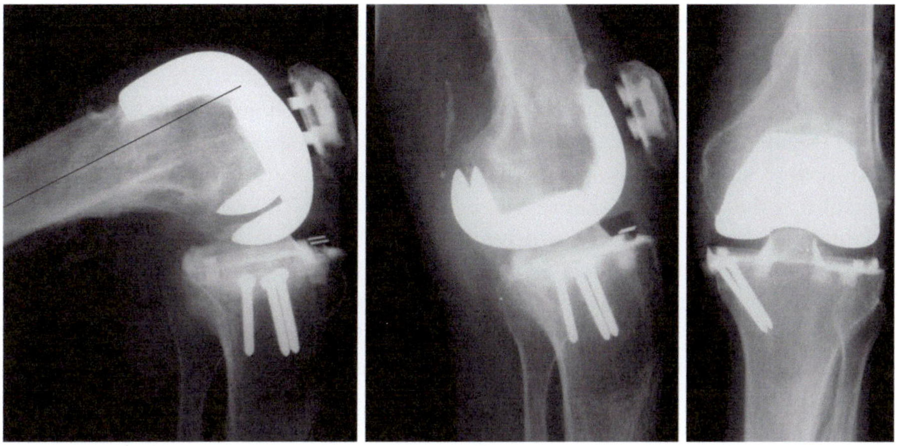

Fig. 8.3 Long-term follow-up of a Townley Anatomic knee. The patient's knee was in severe varus with a medial bone defect. The defect was filled with a graft and fixed with screws, prior to the cementing of the entire component. The tibial component was metal-backed in the shape of a horseshoe for preservation of both cruciate ligaments. A number of small drill holes can be seen in the proximal tibia for cement penetration, to provide improved fixation. The patella component is also metal-backed. (Photos courtesy James W Pritchett MD)

lie in the meticulous attention given to the surgical technique in that the target was to align the knee to the mechanical axis with the valgus angle at the knee set on an individual basis, and the joint line in the frontal plane set parallel to the ground. As for the cement technique: "small one-eighth inch anchor holes are punched into the supporting bone surfaces of the femur and tibia." The radiographs shown by Townley in articles do show substantial cement penetration into the trabecular bone, shown in experiments by Krause many years later to provide a major increase in fixation strength. Another factor was that there was only a few millimeters of proximal tibial bone resection, preserving the strongest trabecular bone near to the surface. Townley used his engineering knowledge and careful observation to formulate solutions which worked.

Cloutier's total knee design was similar to that of the Townley, but in this case, the tibial component consisted of a metal baseplate where individual plastic bearings were snap-fitted laterally and medially (Cloutier 1983). The bearing surfaces were again shallow. The anterior bridge being made of metal could be much smaller than for the Townley all-plastic design, although in a metal-backed construct, the total thickness of the component is elevated due to the need for 6 mm minimum thickness of plastic and 2–3 mm of metal-backing. Certainly, the load distribution on the underlying trabecular bone is more uniform than for an all-plastic component, which has generally been considered to be an advantage for long-term fixation. Cloutier emphasized that the preservation of the ACL, as well as the PCL, was the only way in which normal kinematics could be achieved. He also pointed out that in normal knees, when the ACL had been torn, posteromedial wear was often seen, as well as AP instability in function. The same could occur in an artificial knee where the anterior cruciate was resected. He used an advanced surgical technique, incorporating ligament releases, making bone cuts perpendicular to the mechanical axis, and tensing the ligaments with a distractor.

Total knee designs similar to those of Townley and Cloutier have been in continual use to this day, and in recent years, there has been some increased interest due to improved surgical techniques where greater accuracy could be achieved. It is logical that the best functional results can be obtained if the knee is restored to its original anatomical condition, which requires both accurate shapes of implants and a high degree of surgical precision, as well as adequate means of fixation. Hence this type of tibial component with cruciate preservation is a viable design for achieving optimal results, at least for those patients without severe deformity and where the cruciate ligaments are preserved and functional.

Development of the Central Peg

So far, three types of tibial components have been described: a one-piece component covering the entire tibial surface, two separate components replacing the lateral and medial plateaus, and two separate plateaus joined anteriorly with a bridge. Yet another scheme, introduced in the early 1970s, was to increase the size of the anterior bridge in the anterior-posterior direction, at the expense of resecting the anterior cruciate ligament. This work took place at the Hospital for Special Surgery, where Chit Ranawat, John Insall, and Allan Inglis had been using the Duo-condylar knee for 1–2 years. Already, the deficiencies of separate plastic plateaus had been observed, and while there were potential advantages of a one-piece component with a large surface area such as in the Freeman-Swanson design, even there, reliable fixation had not been achieved. Moreover, there was no desire at that stage to sacrifice both cruciate ligaments. Because of the location of the posterior cruciate ligament, all that was required for its preservation was a central notch about 15 mm in depth at the posterior of the component. This meant that the tibial component would cover most of the resected surface of the tibia, increasing the stiffness of the component and enhancing fixation. It was generally assumed that the posterior cruciate was more important to preserve because it was thicker and stronger than the anterior cruciate and prevented the femur from sliding anteriorly on the tibia, whereas the anterior cruciate was often absent or deficient in the arthritic knee. Another strong motivation for preserving only the posterior cruciate was to simplify the technique. When both cruciates were preserved, it was difficult to access the bone surfaces for preparing keyholes for pegs in the components, removing soft tissue around the edges of the tibia, and removing excess cement which may have squeezed out posteriorly. With the anterior cruciate resected, the tibia could be subluxed anteriorly affording improved exposure. One of the earliest such designs of this type was the Duo-patella, designed collaboratively between the Hospital for Special Surgery and the Robert Brigham Hospital in Boston (Sledge and Ewald 1979). Artificial knee designs which preserve only the posterior cruciate are termed "cruciate retaining," or CR, and have been widely used, initially all-plastic, but, in recent years, predominantly metal-backed.

From the outset, the CR tibial component incorporated one vital feature, a central fixation peg. Most other tibial component designs had various features on the base for fixation to the proximal tibia, such as serrations or dovetails so that the cement would lock to the component. Other designs used short projections requiring holes or slots to be cut into the bone. The principles were explained by Swanson et al. (1973), in terms of the various forces acting on the component: "An axial force acting on the center of the component would be supported by compression stresses on a resected surface of trabecular bone. Hence the largest surface area possible would be preferable. Another way in which an axial force can be supported is by a tapered peg in which case some of the axial force is supported as shear down the sides of the peg. Indentations of some sort would increase the shear force that could be transmitted. However an excessively rigid intramedullary stem may raise the danger of localized disuse-osteoporosis, or stress protection. An anterior force on the component would require a means of preventing the posterior of the component from distracting upwards." Swanson correctly pointed out that on the medial side at least, the strongest trabecular bone was located close to the center of the lateral and medial tibial plateaus such that in the sagittal plane: "there would be a tendency for the component to rock about a fulcrum of relatively stiff bone." Torque acting on the surface of the component would produce shear stresses at the cement-bone interface, but such stresses could be reduced by projections into the bone which would transmit forces on the sides. Another important point made by Swanson was that: "tensile and shear stresses at the interfaces be as small as possible…and compressive stresses are at a level that will not cause fatigue failure in the bone." Systematic thinking such as this had seldom been evident in total knee design. In the case of design features for optimal fixation of the tibial component, it was scarcely raised as a design problem requiring special attention.

The Special Surgery group was likely the first to carry out experiments to demonstrate the efficacy of a central peg. There were several factors that led to this solution. Observations of their own designs, the Unicondylar and Duo-condylar, as well as of other early design such as the Freeman-Swanson, Polycentric, and Geometric, showed that short projections into the resected proximal tibia did not provide sufficient fixation, evidenced by frequent development of radiolucent lines at the bone-cement interface. The lines would often progress over time to cover the entire interface, such that a revision procedure was often necessary. A recommended technique for fixing compartmental components, based on laboratory experiments, was to drill holes about 10 mm in diameter in the anterior and posterior of the resected tibial surface (Walker et al. 1976). The cement would fill these holes and penetrate the surrounding trabeculae, providing resistance to distraction as well as carrying shear forces. However a reliable method was needed for rigidly fixing a one-piece all-plastic tibial component as used for the Total Condylar or Duo-patella. Previous studies of the density and strength of the trabecular bone in the proximal tibia had shown that the bone in the center was the weakest, whereas the strongest bone occurred in the central regions of the lateral and medial plateaus, the major areas of load transmission (Behrens et al. 1974). Hence if the weakest bone at the center was removed, it could provide access for a central stem. Metallic stems had of course been used for decades in the hinged replacements as well as the more recent Eftekhar knee, but these were intended to fix to the cortical bone along a length of 120 mm or more below the tibial surface. There was however one example of an all-plastic tibial component with a central stem only about 60 mm in length, the Attenborough Stabilized Gliding prosthesis (Attenborough 1976). The rationale for the stem in that design was to provide varus-valgus stability, but in an unlinked design, this would not be a major requirement. However, if a central peg was designed with a rectangular section and cemented into a central cavity, it could possibly transmit anterior-posterior shear forces as well as axial rotation forces. In addition it would also transmit vertical shear forces down the trabecular bone at the sides of the cavity.

The initial central peg designed by the HSS group was 40 mm in length, with a rectangular section. The peg was tapered posteriorly as seen in the sagittal view, so that the posterior distal corner of the stem would not impact the posterior tibial cortex. The length was based on the observation that the density of the trabecular bone reduced steadily with depth, reaching the hollow intramedullary cavity at about 60 mm depth. Another important feature of the peg was the rectangular cavities cut into the sides. These cavities would fill with cement and transmit the vertical shear forces. It was proposed that even if the bone-cement interface on the horizontal surface of the tibia became loose, the central peg was likely to remain firmly fixed and hence maintain strong enough fixation of the entire component. An advantage of the central peg was that it did not invade the strong bone on the lateral and medial sides of the tibia. For this reason, smaller side pegs to augment the central peg were not added.

While it seemed likely that a central peg would afford stronger fixation than previous configurations, experimental validation was needed. The most direct method for this was mechanical testing, but machines which simulated the variable loading conditions of everyday use had not yet been designed. Moreover the test would require cyclic loading of high enough magnitude over an extended time period. Using a single station would take a great deal of time to test sufficient samples. This was the motivation for the design of a multichannel test machine. "A 9-channel machine was designed and constructed which oscillated the femoral component back and forth through an arc of 45° in a flexion-extension plane. A force of twice body weight was applied for one half of the cycle by air cylinders mounted above the femoral components. The tibial components were cemented to cadaveric tibias which were fixed to the machine base" (Walker and Hsieh 1977). Anterior-posterior shear force components were applied to the tibial components when the femur was in a flexed position, because the force was applied down the axis of the femoral component itself. The test was designed to compare separate condylar components with anterior and posterior holes for cement and a one-piece component with a central peg. The tests showed the clear superiority of the central peg design which remained rigidly fixed in all specimens. The separate plateaus failed by compressive failure of the trabecular bone at the interface. Where there were several keyholes for cement: "the islands of bone (between the key holes) thus created were susceptible to weakening." "The logical provision of a central peg, introduced into the weak central area but flanked by strong cancellous bone, was shown to provide the necessary strength…"

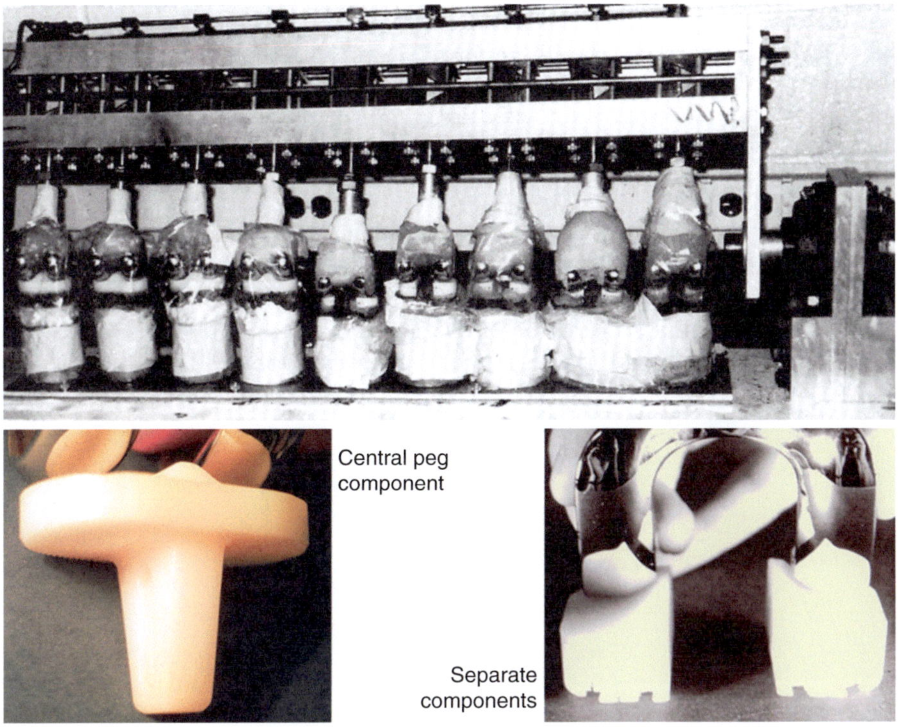

Fig. 8.4 Testing of the fixation of tibial components using a nine-channel knee simulating machine, at Hospital for Special Surgery. The machine flexed-extended with cyclic loading for up to 1 million cycles. The load included shear forces during the flexed phases. All central peg components remained well fixed. The separate components failed at different times due to failure of the trabecular bone beneath the components and between cement holes drilled to enhance the fixation (Walker and Hsieh 1977). (Top, Reprinted with permission from Journal of Bone & Joint Surgery A)

The all-plastic tibial component with a central peg was accordingly applied to the Total Condylar and Duo-patella knees. Follow-up studies of various central peg designs used to this day have attested to the durability of the central peg concept used on all-plastic components. However certain deficiencies have been noted. Radiolucent lines have frequently developed at the sides of the horizontal tibial surface as seen in the anterior-posterior view, signifying loss of rigid cement-bone fixation. This has been most commonly seen on the medial side, likely due to the higher axial forces occurring on that side. From radiographs the radiolucency has often been seen to be associated with inadequate cement penetration. As the component is seated at surgery and pressed down on the soft cement layer, the pressure at the sides is much less than at the interior because the cement can readily flow out sideways. This is a well-known characteristic of a squeeze film. Another situation has been where the medial side of the knee has been overloaded, and there has been gradual collapse of the trabecular bone. The plastic has permanently bent downward due its lack of stiffness. Cement has often extruded beyond the tip of the stem into

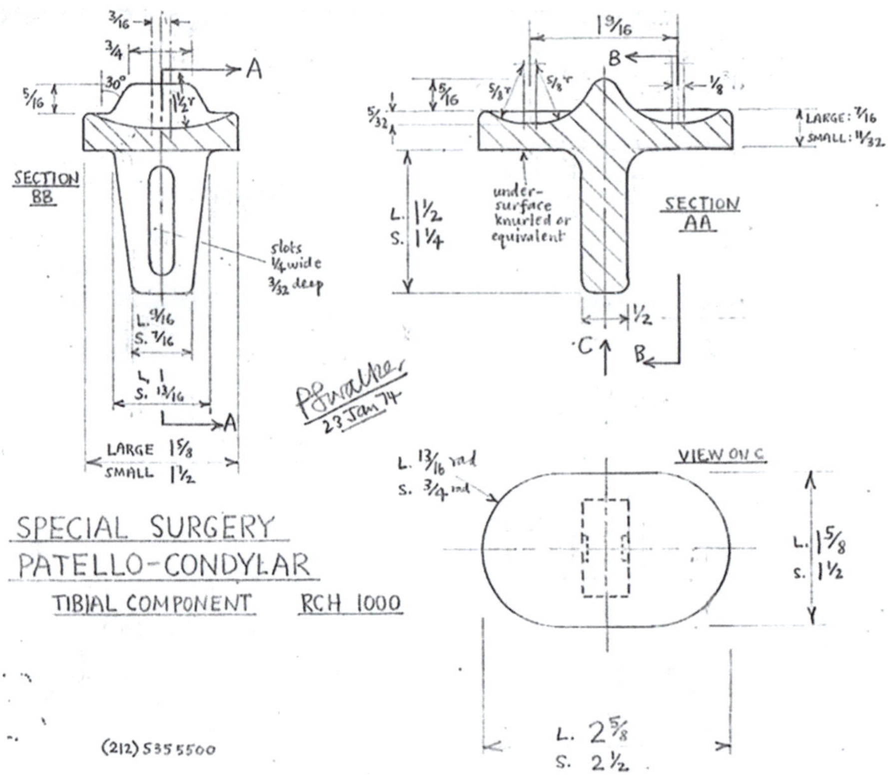

Fig. 8.5 The design drawing of the first Total Condylar central peg tibial component dated January 1974. The radii of the condyles in frontal and sagittal planes were slightly larger than those of the femoral component, calculated to provide the anatomic values of laxity and stability under functional weight-bearing conditions. The component fitted both right and left knees, and there were two sizes. The lower surface of the component was knurled to provide shear transmission of forces on the cement. The sides of the peg had pockets to transmit shear forces. This one-piece central peg was designed to provide more durable fixation than had been experienced with separate lateral and medial components used in earlier condylar designs. The central peg design was an equal group effort between Chit Ranawat, John Insall, and Peter Walker

the canal beneath, and while this has not caused any problem, it does signify some loss of cement pressure and reduced penetration around the lower part of the stem. A surgical technique introduced to prevent that was to use an impactor the same size as the peg to punch the central bone downwards to form a bone plug. A further observation has been that in some cases the cement has interfaced with the posterior tibial cortex, providing a rigid axial support to the distal part of the peg. This would tend to unload the bone at the lateral and medial sides, causing stress protection and bone resorption. However for an all-plastic component, this effect would be small due to the low stiffness of the plastic, but could certainly be a problem with metal-backed components. Despite the deficiencies, fixation of the central peg tibial components has been very reliable in the large majority of cases.

All-Plastic vs Metal-Backing

By the late 1970s, most artificial knee systems, where central pegs were used for fixation, had shifted away from all-plastic components to metal-backed components with tibial inserts. The main reason was the advantages of modularity and the ability to add extension stems to the metal-backing. There was also the general assumption that the metal-backing would transmit the forces more uniformly to the proximal tibial surface, thus avoiding areas of high stress beneath the lateral and medial contact points which could occur with all-plastic components. This seemed both intuitive and self-evident which probably accounts for the lack of need to carry out any verification. Nevertheless, around 1980 there was a sudden interest in using finite element analysis to justify the widespread use of metal-backing (Bartel et al. 1982; Lewis et al. 1982; Murase et al. 1983). A typical finding was: "...in general, metal components provide lower system stresses than polyethylene components, particularly in the methacrylate and the cancellous bone, and that one-piece designs gave lower cement-bone interface stresses compared with those with separated condylar components" (Lewis et al. 1982).

As a result of such data, all-plastic components were used mainly for older and less active patients. But surprisingly, several recent long-term follow-up studies have shown that the survivorship is at least as good as for metal-backed components (Houdek et al. 2017): "...in a large cohort of patients...all-polyethylene components significantly outperform modular and monoblock metal-backed components in terms of survival...across all age groups and a majority of BMI's." This outcome data seems to contradict what would be expected from the theoretical and experimental studies cited above. One possible explanation is that when plastic inserts are snapped into a metal-backing, micromotion occurs at the interface due to the cyclic forces applied, generating backside wear of the plastic (Sisko et al. 2017). The microscopic particles so generated have been implicated in causing osteolysis of trabecular bone at the cement-bone interface, eventually leading to loosening. This explanation does not however apply to monoblock metal-backed components where there is no escape route for wear particles. Another possible explanation is that the stresses with metal-backing, spread over a wide area, are much lower than in the normal anatomic knee in certain areas, causing stress protection with resulting bone resorption. A stiff metal central peg would exacerbate this effect, especially if the tip was in close proximity to the posterior cortex of the tibia.

But whether all-plastic or metal-backed, the one-piece tibial component with a central peg has been successful. In a review of no less than 27,000 cases of artificial knees performed since 1999, the Swedish registry data showed a survivorship of the tibial components, whether metal-backed or all-plastic with central peg fixation, to be 97% at 10 years follow-up (Gudnason et al. 2014). This is not to say that other design configurations did not have similar success. A bi-cruciate preserving Townley design, where the tibial component consisted of a plastic insert in a metal-backed anteriorly bridged construct, was followed

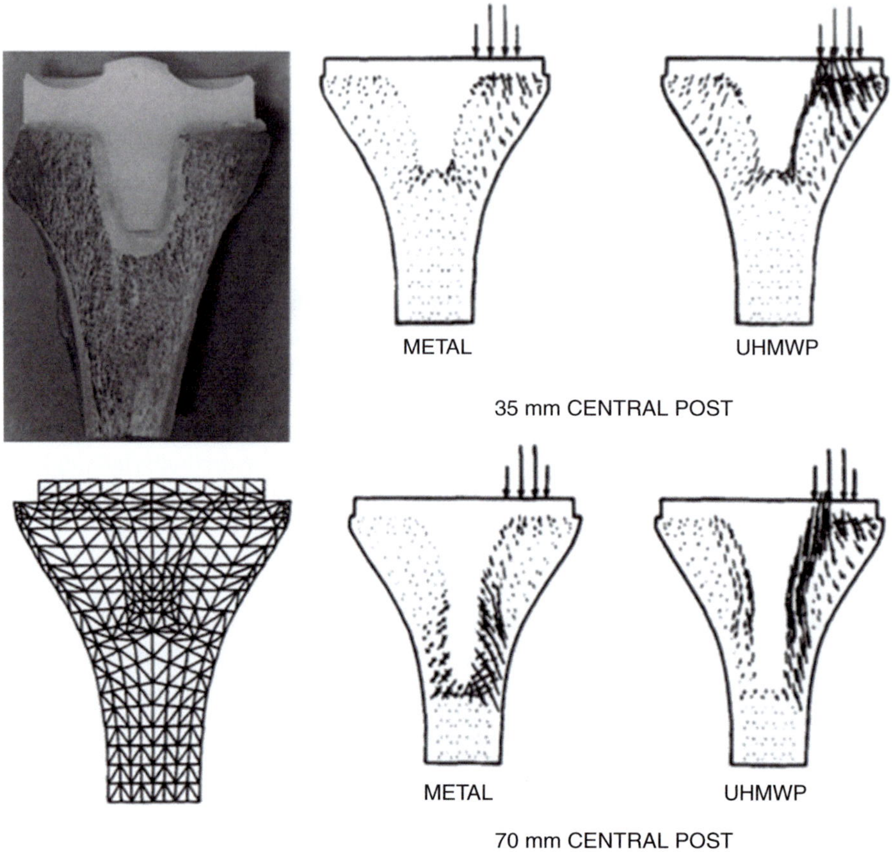

Fig. 8.6 Finite element analysis was used to compare the maximum stresses in the bone adjacent to the tibial components. This study compared the stresses with an all-plastic component and with a short and a long central peg. Eccentric loading was chosen to model varus loading. For the short peg, the flexible plastic produced high stresses under the load, whereas the stresses for the metal-backing were much less. For a longer central peg, however, the metal back produced stress protection at the tibial surface under the load, due to transfer of high loads at the lower end of the peg. Analyses such as these accelerated the shift from all-plastic to metal-backed components starting in the late 1970s (Murase et al. 1983). (Reprinted with permission from Journal of Biomechanics)

for 23 years in 214 knees (Pritchett 2015). The surgeon, Jim Pritchett, was an expert in the use of this device. There were only 18 failures of the tibial component for all causes including excessive wear, loosening, and fracture. These levels of success of the central peg type of tibial component, as well as certain other designs, have been the result of a steady improvement in design, technique, and materials. The application of basic engineering principles, design methodology, and experimental, and theoretical and clinical studies, consistent alignment, attention to adequate cement penetration, and retrieval analysis, have all played a role.

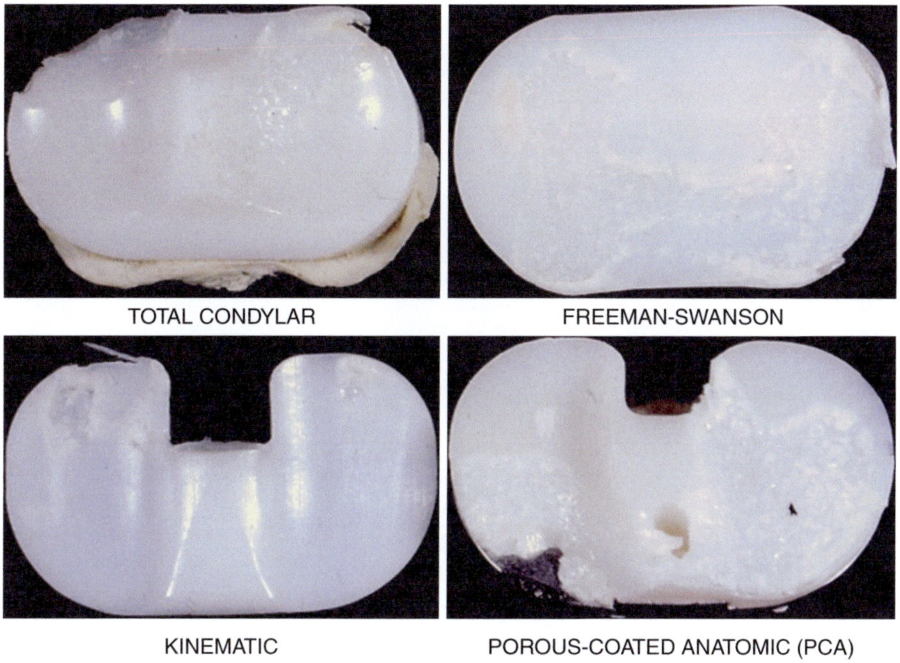

Fig. 8.7 Wear and damage of plastic inserts seen on retrieved tibial components of early artificial knees. Total Condylar, large fatigue crack posteriorly resulted in corner dissociation. Some delamination medial side. Freeman-Swanson, internal-external rotation about the center has produced bow-tie delamination wear. Kinematic condylar, excessive posterior-lateral contact. PCA predominantly anterior delamination wear, possibly due to lack of posterior slope

Bone Strength Under Component

For all tibial component designs, the load is transmitted between the base of the component and the underlying trabecular bone. The strength of this bone varies considerably across the surface and with depth. The strength is highest over patches medially and laterally, reflecting the regions of highest load transmission. As mentioned above, the strength in the central region is the lowest. The load distribution across the surface will be in proportion to the stiffness which will be related to strength. Load follows stiffness. Hvid and Hansen (1985) demonstrated that the strength of the bone falls off rapidly with depth below the surface of the tibia. Hence it is an advantage to minimize the depth of the bone resection. At a certain level, the trabecular bone will be unable to withstand the stresses which are imposed upon it, suggesting the minimum level of resection. Using CT scanning, Hvid also studied whether the bone density changed over time after an artificial knee. He studied cases where the knee had been in varus prior to the procedure, and hence the medial bone was more dense than normal and the lateral bone less dense. It would be expected

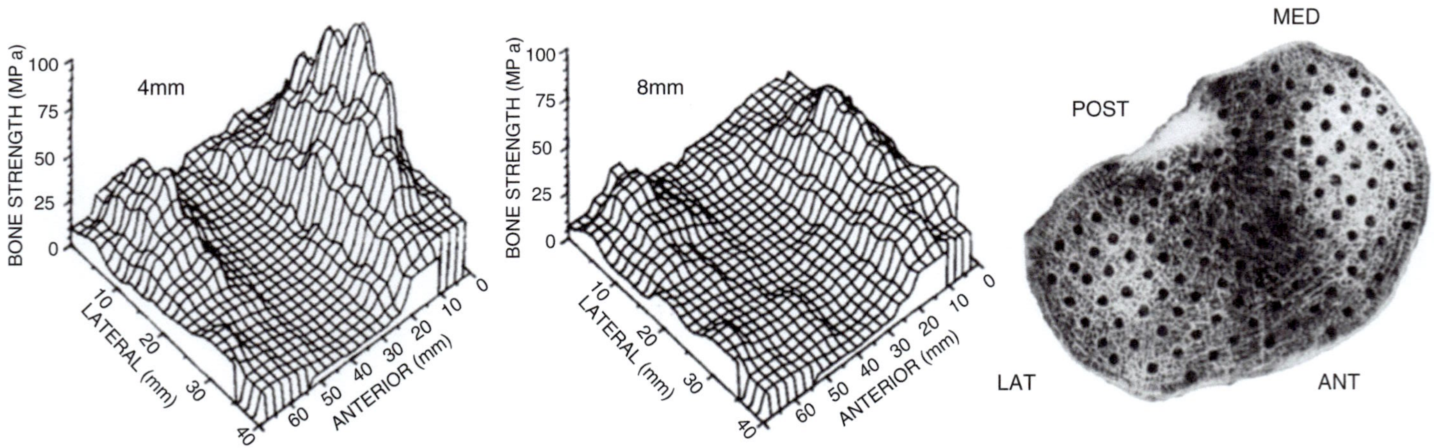

Fig. 8.8 The strength of the trabecular bone across the tibia as a function of depth below the surface. The 4 and 8 mm are depths below the bottom of the subchondral plate which was removed. The locations of highest strength approximate to the bone under the menisci. The strength reduces considerably with depth. The white dense bone on the proximal cut surface corresponds to the highest strength (Hvid and Hansen 1985). (Reprinted with permission from Journal of Orthopaedic Research)

that when the alignment was corrected at surgery, this would restore the normal lateral to medial force distribution, causing the bone density to revert to normal. While this did in fact occur, it took a considerable time, more than expected. The reduction in strength with depth has a particular significance to unicompartmental knees, where the surface area is relatively small. The knee that Charnley designed, the Load Angle Inlay (described in Chap. 9), used a thin metal plate for the tibial component, which had the advantage of being seated on the strongest bone possible.

Peripheral Shape

One of the issues in tibial component design has been the peripheral shape; is a symmetric shape satisfactory, or would an asymmetric shape have advantages? The aim should be to minimize the stresses on the proximal tibia by obtaining as close a contact to as much of the periphery as possible, thus maximizing the percentage coverage. At the same time, there should be no overhang, especially posterolaterally where popliteus irritation can occur or medially which can irritate the medial collateral ligament. One of the first studies to investigate coverage, the fit of asymmetric and symmetric components was measured on the resected bone pieces from surgical cases (Westrich et al. 1994). The peripheral fits were found to be from 81 to 85% with no difference between symmetric and asymmetric components. A more elaborate study was carried out on the fit of contemporary designs based on CT scans at the resection level of 100 surgical cases (Meier et al. 2018). The components were from 7 to 10 size systems and included symmetric and asymmetric designs. The components were fitted based on the rotational axis: the ML axis, the medial third axis, or the rotation of best fit. Their conclusions were: "Tibial coverage is similar for symmetric and asymmetric designs, but depends on the rotational landmark for which the implant is designed. The surgeon has the option to improve tibial coverage by optimizing placement between the two anatomic rotational alignment landmarks, the medial 1/3 and the ML-axis." Most of the percentage coverage values were between 79 and 88%, except for one design aligned along the medial third axis which dipped to 73%. In all cases, the standard deviations indicated that there would be an incidence of undercoverage. The ideal situation is that the surgeon obtains the best fit regardless of rotation. This would be acceptable for a rotating platform knee, whereas for other knee designs, it would depend how much rotational laxity was built in. For practical reasons, there should be enough laxity to accommodate variations in placement and between individuals, although the exact value of laxity needed is unknown.

What Are the Best Configurations for Durability?

The most durable fixation is obtained with components which cover the entire proximal tibia or which have only a small area of relief for retention of the posterior cruciate ligament. A central post has been shown to provide durable fixation even if the lateral and medial plateau areas become debonded. Two side posts, or keels, transmit rotational forces for added fixation. All-plastic components and metal-backed components have been equally durable. All-plastic components are not indicated if the underlying bone is deficient, such as in cases of severe deformity. A plastic insert must fit into the metal-backing tightly to minimize micromotion which causes backside wear, generating small wear particles which may lead to areas of osteolysis. Minimizing the depth of cut will result in the component being seated on stronger bone, but care must be taken to still achieve the required cement penetration. Whether the cement needs to bond rigidly to all the surfaces of the tibial component needs further research.

References

Abernethy PJ, Robinson CM, Fowler RM. Fracture of the metal tibial tray after kinematic total knee replacement. A common cause of early aseptic failure. J Bone Joint Surg Br. 1996;78(2):220–5.

Ahir SP, Blunn GW, Haider H, Walker PS. Evaluation of a testing method for the fatigue performance of total knee tibial trays. J Biomech. 1999;32(10):1049–57.

Attenborough CG. Total knee replacement using the stabilized gliding prosthesis. Ann R Coll Surg Engl. 1976;58(1):4–14.

Bartel DL, Burstein AH, Santavicca EA, Insall JN. Performance of the tibial component in total knee replacement. J Bone Joint Surg Am. 1982;64(7):1026–33.

Behrens JC, Walker PS, Shoji H. Variations in strength and structure of cancellous bone at the knee. J Biomech. 1974;7(3):201–7.

Cloutier JM. Results of total knee arthroplasty with a non-constrained prosthesis. J Bone Joint Surg Am. 1983;65(7):906–19.

Eftekhar NS. Adjustable intramedullary replacement of the knee: evolution of surgical technique and prosthesis. Clin Orthop Relat Res. 1978;(137):235–43.

Freeman MA, Swanson SA, Todd RC. Total replacement of the knee using the Freeman-Swanson knee prosthesis. Clin Orthop Relat Res. 1973;(94):153–70.

Gudnason A, Hailer NP, A WD, Sundberg M, Robertsson O. All-polyethylene versus metal-backed tibial components-an analysis of 27,733 cruciate-retaining total knee replacements from the Swedish knee arthroplasty register. J Bone Joint Surg Am. 2014;96(12):994–9.

Gunston FH. Polycentric knee arthroplasty. Prosthetic simulation of normal knee movement. J Bone Joint Surg (Br). 1971;53(2):272–7.

Houdek MT, Watts CD, Wyles CC, Martin JR, Trousdale RT, Taunton MJ. Metal or modularity: why do metal-backed tibias have inferior outcomes to all-polyethylene tibial components in patients with osteoarthritis. J Arthroplast. 2017;32(3):836–42.

Hvid I, Hansen SL. Trabecular bone strength patterns at the proximal tibial epiphysis. J Orthop Res. 1985;3:464–72.

Lewis JL, Askew MJ, Jaycox DP. A comparative evaluation of tibial component designs of total knee prostheses. J Bone Joint Surg Am. 1982;64(1):129–35.

Meier M, Webb J, Collins JE, Beckman J, Fitz W. Do modern total knee replacements improve tibial coverage? Knee Surg Sports Traumatol Arthrosc. 2018;26:3219–29.

Murase K, Crowninshield RD, Pedersen DR, Chang TS. An analysis of tibial component design in total knee arthroplasty. J Biomech. 1983;16(1):13–22.

Paganelli JV, Skinner HB, Mote CD. Prediction of fatigue failure of a total knee replacement tibial plateau using finite element analysis. Orthopedics. 1988;11(8):1161–8.

Pritchett JW. Bicruciate-retaining Total knee replacement provides satisfactory function and implant survivorship at 23 years. Clin Orthop Relat Res. 2015;473(7):2327–33.

Ranawat CS, Shine JJ. Duo-condylar total knee arthroplasty. Clin Orthop Relat Res. 1973;94:185–95.
Sisko ZW, Teeter MG, Lanting BA, et al. Current total knee designs: does baseplate roughness or locking mechanism design affect polyethylene backside wear? Clin Orthop Relat Res. 2017;475(12):2970–80.
Skolnick MD, Coventry MB, Ilstrup DM. Geometric total knee arthroplasty. A two-year follow-up study. J Bone Joint Surg Am. 1976;58(6):749–53.
Sledge CB, Ewald FC. Total knee arthroplasty experience at the Robert Breck Brigham hospital. Clin Orthop Relat Res. 1979;(145):78–84.
Swanson SA, Freeman MA, Heath JC. Laboratory tests on total joint replacement prostheses. J Bone Joint Surg (Br). 1973;55(4):759–73.
Townley CO. The anatomic total knee resurfacing arthroplasty. Clin Orthop Relat Res. 1985;(192):82–96.
Walker PS, Hajek JV. The load-bearing area in the knee joint. J Biomech. 1972;5(6):581–9.
Walker PS, Hsieh HH. Conformity in condylar replacement knee prosthesis. J Bone Joint Surg. 1977;59(2):222–8.
Walker PS, Ranawat C, Insall J. Fixation of the tibial components of condylar replacement knee prostheses. J Biomech. 1976;9(4):269–75.
Westrich GH, Laskin RS, Haas SB, Sculco TP. Resection specimen analysis of tibial coverage in total knee arthroplasty. Clin Orthop Relat Res. 1994;309:163–75.

9 Condylar Replacements

What Were the Steps Leading to the Basic Condylar Replacement Knees?

When the cemented metal-polyethylene artificial hip joint began to show promising results in the mid-1960s, it was only a matter of time before the same materials would be used for the design of an artificial knee. From the start, it was realized that there were significant design problems involved. In the hip, there had been many years of experience with components which replaced the femoral head and the acetabulum. For the artificial hip, it was a matter of combining the components in such a way that the capsular structures still provided sufficient stability. Charnley achieved this by removing the greater trochanter at the start of the procedure and refixing it in a tightened position after the components were cemented in place. The ball-in-socket joint itself provided considerable stability with a single rotation point. For the knee, a similar problem needed to be solved, how to tension the ligaments such that stability would be restored. However the bearing surfaces were nonconforming, allowing both sliding and rotation to occur with little inherent stability. In addition the arthritis had usually caused an alignment deformity at the knee, with damage to the condyles and the ligaments. These were not easy problems to solve, but by the end of the 1960s, solutions had been reached. The first two designs, the Gunston and the Freeman-Swanson, could not have been more different.

Gunston Polycentric Knee

Frank Gunston FRCS started his career as an engineer before switching to medicine and then took a fellowship with Sir John Charnley at the Hip Center at Wrightington Hospital in England to work on artificial hip joints. Noting that many of the hip patients had severe knee problems which prevented them from returning to normal function, Gunston was motivated to design an artificial knee, the idea receiving Charnley's support. The rationale for the knee design was: "The biomedical principles and experience gained from total hip arthroplasty were combined with an analysis of normal knee movement. The design objective was to provide an articular

P. S. Walker, *The Artificial Knee*, https://doi.org/10.1007/978-3-030-38171-4_9

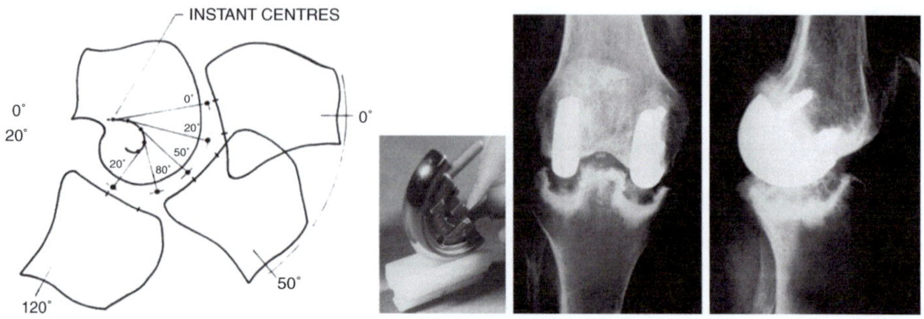

Fig. 9.1 The Gunston Polycentric knee was based on restoring the bearing surfaces only, retaining both cruciate ligaments, and providing sufficient laxity between the femoral and tibial components to allow for the changing instant centers of rotation during flexion. The femoral component was cemented into narrow slots cut in the femoral condyles. The tibial components were set at the correct heights and cemented into slots in the tibial condyles (Gunston 1971). (Reprinted with permission from Journal of Bone & Joint Surgery B)

replacement procedure that would simulate the normal anatomic and functional modalities of the knee joint as closely as possible" (Gunston 1971). Gunston stated that from extension to 10 degrees flexion, the tibia internally rotated, analogous to the "screw-home" movement shown in early anatomic studies, and from 10 to 20 degrees flexion the femur rolled posteriorly on the tibia, after which the same contact points were maintained until full flexion. This constituted a polycentric pathway for the instant centers of rotation, which gave the name to his design, the Polycentric knee. Hence Gunston emphasized that the motion of the knee was not limited to the sagittal plane and that there were different motions on the lateral and medial sides. The idea that the artificial knee should be designed to allow for variable centers of rotation and contact point locations was fundamental.

The femoral component as seen in the sagittal view was an arc of constant radius, in contrast to the anatomic shape where the distal femur was of larger radius than the posterior, particularly on the medial side. This compromise was made because the component was made easily in Charnley's Biomechanical Laboratory. The narrow femoral disc in the wider plastic tibial runner allowed for 20 degrees of internal-external rotation as well as freedom of anterior-posterior displacement. The heights of the tibial components above their respective joint surfaces were adjusted at surgery to provide the correct ligament tensions and allow for a full range of flexion. Gunston did not elaborate on how the overall leg alignment was evaluated. In essence, the Polycentric knee aimed to restore the original profiles of the bearing surfaces, with appropriate ligament tensions, in an effort to restore the normal kinematics.

While only small numbers of the Polycentric knee were carried out at Wrightington from 1968 to 1969, after Gunston's return to Winnipeg in 1970, surgeons at the Mayo Clinic started using the knee after making modifications to widen the bearing surfaces. Up to 1973, Mark Coventry and Richard Bryan carried out 713 cases but found that the technique could be exacting and difficult, mainly due to the lack of instrumentation (Coventry & Bryan 1974). This explained the problems they encountered of postoperative instability and misalignment of the limb. Ed Chao PhD, Director of the Biomechanics Laboratory at the Mayo Clinic, while not involved with the design itself, studied the wear and deformation of the polyethylene as well carrying out gait analysis on patients. Chao's interest was in developing basic science methods for the clinical evaluation of artificial knees. His elaborate methods of analysis of the gait patterns were a model for future studies in other laboratories. Longer-term results were published of the earliest Polycentric cases, showing that only 66% could be considered successful at 10 years follow-up, the main problem being instability and tibial loosening, with some cases of excessive wear and femoral condylar fractures (Lewallen et al. 1984). The tibial loosening was evidently due to excessive stresses on the underlying trabecular bone, something that Freeman and Swanson had drawn attention to.

Freeman-Swanson Knee

While Gunston was located at Wrightington Hospital in a small village in the north-west of England, Michael Freeman FRCS and Professor Alan Swanson PhD were at the London Hospital and Imperial College, affiliated with the University of London. They had set up a Biomechanics Unit in the Department of Mechanical Engineering in 1965, with the major purpose of developing an artificial knee. Their first implant design was relatively simple, consisting of a circular-sectioned metal femoral component and plastic tibial blocks shaped after the MacIntosh plateau, on the lateral and medial sides. After a small number of cases, it was found that obtaining correct leg alignment and adjusting the heights of the separate tibial plateaus were too difficult and time-consuming, especially for knees with severe varus or valgus deformities. They soon produced the new Freeman-Swanson design based on the following design criteria (Freeman et al. 1974):

- Stability from the bearing surfaces and the collateral ligaments, with excision of the cruciate ligaments.
- Any degree of deformity can be corrected.
- Soft tissue releases to be carried out of the collateral ligaments to correct for varus or valgus deformities.
- Large areas of contact between the components and the cut surfaces of the bone to minimize bone stresses.
- Large contact areas on the bearing surfaces to minimize wear.
- Full width of the bearing contact seen in the frontal plane to maximize varus-valgus stability.
- Square bone cuts to facilitate alignment to the long axes of the femur and tibia.

The main concern was to design an artificial knee that was mechanically sound, with a simple reproducible technique that could be used by any surgeon to treat cases of severe arthritis. Freeman and Swanson claimed that their design had major

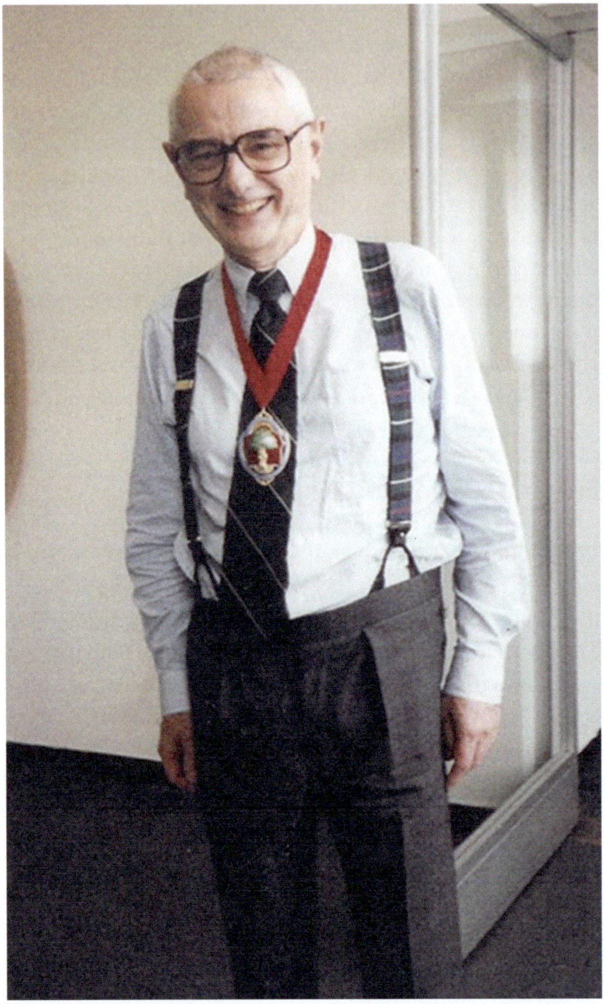

Fig. 9.2 Michael A R Freeman FRCS, at the first European Federation of Orthopaedics & Traumatology EFORT meeting held in Paris in 1993. He was one of the founding members of the organization. Freeman and Alan Swanson PhD developed one of the first metal-plastic artificial knees, in London, UK, in the late 1960s. Freeman was an active figure at conferences around the world for many decades. (© Peter S Walker)

advantages over both the fixed-axis metal hinges that were still being widely used and condylar designs where separate tibial components were used medially and laterally. For such designs, the surface area of fixation of the components to the bone was too small, which could cause compressive failure of the supporting bone. In addition, flat or shallow bearing surfaces would produce excessive contact stresses and wear.

From the first cases in 1970, the Freeman-Swanson knee was used by an increasing number of surgeons such that over 1000 cases had been carried out by the time of the Institution of Mechanical Engineers Conference on Total Knee Conference in 1974. The majority of the patients were said to be "free of complaint," but few other details were available. In a retrospective review (Bargren et al. 1983), it was reported that the major determining factor for success or failure was the overall leg alignment. For cases that were in valgus, relative to an in-line femur and tibia, 89% were

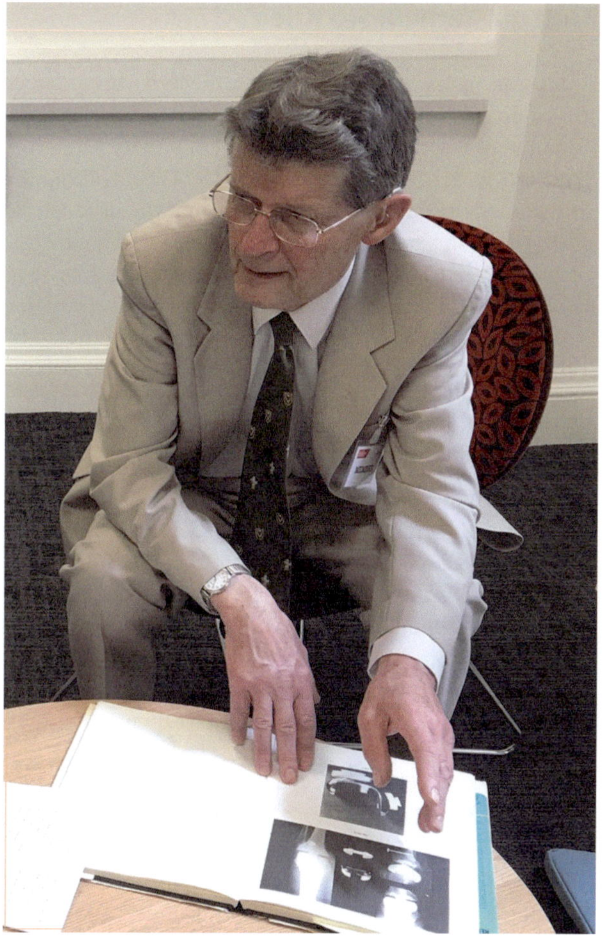

Fig. 9.3 Professor Alan Swanson PhD and Michael Freeman FRCS designed the Freeman-Swanson knee in the late 1960s and went on to design several improved versions. Alan Swanson was a Professor at Imperial College London. He now devotes much of his time to locating and refurbishing woodworking tools for an organization which sends these to disadvantaged regions of the world. (Photo of Alan Swanson taken during an interview in 2017 at the Institution of Mechanical Engineers in Birdcage Walk, London, England) (© Peter S Walker)

successful. For varus cases, only 14% were successful. This can be attributed to the early surgical technique where the distal femoral and proximal tibial cuts were made perpendicular to the long axes of the bones themselves. In the case of the femur, the cut should have been at 85 degrees, providing the normal 5 degrees of valgus. This could explain the tendency to varus alignment which would have caused excessive loading on the medial side.

By 1974, Freeman and Swanson had designed two other versions of the knee, one with a patella flange, the other with slots for retention of the cruciate ligaments. Yet other design variations were introduced in succeeding years, based on limitations of preceding designs, as well as incorporating entirely new ideas. This process, while progressing the design itself, had the negative effect of making it difficult to conduct orderly clinical follow-up studies. In addition, other surgeons became uncertain about which design they should be using, which resulted in some loss of credibility even though a number of the design features were both innovative and beneficial.

Kodama-Yamamoto Knee

While this work on artificial knee design was proceeding in England, in the late 1960s, development was taking place in Okayama in Japan (Yamamoto 1979). Drs. Kodama and Yamamoto, from the University Department of Orthopaedics, used a Sbarbaro femoral shell (Sbarbaro 1974) in combination with a horseshoe-shaped polyethylene tibial component such that the cruciate ligaments could be preserved. The interior surface of the femoral shell fitted against surgically shaped distal femoral condyles, fixation being with thin metal fins. The shell included the patella flange. The tibial component was fixed anteriorly with two staples, preventing anterior lift-off. Although they were aware of the availability of acrylic cement, they considered that it was harmful to the bone and soft tissue. After some experience with a congruent tibial design, they stated that "there should be some incongruity between the femoral and tibial components, with sufficient rotatory movement allowed in flexion, slightly restricted in extension." Also, posterior femoral rollback was necessary to achieve high flexion, essential for Japanese patients. In their follow-up studies starting in 1970, they indicated that there was no problem with the uncemented press-fit fixation. They did note however that complete coverage of the tibial surface was necessary to avoid some sinkage, addressed by providing several sizes. By the time of the 1979 review, the authors reported few problems, including no loosening or radiolucent lines, implying the uncemented fixation was satisfactory. Even so they made several design changes, partly influenced by Freeman in London with whom Sumiki Yamamoto spent a Fellowship.

Townley Anatomic Total Knee

Charles O Townley MD, from Port Huron in Michigan, had been experimenting with anatomically shaped components since 1953, when he started using his metal tibial resurfacing component. Even before then he had devised a metal femoral component, but metal-on-metal was not considered to be a viable bearing. Why a metal-plastic version of Townley's design was not made until 1972 is surprising, considering that total hips were made with those materials from the early 1960s, and by the late 1960s, the Freeman-Swanson and Gunston knees were in widespread use, although mainly in England. The main reason was the difficulty of finding a manufacturer who was interested. Nevertheless Townley was quite clear about the basis of his design: "provide an articular replacement procedure that would simulate the normal anatomic and functional modalities of the knee joint as closely as possible" (Townley 1988). His design criteria were:

- Nonconstrained articulation in all planes of motion.
- Reconstitution of the normal synchronized articular motion patterns.
- Minimization of abnormal shear and tension stresses by accurate alignment.
- Thinnest possible implants.
- Total resurfacing including patella.

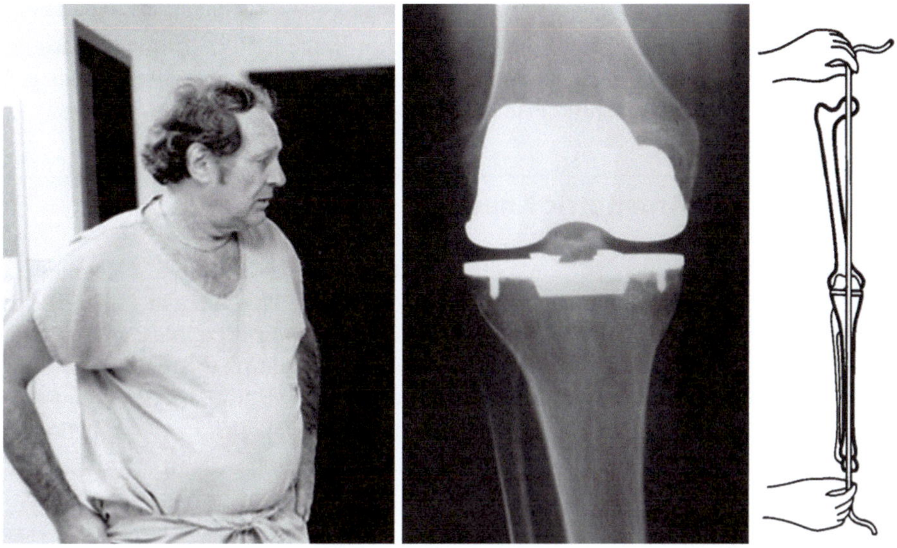

Fig. 9.4 In an article called “Charles O Townley: Design by Reason,” James Pritchett MD described the principles behind Charles Townley’s artificial hip and knee designs. The Anatomic total knee originally had an all-plastic tibial component; later a metal-back was added. An eminence of the bone was preserved in the center of the tibia so that both cruciates could be retained (radiograph). The joint line was tilted medially by 2–3 degrees, as in the normal knee. To check the limb alignment, Townley used a cord stretched between a marker over the center of the femoral head, radiographically placed, and the center of the ankle (Pritchett 1988, 2015). (Photos courtesy James Pritchett MD, Interview with James Pritchett 2017)

It was obvious that Townley regarded his new Anatomic total knee as a major advancement over the metal tibial plate he had been using up till then, based on the numbers used in patients. In the 17 years from 1953 to 1972, he used only 170 plates, about one every 6 weeks. Between 1972 and 1988, he had used 1700 total knees, an average of two each week. His proposition that good results could only be obtained by meticulous attention to accurate surgery was expressed in his statement: “Significant abnormalities in either the size, contour, or placement of the femoral component will distort or misplace the condylar articular outlines and place it out of tune with the holding pattern of motion sustained by the ligaments.” His technique emphasized accurate alignment of the components to achieve the two degrees medial slope of the joint line with the patient standing, as well as the mechanical axis (the line joining the center of the hip to the center of the ankle) passing 10 mm medial to the center of the knee itself. This was tested with a length of rope, possibly the simplest instrument ever invented! In a long-term follow-up of the Townley Anatomic Total Knee, James Pritchett achieved 89% survivorship at 23 years follow-up, with a mean flexion angle of 117 degrees (Pritchett 2015). It is not easy to find any results which surpass these with any design of artificial knee. Undoubtedly the surgical expertise of Pritchett was a factor in these results. The article entitled “Design by Reason” (Pritchett 1988) was a strong tribute to Townley, written by a surgeon who had trained under Townley and was a close colleague for his entire surgical career. Pritchett himself was an innovator in the field of artificial knees, in carrying out extensive clinical studies of bilateral cases to determine which designs gave the best functional results (Pritchett 2004, 2011).

Geometric and Anametric Knees

The Geometric knee was in marked contrast to Townley's design. Designed in 1969–1970 by Bob Averill and Alex Khowayla, design engineers at Howmedica, Rutherford, New Jersey, it focused mainly on engineering principles, minimizing the contact stresses on the polyethylene and providing complete anterior-posterior and rotary stability. In these design criteria, there is a close similarity with those of Freeman and Swanson. When the Geometric design was close to completion, a

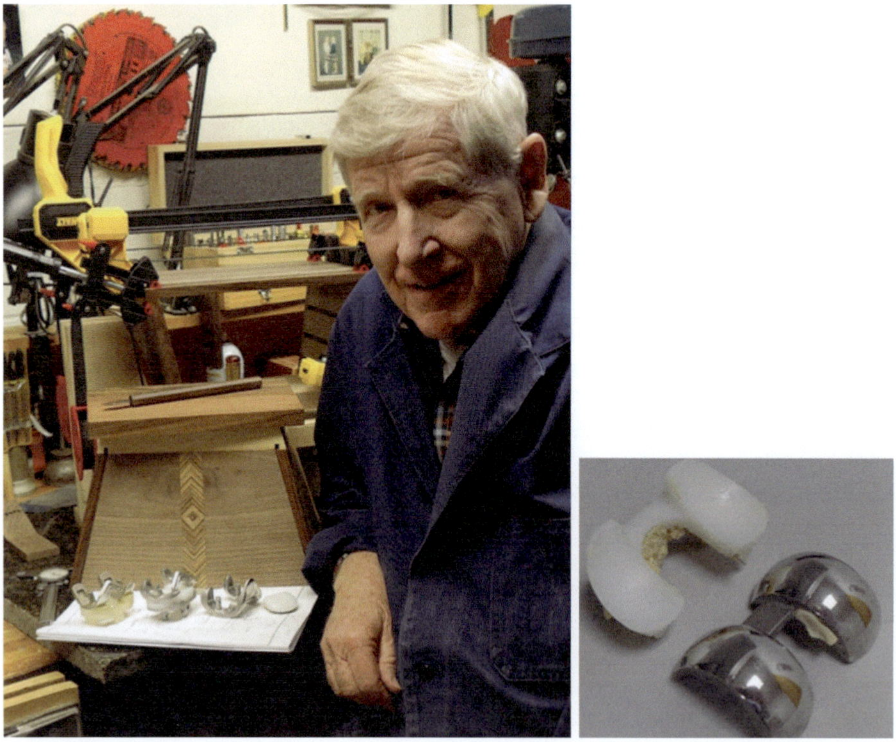

Fig. 9.5 Robert Averill at his home in New Jersey. He and Alex Khowayla, design engineers, developed the Geometric knee while working at Howmedica, starting in 1969. After an exhibit at the AAOS in 1972, the knee became widely used. At bottom right, the spherical femoral runners and matching plastic tibial condylar surfaces can be seen. Later Averill and Khowayla founded their own company called Osteonics, which became a significant force in orthopedics. (Photo courtesy Robert Averill)

group of prominent surgeons was invited to form a user's group, with the main goals of developing the instrumentation and technique and carrying out initial surgeries. This was a remarkable way to implement an initial introduction, in that it would have been easier to identify a single "product champion" from a well-known institution. Averill chose to form a group for several reasons. They could form a consensus on the design and recommend modifications. They would be able to develop the instrumentation and technique, again with a consensus. Finally, there would be a larger volume of knees used, and a greater exposure at conferences. There was little competition from other knees at the time; the first implantations were made in 1971. Consequently the Geometric became widely used in the USA soon after its introduction at the AAOS in 1972.

But even as early as the 1974 Total Knee Conference in London, there were some problems reported in an article entitled "Technical pitfalls in the Polycentric and Geometric total knee arthroplasties" authored by Mark Coventry and Richard Bryan from the Mayo Clinic (1974). The main pitfalls concerned the technique, mainly misalignments, lack of soft tissue balancing, and improper cementation (Coventry et al. 1973). These problems are understandable because at that time, there was little appreciation of the consequences of these factors, and hence the instrumentation was not designed appropriately. In addition, due to the limited knowledge of knee forces and kinematics, there was no accommodation in the design for anterior-posterior and rotary laxity, which evidently led to kinematic conflict with the cruciate ligaments, producing high tensile and compressive stresses at the cement-bone interface. Even though the Geometric was subsequently modified in several ways by more than one company, it was not regarded as easy to insert or reliable in function. The group of surgeons recognized that fundamental changes were needed to the Geometric, and as a result, the anametric knee was designed (Finerman et al. 1979). The femoral-tibial conformity was reduced to increase flexion and to reduce the shear forces on the tibial fixation. A central tibial peg and a patella flange were added. These changes resulted in improved clinical results compared with the Geometric.

Anatomic Designs of Seedhom and Ewald

Soon after the above developments, efforts were under way in both England and the USA to design a truly anatomic artificial knee. Bahaa Seedhom, a mechanical engineer who had just completed a PhD at Leeds University in England, was offered a position at the newly formed "Bioengineering Group for the Study of Human Joints" which had been formed by Professors Duncan Dowson and Verna Wright. He was asked to suggest a research topic and chose to design an artificial knee. He spent much of his time in the Anatomy Laboratory at the Leeds General Infirmary dissecting knees, determining how they functioned and how best to design an artificial knee replacement. He concluded that the implant should be a thin shell which required only a removal of a surface layer and hence the bearing surfaces of the implant had to be close to the anatomic shape. Seedhom realized that the relative geometry of the femoral and tibial condyles was the determining factor for both kinematics and stresses (Seedhom et al. 1972). A patella flange was necessary to provide a smooth unbroken track for the patella, which was known to carry high forces especially in higher flexion.

The shape of the tibial surface was generated by flexing and extending the femoral component to allow a range of flexion from 0 to 120 degrees, together with sufficient laxity. Seedhom designed the knee based on anatomic considerations and developed effective shape molding techniques by working with a dental technician in the Leeds General Infirmary. Molds were used to produce femoral castings in cobalt-chrome alloy in several sizes, right and left. After polishing of the bearing surfaces, the appearance was exactly like an anatomic femoral condyle. Similar meticulous methods were used for designing the tibial components, including a technique for molding the polyethylene to improve its wear resistance (Seedhom et al. 1973). After producing prototypes of the final design, he worked with Eddie Longton, an orthopedic surgeon at Leeds General Infirmary, on the technique of implanting the components into the knee. With little precedent for collaboration between engineers and surgeons, Seedhom felt that there was a considerable barrier to communication, because the surgeon was unfamiliar with even the basic concepts of mechanics and materials, while Seedhom had little notion of surgical realities. The Leeds Knee was finally manufactured and first implanted in 1972. However after about a year, only ten cases had been performed, and the results were not promising: "The extreme variability and sometimes disastrous results obtained have necessarily inhibited extensive employment of this prosthesis" (Seedhom et al. 1974). This was unfortunate because the design was more sophisticated than others at that time, and possibly if it had received sufficient priority, it could have succeeded. As a result of this situation, the manufacturer changed several times causing delays and eventually the project became sidelined.

In the same time frame as Seedhom's work, Fred Ewald MD, a surgeon at the Robert Breck Brigham Hospital in Boston, developed an artificial knee almost identical to that of Seedhom, although there was no evidence of any connection between the two projects. Ewald's femoral component, a shell with an anatomic surface and an intramedullary stem for fixation, was modeled after the Massachusetts General Hospital (MGH) femoral condyle designed in Boston in the late 1950s. However Ewald's idea for forming the tibial surface was unique and original. He flexed and extended the femoral component in a mechanical jig through a container of soft wax. When the wax hardened, the surface was the most conforming surface possible which would accommodate the relative motion between the femur and tibia, allowing ".... constantly changing instantaneous centers of rotation during flexion" (Ewald 1974). Implants were produced by Zimmer after which Ewald performed 23 cases (Ewald 1975). However Ewald decided to discontinue the use of the design even though the early results were promising. One difference between the Seedhom and Ewald designs was that the former retained the cruciates and the latter did not.

Even though the appearance of these designs was closely anatomic, which seems the logical shape to make an artificial knee, it may be more than a coincidence that neither of these designs became widely used nor were implanted in patients for more than a few years. At that time, manufacture of the anatomical shapes was difficult and expensive because the femoral components had to be hand ground and polished. The tibial components required a molding process which was much slower than machining. Forming the distal end of the patient's femur at surgery to be a sufficiently accurate fit, even allowing for cement filling of any gaps, was very challenging for the surgeon requiring repeated trial and error. Even though reaming had been used to produce accurate spherical surfaces in the hip, that could not be translated to the knee, so handcrafting with osteotomes was necessary. Also, ligament balancing was difficult due to the relatively high femoral-tibial conformity. Finally, even though the surfaces were anatomic in shape, for a particular knee, there could still be a mismatch of both size and shape, especially because in Seedhom and Ewald's designs, only a few sizes were made of the components.

Hospital for Special Surgery (HSS): Duo-condylar, Duo-patella (CR), and Total Condylar

The groundwork for artificial knee design started at the Hospital for Special Surgery (HSS) in New York during the late 1960s. Lee Ramsay Straub MD, an Attending Surgeon at HSS, had alerted Chit Ranawat MD to the possibilities of joint replacement, not only for the hip which was already being used but for the knee. They started by using MacIntosh spacers and used that as a starting point to fabricate a custom-made metal-plastic unicompartmental knee. This set the stage for artificial joint developments. During the 1960s, Harlan Amstutz MD had established a Biomechanics Laboratory to carry out research on materials for artificial hip joints. Development of artificial joints in general was seen by the Surgeon-in-Chief, Robert Lee Patterson, to be an area of considerable potential, so it was decided to expand the staff of the laboratory. There were already several Universities in England where such work was in progress. Harlan Amstutz visited Leeds University where Peter Walker was just completing a PhD on the lubrication of joints. Walker was offered a position at HSS which he started in late 1969. But in 1970, Harlan Amstutz was appointed Chairman of Orthopaedics at UCLA, and the other biomechanics staff moved there. On the other hand, Walker felt that California was too far from London, and he asked the Director of Research at HSS, Robert Mellors, if he could continue to work in the Biomechanics Laboratory. Accordingly he was given the opportunity to start a new activity focused on the knee and was assigned support staff. Coincidentally an orthopedic Resident, Joe Hajek, proposed a project to determine the contact areas in the knee. Hajek and Walker thought that this work could have an important application: "The significance of the study can relate to….the design of total knee prostheses which seek to imitate the load-bearing surfaces in the natural joint" (Walker & Hajek 1972). Hence the underlying concept was to carry out basic research first and then use the results for a practical purpose. The study that was devised was to position a knee specimen into an Instron loading machine, pack soft acrylic cement inside the joint, apply load, and, when the cement had hardened, remove the acrylic casting. The castings had lateral and medial apertures showing

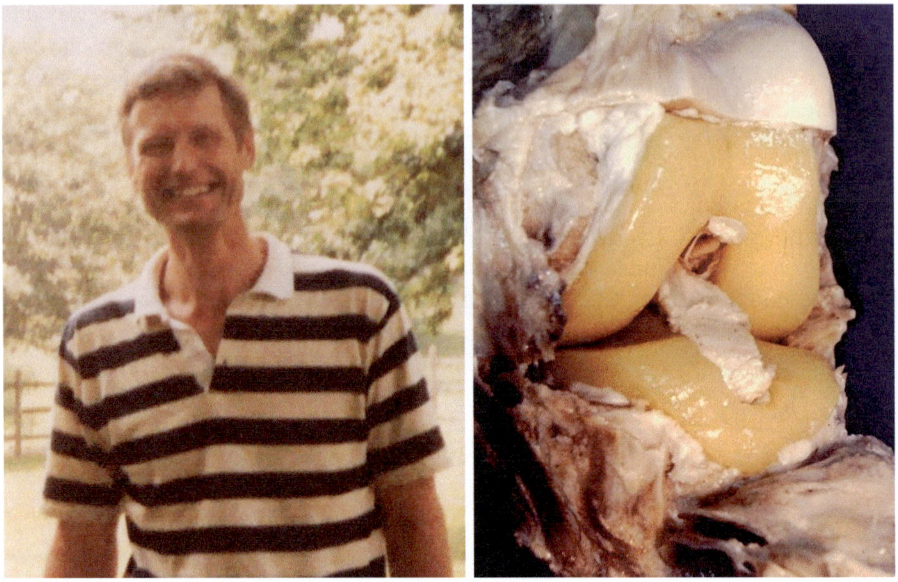

Fig. 9.6 Joe Hajek MD, at his home in Sharon CT where he was a practicing orthopedic surgeon after his residency at the Hospital for Special Surgery in New York. He carried out studies with Peter Walker on the contact areas in the knee, from which the Duo-condylar artificial knee was designed in 1971. (Photo taken c 2010) (© Peter S Walker)

the contact areas and were obtained at a range of flexion angles. The castings were then placed over the tibia and the femur and the outlines of the contact areas drawn on the condyles (Walker & Hajek 1972). It was then possible to produce shapes which would be suitable for condylar resurfacing components. Anterior bridges were included so that the femoral and tibial components were one-piece. These shapes were used in the design of the Duo-condylar artificial knee manufactured using cast cobalt-chrome alloy and high-density polyethylene, which started to be used in 1971.

Ongoing basic research on knee mechanics had confirmed that there needed to be freedom of motion in anterior-posterior and rotation between the components, with the stability being provided by the retained cruciate ligaments (Walker et al. 1972; Walker 1973; Wang & Walker 1973; Wang & Walker 1974). Input in theoretical kinematics was provided by a collaboration with Professor Barry Wolf from Brooklyn Polytechnic Institute (now NYU Tandon School of Engineering), including the calculation of ligament length patterns from measurement of external reference points. By now, several surgeons including Chit Ranawat, John Insall, and Alan Inglis were using the Duo-condylar and were interested in further developments. Two surgeons from Europe, Yann Masse from Paris, France, and Adrian Bain from Durham, England, also carried out surgeries and gave valuable input on technique and follow-up. From this early experience, it was determined that cases with severe deformities were contraindicated with the Duo-condylar due to the difficulty

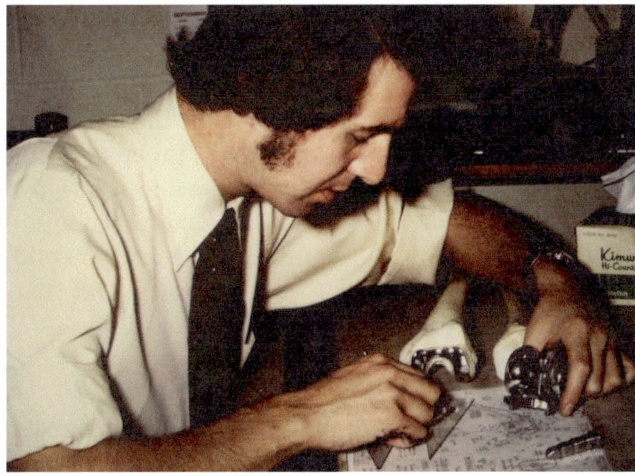

Fig. 9.7 Peter Walker PhD in the Biomechanics Laboratory at Hospital for Special Surgery, working on early knee designs including the Duo-condylar and an all-metal-linked hinge. (Photo taken 1972)

of balancing ligaments. Improvements were needed in several areas. Patellofemoral resurfacing was required. The fixation of the tibial component needed enhancement.

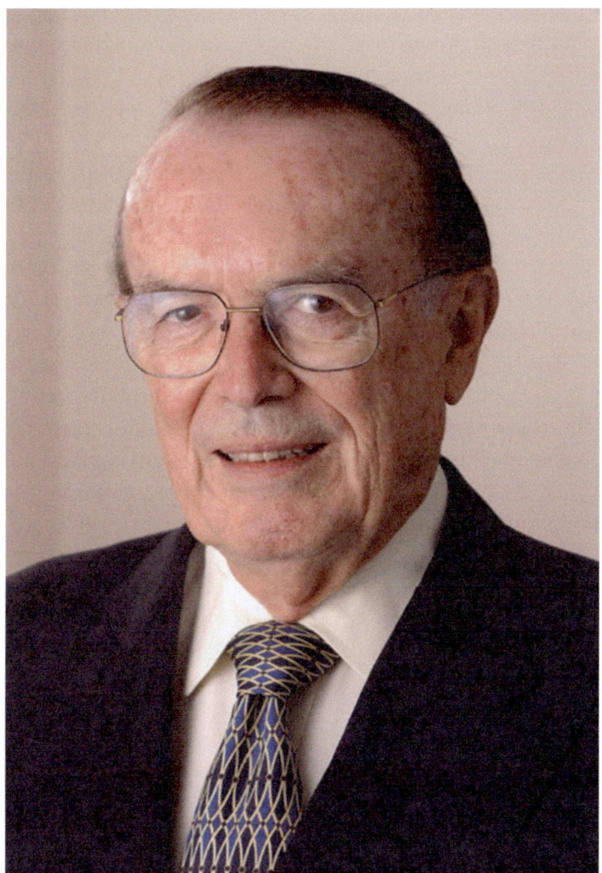

Fig. 9.8 Alan Inglis MD was Director of the Comprehensive Arthritis Service (CAP) of the Hospital for Special Surgery in the 1970s. He took part in the early studies of the kinematics of the knee before and after artificial knees. He participated in the developments of the Duo-condylar and Duo-patella artificial knees and with the surgical techniques. (Photo courtesy Alan Inglis Jr.)

Instrumentation was required to accurately fit the femoral component and achieve correct alignments (Ranawat et al. 1976).

During this time at HSS, it was evident that artificial knees were a potential breakthrough in treating the arthritic knee, and Philip D. Wilson, Jr. was assigned to coordinate this activity. He organized a group consisting of Ranawat, Insall, Inglis, and Walker. The group held regular meetings, as well as numerous ad hoc meetings in the Biomechanics Laboratory. Several research projects were initiated and carried out with the aid of orthopedic Residents and Fellows, including Hiromu Shoji, Jack Shine, Paolo Aglietti, Ching-jen Wang, and Hua Hsieh. Design criteria for a new design of artificial knee were formulated.

- Applicable to all levels of arthritis.
- Stability in anterior-posterior and internal-external rotation provided entirely by the condylar surfaces.
- Varus and valgus stability from the collateral ligaments but with stable pivot points in the condylar surfaces in case of lift-off.
- Normal laxity to provide similar freedom of motion as the anatomic knee.
- Sufficiently large areas of contact to avoid excessive wear.
- A patella flange on the femoral component and a patella resurfacing component.
- A one-piece tibial component which fixed rigidly to the tibia.
- Components requiring "square cuts" on the bone for ease and accuracy of surgery.
- Instrumentation which would achieve accurate component placement and alignment, as well as equal tensions in the ligaments in both extension and flexion.

Some of these criteria were influenced by Michael Freeman, with whom John Insall kept closely in touch with, having gone through Medical School together in Cambridge and London in England.

The design of the bearing surfaces of the new knee design, to be called the Total Condylar, resulted directly from basic research studies of the stability of the knee. The studies were planned by Peter Walker and carried out by Ching-jen Wang, Yann Masse, and Hua Hsieh in the Biomechanics Laboratory (Wang & Walker 1974; Hsieh & Walker 1976). The most important finding was that while the unloaded knee joint had considerable laxity in anterior-posterior and rotation, the laxity was substantially reduced under axial load. This was shown to be due to an "uphill mechanism," whereby as the femur was displaced from the neutral position, there was an upward displacement. Hence stability was achieved by gravity forces. Theoretical analysis was used to define the radii of double-dished partially conforming bearing surfaces which provided similar stability and laxity as the anatomic knee (Walker et al. 1974). The basic principle was that if a combined vertical and shear force was applied to the knee during an activity, the femur would displace horizontally on the tibial surface, reaching an equilibrium position. The displacement represented the laxity which occurred. These bearing surfaces provided anatomic stability without the cruciate ligaments although the collateral ligaments, if taut, would increase their tension due to the vertical displacement of the femoral components and further reduce the laxity.

The balance between the laxity and the stability was an essential requirement of the bearing surfaces: less laxity and more stability than provided by shallow tibial surfaces, but not as constrained as with fully congruent femoral and tibial surfaces. The sagittal profile of the femoral bearing surfaces was similar to anatomic values. Calculations were made for the radii of the tibial bearing surfaces which would result in anatomic laxity and stability. In the frontal plane, the tibial surfaces were dished to provide medial-lateral stability and to provide a pivot point should lift-off occur. The final surfaces were termed "double-dished bearing surfaces with partial femoral-tibial conformity". With these surfaces, the contact areas on the tibial bearing surfaces were also much larger than in the Duo-condylar and other knee designs which had relatively flat tibial surfaces, which would result in reduced polyethylene wear.

The tibial fixation requirement was solved by focusing on how best to resist the combination of forces and moments, without requiring excess invasion of tibial

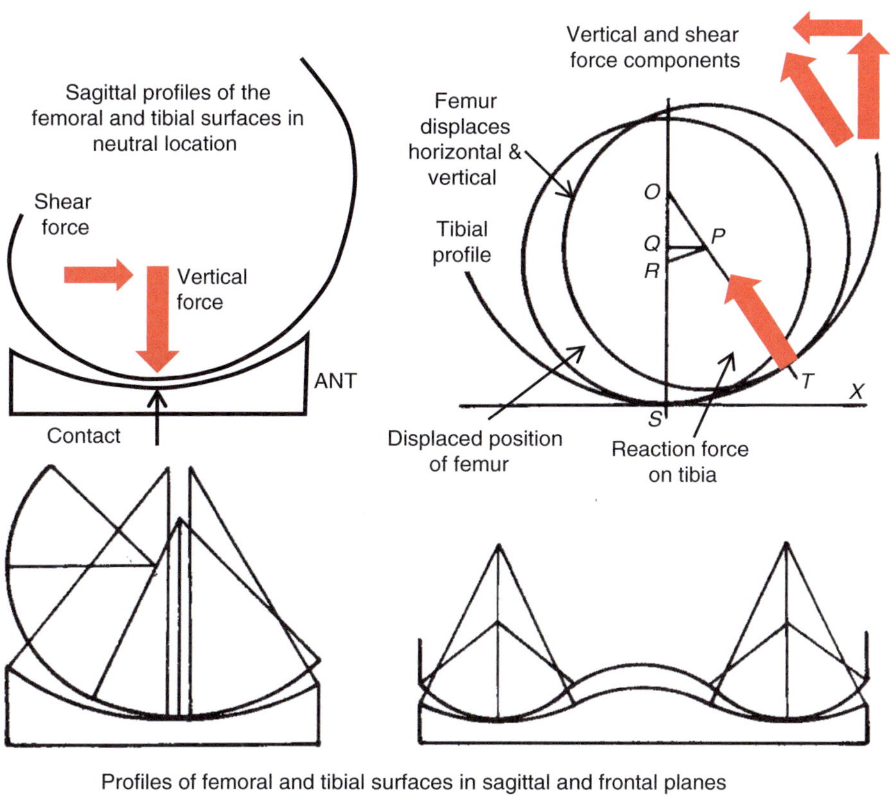

Fig. 9.9 The design of the bearing surfaces of the Total Condylar knee. Based on a theoretical analysis using force data during activities from Morrison (1970), the radii of the tibial bearing surfaces were calculated to provide similar AP laxities and internal-external rotations as determined for the anatomic knee in laboratory experiments. The stability obtained from the bearing surfaces was independent of any contribution from ligaments (Walker et al. 1974). (Below, Reprinted with permission from Institution of Mechanical Engineers, London, England)

bone. The solution was a one-piece all-plastic component with a central peg, which had a rectangular cross section. The efficacy of the central peg was demonstrated using a specially constructed nine-channel simulating machine (Walker & Hsieh 1977). The design and testing of the central peg was described in Chap. 8.

The artificial knee design was called the Total Condylar in that it replaced all of the bearing surfaces. To complete the design, a patella resurfacing component was required. This was designed by Paolo Agletti MD, a Fellow from Florence, Italy. The design was based on anatomic studies and mechanical testing. This is described in Chap. 7. The instrumentation for the Total Condylar was designed mainly by John

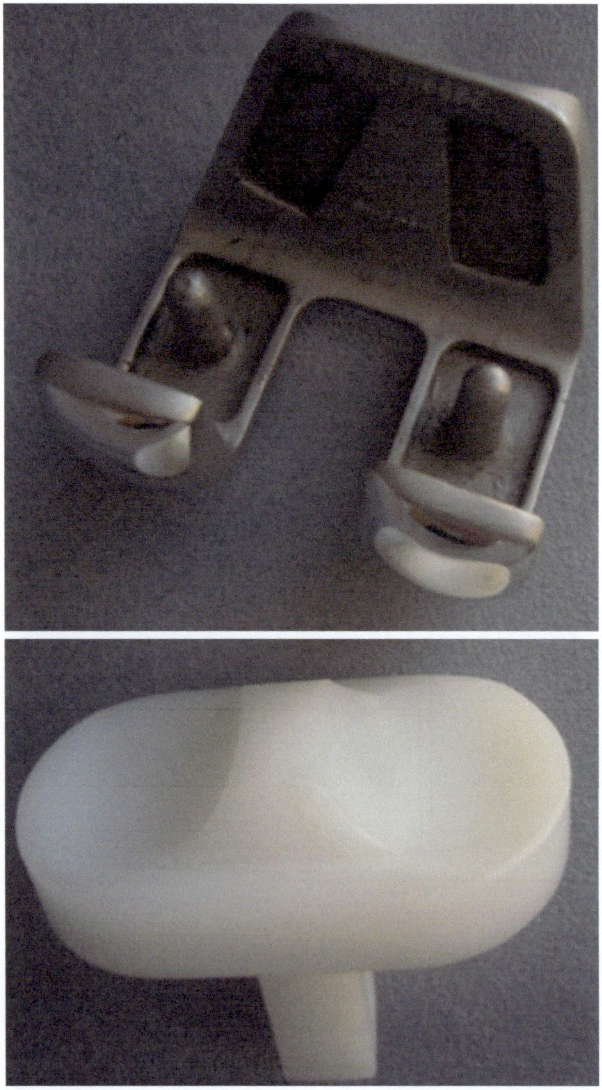

Fig. 9.10 The original Total Condylar knee designed equally by Peter Walker PhD, Chit Ranawat MD, and John Insall MD in 1973. The design was an evolutionary step from the Duo-condylar and Duo-patella knees. This knee was designed with double-dished bearing surfaces which under weight-bearing conditions provided similar laxity and stability as the anatomic knee

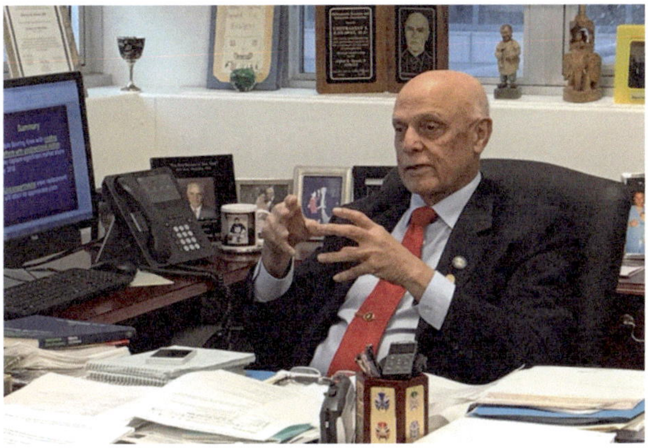

Fig. 9.11 Chitranjan Ranawat MD in his office at the Hospital for Special Surgery (HSS) in 2019. In the early 1970s, he was a principal participant in the group who designed some of the first artificial knees in the USA. Since that time, he has been a major influence in the orthopedic world, primarily for the knee but also for the hip and other joints. His innovative contributions have been wide ranging. He has been recognized at HSS for his outstanding teaching contributions and has been an authoritative participant at major conferences around the world. (© Peter S Walker)

Insall working with his Fellow, Norman Scott, and by Chit Ranawat. They devised methodologies for achieving square cuts aligned relative to the femoral and tibial axes. The levels of the cuts were determined by distracting the knee in extension and flexion such that the collateral ligaments would be tightened. But despite the fact that the tibial bearing surfaces could provide all of the necessary stability without the cruciate ligaments, Chit Ranawat and Alan Inglis still preferred to retain the cruciates in cases with only small amounts of deformity, which applied to many rheumatoid arthritis cases. However the one-piece tibial component with a central peg was incompatible with cruciate preservation where a long central slot would be required. A compromise was made by preserving only the posterior cruciate, requiring only a small notch at the posterior center of the tibial component, just behind the peg. This was considered an acceptable solution because the posterior cruciate was thought to cause posterior femoral rollback in flexion, necessary for obtaining a high flexion range, whereas the anterior cruciate played a less important role.

The end result was that two new artificial knees were designed, the Total Condylar where the cruciates were resected and the Duo-patella which retained the posterior cruciate. The Duo-patella represents the CR type of artificial knee. The posterior tibial surface in the Duo-patella was made shallower than the Total Condylar to allow the extra posterior displacement of the contact points in high flexion. Each of these designs was very successful clinically in long-term follow-up, although the Total Condylar became the more widely used (Insall et al. 1976; Sledge & Ewald 1979; Ranawat & Boachie-Adjei 1988; Rodriguez et al. 2001). In the late 1970s, these two types of knees, posterior cruciate retaining (CR) and cruciate sacrificing (TCP), would be combined with the Duo-condylar and Unicondylar knees and a

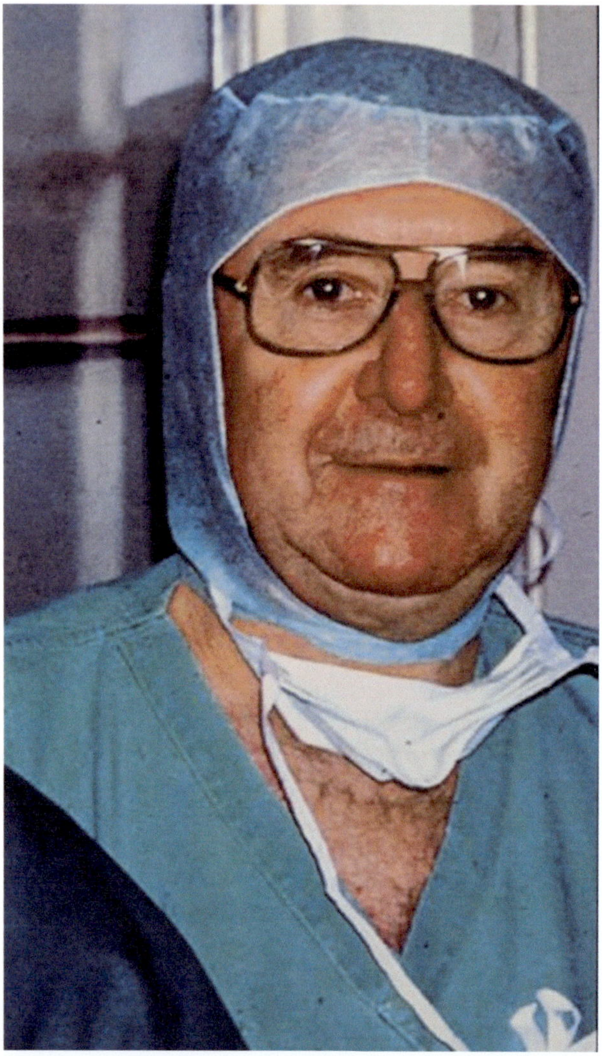

Fig. 9.12 John Insall in the operating room at the Hospital for Special Surgery in c 1974. Working with Fellows including Paolo Aglietti and Norman Scott, John Insall was one of the main developers of the instrumentation for the Total Condylar knee replacement. He later went on to design the posterior stabilized knee with Al Burstein. His unique legacy in knee replacement is well-known in orthopedics. (Photo courtesy The Knee Society)

Stabilo-condylar design, to form a "Graduated Knee System," the idea being that such a range was the solution to satisfying the full scope of severities of arthritis.

The role of the manufacturers was important in the introduction of these artificial knee designs. In the early phase, Walker had chosen a small company in Boston, called Cintor (later acquired by Johnson and Johnson), to be the manufacturer. However their lack of in-house metal casting and other processes led to frequent supply delays. To solve this problem, Howmedica, located in New Jersey close to New York, was asked to manufacture the Total Condylar. Howmedica gave the knee a high priority in their marketing efforts. As a result, the Total Condylar rapidly gained in clinical use, although the Graduated Knee System still retained a substantial following. This reflected the general view of the surgical community that cruciate retaining and sacrificing knees were both needed to treat a range of patients.

Other Designs of the 1970s and beyond

A number of other designs played an important role in the early development of the basic condylar replacement knee. The UCI design by Ted Waugh, used from 1972, was a condylar replacement without a patella flange. The problem of accurately matching the metal crossbridge, joining the lateral and medial condylar to the femoral trochlea, was solved in an ingenious way. A thin triangular metal blade joined the condyles and was imbedded in the bone, creating only a small surface discontinuity, but substantially enhancing the fixation. Late in the 1970s, the first porous-coated knees were introduced, the Miller-Galante and the PCA, both cruciate-preserving with low femoral-tibial conformity. Another "first" was the low-contact-stress (LCS) mobile-bearing knee designed by Buechel and Pappas to be discussed in Chap. 11. Also at that time, the posterior stabilized (PS) knee was designed by John Insall and Al Burstein, the design described in the next chapter.

It can be seen that during the 1970s, the condylar replacement artificial knee had evolved into three separate paths: designs with low femoral-tibial conformity which preserved both cruciates; moderate femoral-tibial conformity, preserving only the posterior cruciate; and designs with moderate to high conformity where only the collateral ligaments were preserved. In the first type, the cruciates provided anterior-posterior stability, while the bearing surfaces allowed freedom of motion. In the second type, the posterior cruciate prevented excessive anterior femoral displacement and produced progressive femoral rollback in flexion. In the third type, the bearing surfaces provided both anterior-posterior and rotary stability, but there was no specific mechanism for inducing femoral rollback in flexion. The first type usually used several small pegs for tibial fixation, the second and third types, a large central peg. Overall the clinical results of the three types were similar. The range of flexion was higher in the cruciate retaining designs, which achieved averages of 100 to 110 degrees. However these designs showed more instability due to the low constraint and the difficulty of accurate ligament balancing at surgery. Tibial loosening was more prevalent in the designs with only small fixation pegs, whereas the central peg proved to be more durable. The lower constraint designs showed more polyethylene wear due to the higher contact stresses and increased sliding. Another factor claimed by some surgeons was that cruciate preservation and lower constraint led to a more natural feel to the knee. With these different factors at play, by 1980, it was not possible to definitively favor one type of design over the other. But the achievement of the 1970s was to produce design types that worked well, covered a wide span of indications, and were a sound basis for any future developments.

Combining the different design concepts into one system was a reasonable step at that time. In the mid-1970s, Peter Walker worked in Boston for a year prior to working at Howmedica. Surgeons at the Robert Breck Brigham Hospital including Clem Sledge, the Department Chairman, Fred Ewald, Bill Thomas, and Bob Poss invited Peter Walker to join clinical meetings and expressed an interest in further artificial knee developments. By the time Walker started working at Howmedica soon after, it had been decided to design a unified system, to be called the Kinematic Knee System. This would include an ACL + PCL, a PS, and a CR, as well as a stabilizer. Fred Ewald was the main collaborator on this project, including the design of the instrumentation, with an all-in-one cutting guide called the Gobot. This instrument included distraction arms for tensioning each sides of the joint equally. By the late 1970s, the Kinematic had become Howmedica's flagship knee, and the system became popular in the USA and in Europe. This relationship between Howmedica and the Brigham and Women's Hospital progressed further in the 1980s. The same group, using computer modeling and biomechanical testing, produced the Kinemax Knee System, a much improved Kinematic.

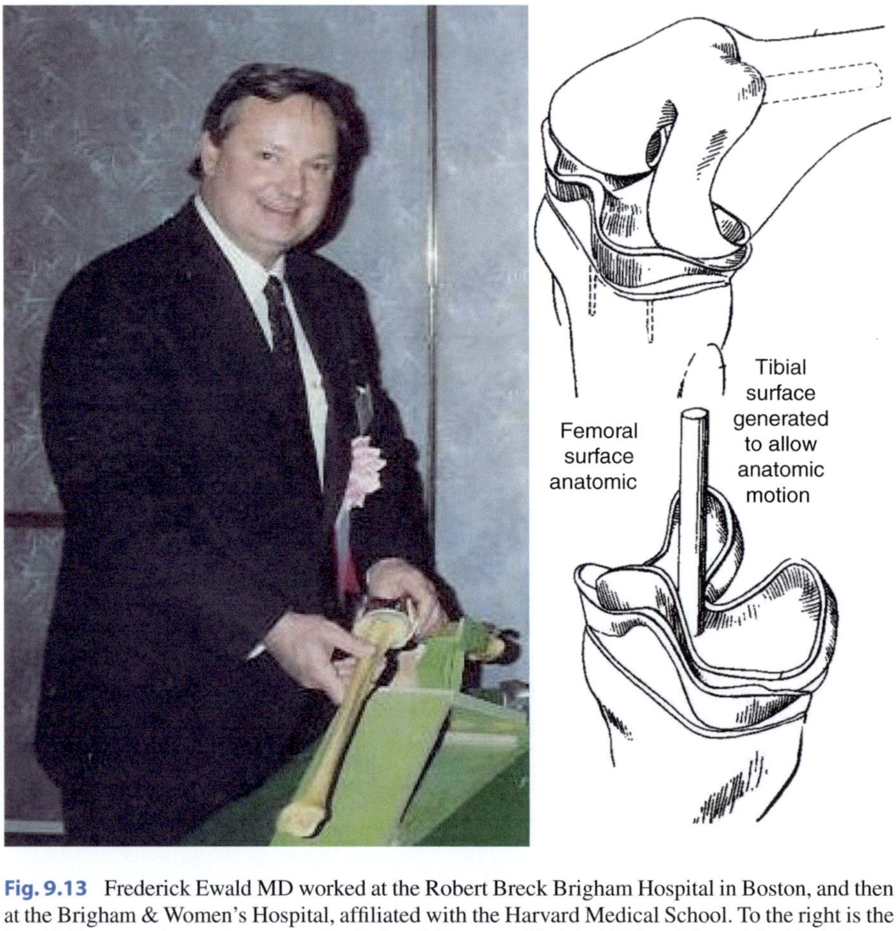

Fig. 9.13 Frederick Ewald MD worked at the Robert Breck Brigham Hospital in Boston, and then at the Brigham & Women's Hospital, affiliated with the Harvard Medical School. To the right is the Ewald Knee, an innovative anatomic design, US patent filed in 1971 and issued in 1974. Later, Ewald worked with Clem Sledge, Bill Thomas, Bob Poss, and Peter Walker, on the Kinematic and the Kinemax Knee Systems. He was one of the founding members of The Knee Society and served as President. He devised the radiographic evaluation system for the Knee Society. He was regarded as a particularly skilled surgeon and teacher, benefiting hundreds of Residents and Fellows. (Photo taken in 1980s) (© Peter S Walker)

Two other surgeons at the Brigham and Women's Hospital in Boston, who were not fully involved with the above developments, had new ideas for implant design and surgical technique. Richard Scott and Tom Thornhill developed the Press-Fit Condylar (PFC) knee with Johnson & Johnson, the first major knee system of that company. One of the features was a bone-preserving cruciate-shaped tibial peg on the metal baseplate for fixation. As a result of the clinical success, the PFC became one of the most widely knees used in the USA (Martin et al. 1997). The long-term results reported by an independent hospital were outstanding up to 25 years of follow-up (Patil et al. 2015). Another knee system of that era was the Vanguard knee, designed by a group of surgeons led by Adolph Lombardi and Keith Berend. The manufacturing company was Biomet based in Warsaw Indiana. The President of the company was Dane Miller, who graduated with a PhD in Materials Science at the University of Cincinnatti in the mid-1970s. Due to his background, he was particularly involved with this knee project. The designers had two particular goals: to design a knee which would continue to perform well into the second decade and provide a "continuum of constraint" so that each patient could be fitted with the best

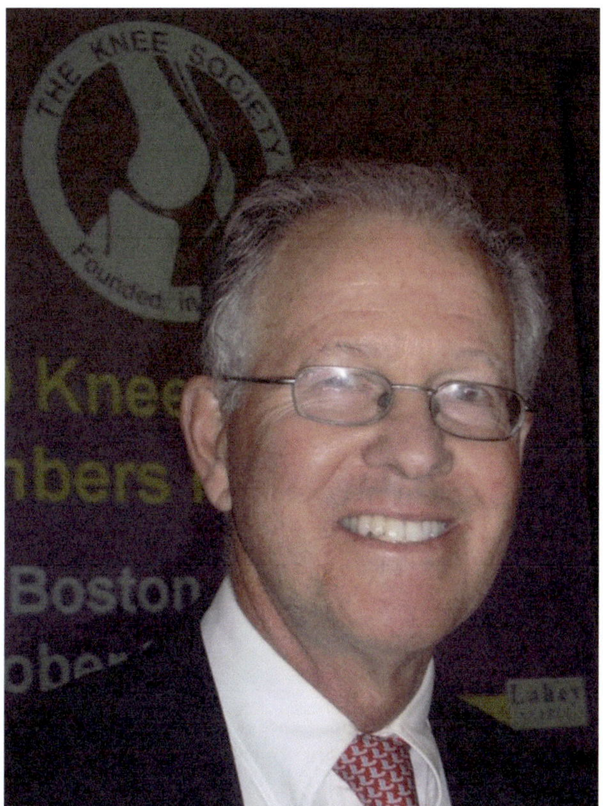

Fig. 9.14 Richard Scott MD and Tom Thornhill MD, who worked at the Brigham and Women's Hospital in Boston until recently, designed the PFC knee system in the 1980s. The PFC became one of the most widely used knee systems worldwide. That design has now been upgraded to produce the Attune system. Richard's recent book *Total Knee Arthroplasty* has been a major success, covering his long experience of knee replacement surgery. (Photo taken 2016 at ISTA Boston, MA) (© Peter S Walker)

possible combination of laxity and stability for their condition. The first goal was eventually realized after a recent follow-up study (Crawford et al. 2019). The second was that tibial inserts with different slopes and conformities were available using the same tibial baseplates, allowing choices to be made at surgery.

It is fitting to complete this chapter with a little-known artificial knee designed by John Charnley himself in the early 1970s. Having been closely involved with the efforts of Gunston on the Polycentric knee, Charnley felt that there were two main deficiencies. Firstly, cutting large slots in the femoral condyles was too invasive, and secondly the tibial components were of insufficient surface area and were subject to loosening. Nevertheless he thought that the concept of small adjustable components was viable. He made the innovative step of reversing the materials, plastic for the femoral component and metal for the tibial component. The femoral component was a plastic runner embedded in a slot in each femoral condyle. Charnley had observed that the arthritic lesions on the femur were most frequently located on the distal condyles only and did not extend posteriorly. Therefore the femoral component was limited in its length so that it embedded only in the distal femoral condyle, which made the component much less invasive and easier to fit accurately. The tibial component was a flat plate with a mesial tab which seated on a minimally resected tibial plateau. Because the plate was less than 3 mm in thickness, only a thin tibial resection was required. This preserved the strongest bone near to the surface for fixation and support of the tibial plate. As in the hip, acrylic cement was used for fixation. Simple but accurate instrumentation was designed including routers for the distal femoral cavity. Hundreds of cases were carried out at Wrightington Hospital, mostly in rheumatoid arthritis patients, when both the lateral and medial sides were resurfaced. The knee was called the load angle inlay (LAI). In 2004, at a bioengineering conference held in Leeds, England, Bodo Purbach presented a 20–28-year follow-up of no less than

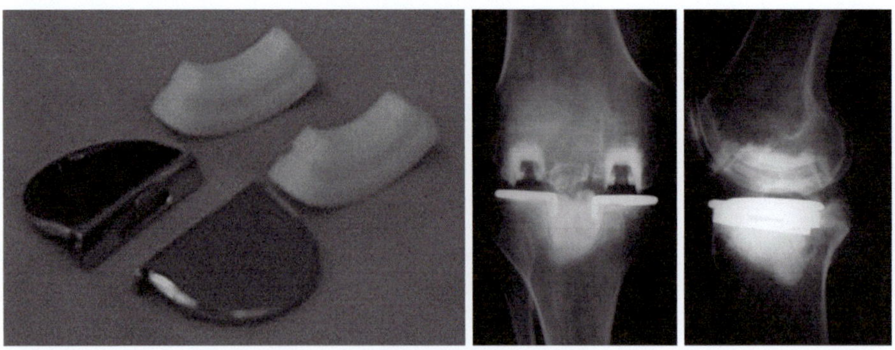

Fig. 9.15 The load angle inlay knee designed by John Charnley in the early 1970s. It was more conservative than the Gunston Polycentric designed just a few years earlier. The plastic femoral component resurfaced only the distal end of the femur, the most frequent site of the arthritic lesions. The metal tibial plates required only a small bone resection. When correctly aligned these implants survived several decades in many patients. (Photos courtesy Martyn Porter FRCS, Wrightington Hospital, England)

746 cases performed by Charnley and other surgeons including Michael Wroblewski (Purbach et al. 2004). The conclusion was "the LAI has given long-lasting success in cases where the leg has stayed in physiological alignment." Only 22 cases were reported to have failed. Most of the failures occurred due to the leg being in excess varus, which caused wear of the femoral component and loosening of the tibial plate. Subluxation sometimes occurred due to the plates being flat without any medial-lateral restraint. It was unfortunate that a full paper on this extensive experience was not published. The only publication was of a study of the failed cases, the authors being Julian Minns PhD, a bioengineer from Durham, England, and Kevin Hardinge FRCS, a surgeon from Wrightington (Minns & Hardinge 1983). The last LAI's were implanted in 1979 after which the knee was discontinued. But to this day, patients with a well-functioning LAI still visit the Wrightington hospital for a long-term checkup.

The load angle inlay design was not pursued beyond the initial cases performed at Wrightington Hospital, possibly due to the perceived limited indications. However unicompartmental knees have retained a place in knee replacement since about 1970. The earliest designs were the St. Georg Sledge from Hamburg, Germany, the unicondylar from HSS, and the Marmor from Los Angeles, California. Jean-Noel Argenson from Marseilles in France was one of the first to explore the possibilities of modular components for the lateral and medial sides as well as the patella trochlea (Parratte et al. 2015). After many years of experience, they found disappointing results except for standard medial unicompartmental, mainly due to design and fixation issues of the modular components. With an improved design and the use of the OrthoPilot Navigation System, improved results were obtained (Confalonieri & Manzotti 2005; Biazzo et al. 2018). In recent years there have been efforts to include compartmental knees as a way to achieve a "custom" solution, where choices are made to replace the patella trochlear, the medial compartment, and the lateral compartment (Romagnoli et al. 2015). Based on gait parameters, simultaneous bi-unis were recommended rather than staged (Marullo et al. 2019). In all of these studies, it was evident that a limitation of the system was that there were not a large number of cases indicated, and the surgery was technically demanding, factors which have limited widespread adoption so far. However the clinical results have been reported as outstanding, probably because the knees had been restored geometrically to a close-to-normal condition, together with preservation of the cruciates.

What Were the Steps Leading to the Basic Condylar Replacement Knees?

Prior to the invention of the first condylar replacement knees, there were a number of examples of metallic components for resurfacing either the femur or the tibia, but not in combination. Once Charnley has succeeded in designing the cemented metal-on-polyethylene hip, it provided the starting point for the first artificial knees. The earliest designs were very different. Each inventor or inventors had their own picture of how the knee worked and what type of components would be needed to restore the knee to a functional condition. In some cases basic research was carried out first, which provided the ideas for the design of the artificial knee itself. Competition between individual designers was certainly a factor, but so too was sharing of ideas and experiences. Progress was rapid, with problems quickly identified and solved; a process aided by the lack of regulations such that new designs could be quickly introduced. By 1975, several basic condylar types of artificial knee had been invented: the ACL + PCL retaining, the PCL retaining (CR), the cruciate sacrificing basic condylar replacement (TCP), and the unicompartmental. By 1980, the posterior stabilizer (PS) had been added. Also, the rotating platform knee was introduced. There had been sufficient clinical experience to show that all of these designs were promising, but the CR and the PS were the most popular.

References

Bargren JH, Blaha JD, Freeman MA. Alignment in total knee arthroplasty. Correlated biomechanical and clinical observations. Clin Orthop Relat Res. 1983;(173):178–83.

Biazzo A, Manzotti A, Confalonieri N. Bi-unicompartmental versus total knee arthroplasty: long term results. Acta Orthop Belg. 2018;84(3):237–44.

Confalonieri N, Manzotti A. Mini-invasive computer assisted bi-unicompartimental knee replacement. Int J Medical Robotics and Computer Assisted Surgery. 2005;1(4):45–50.

Coventry MB & Bryan RS. Pitfalls in the Polycentric and Geometric total knee arthroplasties. Conference on total knee replacement, Institution of Mechanical Engineers, London, 16–18 Sept 1974.

Coventry MB, Upshaw JE, Riley LH, Finerman GA, Turner RH, Turner RH, Geometric total knee arthroplasty. Patient data and complications. Clin Orthop Rel Res 1973;(94):177–178.

Crawford DA, Adams JB, Hurst JM, Berend KR, Lombardi AV Jr. Ten-year minimum outcomes and survivorship with a high flexion knee system. J Arthroplast. 2019;34(9):1975–9.

Ewald FC. Joint Prostheses. United States Patent 3,798,676 filed July 9, 1971, issued March 26, 1974.

Ewald FC. Metal to plastic total knee replacement. Orthop Clin North Am. 1975;6(3):811–21.

Finerman GAM, Coventry MB, Riley LH, Turner RH, Upshaw JE. Anametric total knee arthroplasty. Clin Orthop Rel Res. 1979;(143):85–90.

Freeman MAR, Swanson SAV, Todd RC. Replacement of the knee with the Freeman-Swanson prosthesis. Conference on total knee replacement, institution of mechanical engineers, London, 16–18 Sept 1974.

Gunston FH. Polycentric knee arthroplasty. Prosthetic simulation of normal knee movement. J Bone Joint Surg. 1971;53(2):272–7.

Hsieh HH, Walker PS. Stabilizing mechanisms of the loaded and unloaded knee joint. J Bone Joint Surg Am. 1976;58(1):87–93.

Insall JN, Ranawat CS, Aglietti P, Shine J. A comparison of four models of total knee-replacement prostheses. J Bone Joint Surg Am. 1976;58(6):754–65.

Lewallen DG, Bryan RS, Peterson LF. Polycentric total knee arthroplasty. A ten-year follow-up study. J Bone Joint Surg Am. 1984;66(8):1211–8.

Marullo M, Vitale JA, Stucovitz E, Romagnoli S. Simultaneous bilateral unicompartmental knee replacement improves gait parameters in patients with bilateral knee osteoarthritis. Knee. 2019;26:1413.

Minns RJ, Hardinge K. Failure of one design of surface replacement knee arthroplasty due to loosening deformation and wear of the plastic femoral component. Biomaterials. 1983;4(3):147–52.

Morrison J. The mechanics of the knee joint in relation to normal walking. J Biomech. 1970;3(1):51–61.

Parratte S, Ollivier M, Lunebourg A, Abdel MP, Argenson JN. Long-term results of compartmental arthroplasties of the knee; long term results of partial knee arthroplasty. Bone Joint J. 2015;97-B(10-Suppl A):9–15.
Patil S, McCauley JC, Pulido P, Colwell CW Jr. How do knee implants perform past the second decade? Nineteen- to 25-year followup of the Press-fit Condylar design TKA. Clin Orthop Relat Res. 2015;473(1):135–40. https://doi.org/10.1007/s11999-014-3792-6.
Pritchett JW. Charles O Townley: design by Reason. www.seattlejointsurgeon.com. 1988.
Pritchett JW. Patient preferences in knee prostheses. J Bone Joint Surg. 2004;86(7):979–82.
Pritchett JW. Patients prefer a bicruciate-retaining or the medial pivot total knee prosthesis. J Arthroplast. 2011;26(2):224–8.
Pritchett JW. Bicruciate-retaining Total knee replacement provides satisfactory function and implant survivorship at 23 years. Clin Orthop Relat Res. 2015;473(7):2327–33.
Purbach B, Wroblewski BM, Siney PD, Fleming PA. The Charnley load angle inlay knee replacement: long-term results 20–28 years. Presented at Leeds bioengineering conference, Leeds, 2004.
Ranawat CS, Boachie-Adjei O. Survivorship analysis and results of Total condylar knee arthroplasty. Eight- to 11-year follow-up period. Clin Orthop Relat Res. 1988;226:6–13.
Ranawat CS, Insall J, Shine J. Duo-condylar knee arthroplasty: Hospital for Special Surgery design. Clin Orthop Relat Res. 1976;120:76–82.
Rodriguez JA, Bhende H, Ranawat CS. Total condylar knee replacement: a 20-year followup study. Clin Orthop Relat Res. 2001;388:10–7.
Romagnoli S, Marullo M, Massaro M, Rustemi E, D'Amario F, Corbella M. Bi-unicompartmental and combined uni plus patellofemoral replacement: indications and surgical technique. Joints. 2015;3(1):42–8.
Sbarbaro JL. Press fit implant arthroplasty of the hip and knee. J Biomed Mater Res Symposium. 1974;5(Part 2):285–88.
Seedhom BB, Longton EB, Wright V, Dowson D. Dimensions of the knee. Ann Rheum Dis. 1972;31:54.
Seedhom B, Dowson D, Wright V. Wear of solid phase formed high density polyethylene in relation to the life of artificial hips and knees. Wear. 1973;24(1):35–51.
Seedhom BB, Longton EB, Dowson D, Wright V. The Leeds Knee. Conference on total knee replacement, institution of mechanical engineers, London, 16–18 Sept 1974.
Sledge CB, Ewald FC. Total knee arthroplasty experience at the Robert Breck Brigham Hospital. Clin Orthop Relat Res 1979;(145):78–84.
Townley CO. Articular-plate replacement arthroplasty for the knee joint. 1964. Clin Orthop Relat Res. 1988;(236):3–7.
Walker PS. A comparison of normal and artificial human joints. Acta Orthop Belg. 1973;39(Suppl 1):43–54.
Walker PS, Hajek JV. The load-bearing area in the knee joint. J Biomech. 1972;5(6):581–9.
Walker PS, Hsieh HH. Conformity in condylar replacement knee prosthesis. J Bone Joint Surg. 1977;59(2):222–8.
Walker PS, Shoji H, Erkman MJ. The rotational axis of the knee and its significance to prosthesis design. Clin Orthop Rel Res. 1972;89:160–70.
Walker PS, Wang C-J, Masse Y. Joint laxity as a criterion for the design of condylar knee prostheses. Conference on Total Knee Replacement, Institution of Mechanical Engineers, London, 16–18 Sept 1974.
Wang CJ, Walker PS. The effects of flexion and rotation on the length patterns of the ligaments of the knee. J Biomech. 1973;6(6):587–96.
Wang CJ, Walker PS. Rotatory laxity of the human knee joint. J Bone Joint Surg Am. 1974;56(1):161–70.
Yamamoto S. Total knee replacement with the Kodama-Yamamoto knee prosthesis. Clin Orthop Relat Res. 1979;145:60–7.

10 Posterior Stabilized

What Was the Design Rationale of the Posterior Stabilized Knee?

The earliest artificial knees were of two basic types, those where the cruciate ligaments were preserved and those where their function was substituted by the bearing surfaces. In the first type, the anterior-posterior (AP) stability was provided by the cruciates, while the femoral rollback in flexion, thought to be essential for achieving high flexion, was allowed for by shallow tibial bearing surfaces. This type of artificial knee was most suitable for arthritic knees without severe deformities. In the second type, dishing of the tibial surfaces provided the AP stability, but femoral rollback was limited, reducing the flexion angle in some cases. The advantage of this type of knee was that it could be used for severe deformities. A design problem was how to provide progressive femoral rollback with flexion without making the tibial bearing surfaces too shallow. The answer was to use the condylar surfaces for weight-bearing, but to use the intercondylar region for some type of mechanism which controlled the AP displacement. There were two early examples of this solution, both presented at the 1974 Conference on Total Knee Replacement in London.

Early Designs with Intercondylar Stability

The first was the Deane knee, which actually reversed the materials, plastic for the femoral component and metal for the tibial component (Deane 1974). The femoral condyles blended smoothly with the patella flange, and there was a spherical recess in the intercondylar region. The metallic tibial component had a base which covered the tibial surface, with shallow bearing surfaces on the lateral and medial sides. A sphere projected from the center of the component and entered the recess in the femoral component. The interaction of these features controlled the AP motion, causing posterior displacement of the femur on the tibia with flexion. In addition, Deane considered that it was essential to reproduce the internal-external rotation between the femur and tibia, for balance of the ligament forces, and to reduce stresses on the fixation of the components. This axial rotation was allowed by the tibial sphere in the spherical housing of the

P. S. Walker, *The Artificial Knee*, https://doi.org/10.1007/978-3-030-38171-4_10

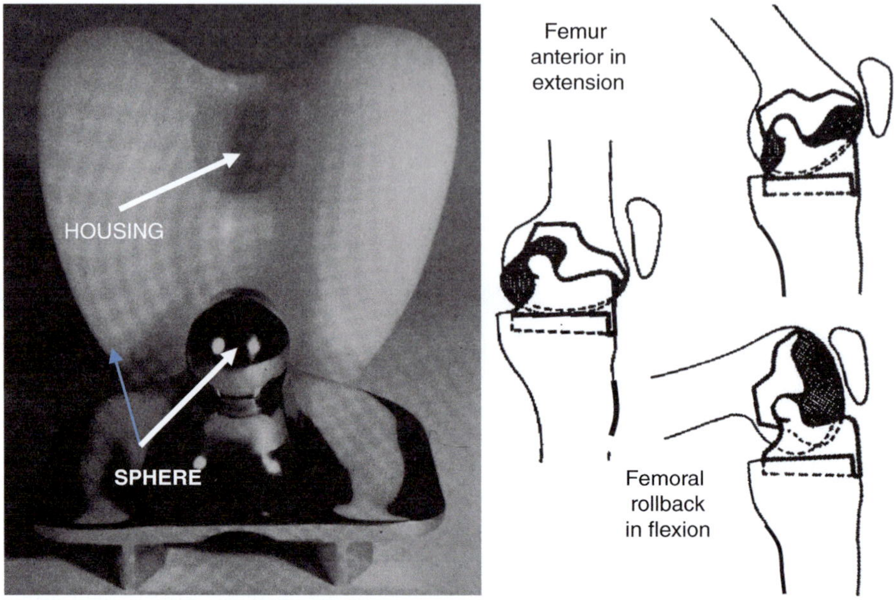

Fig. 10.1 Graham Deane FRCS designed this knee based on contact area and kinematic studies of the anatomic knee. The intercondylar post-in-housing produced progressive posterior displacement of the femur in flexion. At all angles, there was freedom of internal-external rotation due to the sphere-in-housing. The major weight-bearing was across the condyles themselves. This is one of the earliest solutions of a condylar replacement knee which provided unlinked intercondylar guidance to motion (Deane 1974). (Reprinted with permission from Institution of Mechanical Engineers, London, England)

femur. The motion criteria of the artificial knee were based on biomechanical studies of the anatomic knee, carried out by Graham Deane in his Master's Thesis at the University of Surrey in 1970. The knee was used successfully for a number of years; after a period of time, cracks developed in the plastic femoral component. The thickness of the polyethylene was inadequate to withstand the high forces of activity. The Deane knee was the first known example of an unlinked intercondylar mechanism providing femoral rollback and freedom of rotation while weight-bearing on the condyles.

The Attenborough Stabilized Gliding prosthesis similarly used the intercondylar region for a motion-guiding mechanism (Attenborough 1976). Chris Attenborough FRCS was an inventive surgeon who practiced at the Royal East Sussex Hospital in Hastings on the south coast of England. The ingenious mechanism produced posterior femoral displacement with flexion and allowed internal-external rotation. In addition it provided varus-valgus stability. Even though substantial cavities were needed in the center of the distal femur and proximal tibia, the design was considered an advantage over the hinges because the femoral and tibial canals were not invaded and the motion was more anatomic. Advantages were also claimed over the

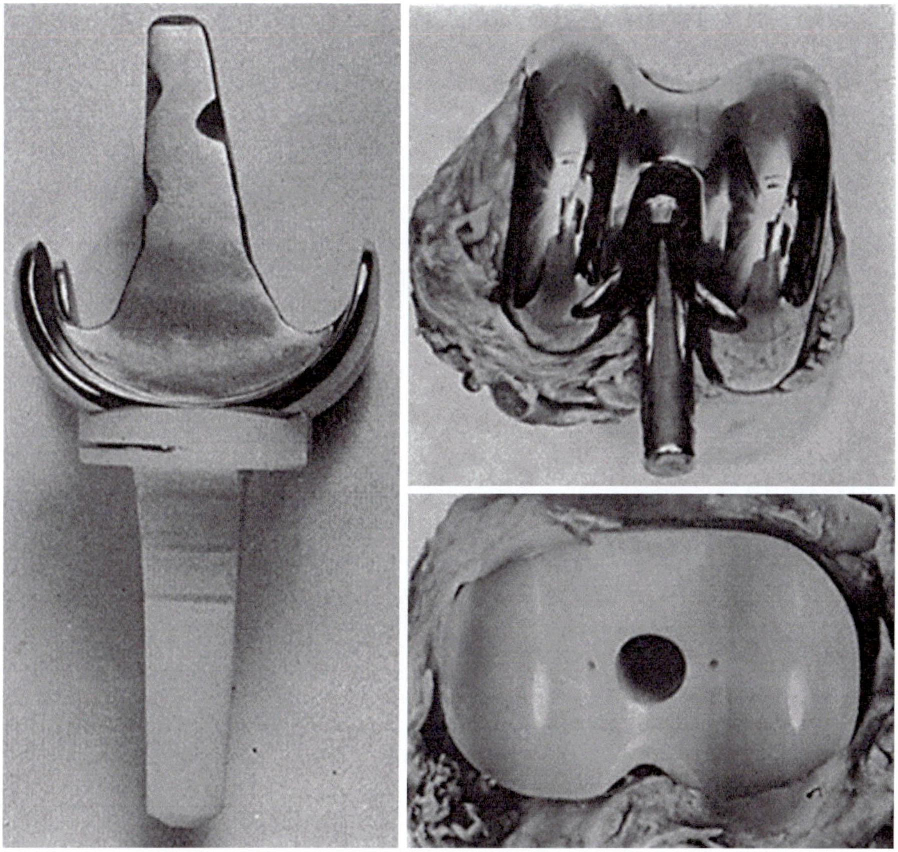

Fig. 10.2 The Attenborough Stabilized Gliding knee. An innovative design with partially conforming condylar contacts, intercondylar AP stability, freedom of internal-external rotation, and varus-valgus restraint. Strong fixation is provided with intramedullary pegs. It was first implanted in January 1973 (Attenborough 1976). (Reprinted with permission from Annals of Royal College of Surgeons of England)

early condylar replacements: "It has an advantage over unlinked condylar prostheses, namely, stability even when correcting severe deformities and in knees with pre-existing ligamentous damage." The Attenborough knee was first implanted in January 1973 and then used extensively in England for a number of years. However, a later follow-up study from Wrightington Hospital showed that there were patella problems due to the absence of a full anterior flange, as well as loosening. Both the Deane and the Attenborough can be credited with the first successful use of the intercondylar space using mechanical guiding means to produce more anatomic motion, particularly causing posterior femoral displacement in flexion and allowing some freedom of internal-external rotation.

Stabilized Designs at HSS

In the process of developing the condylar replacements at the Hospital for Special Surgery (HSS) in the early 1970s, Peter Walker and Hiromu Shoji, an Orthopedic Fellow, had experimented with an intercondylar linked hinge which allowed for some rotational laxity. Remarkably this hinge was almost identical to Gluck's, which he developed in 1890 as described in Chap. 3. Implantations in dogs and sheep showed that the center of rotation of the hinge in the sagittal plane was close to the average center of rotation in the intact joint (Walker and Shoji 1973). But at only 6 months follow-up, the femoral and tibial condyles appeared to be arthritic with degenerate cartilage and osteophytes, probably due to being unloaded. This resulted in the following solution: an artificial knee design with intercondylar stability, but where the axial load-bearing was carried on metal-on-plastic condylar surfaces. In other words, combine a condylar replacement knee with an intercondylar stabilized mechanism. The first design which using this concept was called the stabilo-condylar, made entirely in cobalt-chrome. It was implanted into a patient by John Insall, and while it performed well functionally, it did make clicking noises. After further development, a metal-plastic version of the knee was designed where the tibial component had a vertical plastic post in the center, housed in a cavity in the center of the femoral component, the objective being to provide varus-valgus stability during the full range of flexion.

This project now became a group effort with John Insall and Chit Ranawat. After a few refinements to the shape of the peg and housing, the femoral component was not only prevented from sliding anteriorly but gradually displaced posteriorly with flexion. Varus-valgus stability was still provided. The plastic peg was rounded off at the sides to allow some freedom of axial rotation, rather than allowing only sagittal plane motion which would make the device little different from a fixed hinge. This design was called the Total Condylar 2, or TC2. It was not seen as a substitute for the Total Condylar knee, but for knees where varus-valgus constraint was required, usually arthritic knees with high preoperative deformities or where both collateral ligaments were deficient. Extra fixation was provided by elongating the central stems of both components.

In 1976, when Peter Walker went to work at Cintor, a small implant company in Boston, he consolidated all of the Hospital for Special Surgery knee designs into a Graduated Knee System with the intention of making this a major HSS knee system. This included the Stabilo-condylar which was a modification of the TC2. The main change was that a metal axle was fixed in the metal housing and through the plastic post, linking the two components together. This axle was added to prevent dislocation or hyperextension from occurring although it was probably not necessary and made the surgical insertion more difficult.

After only a year in Boston, Peter Walker started in 1977 as Director of Product Development at Howmedica, a well-established orthopedic company with extensive manufacturing capabilities. One of the first goals was to develop a new knee system, because the company was only making the Total Condylar knee and a few small-volume designs in the custom products section. While in Boston, Walker had

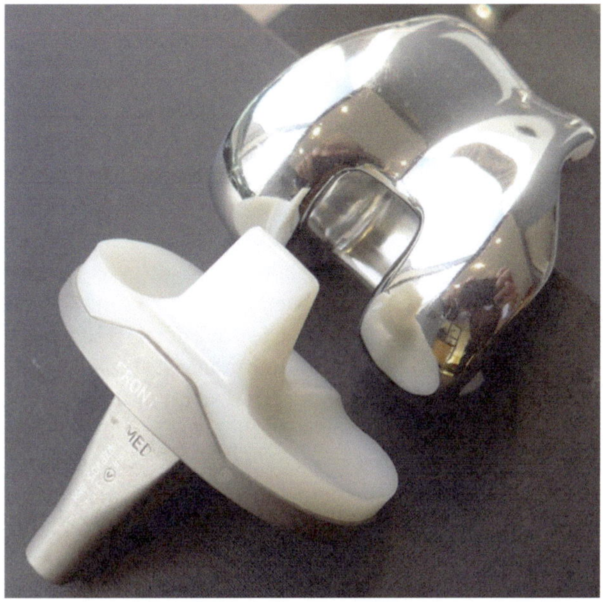

Fig. 10.3 The Kinematic Stabilizer, designed by Peter Walker, maintains the cam and the posterior of the housing in contact throughout flexion to produce progressive femoral rollback. It was a derivative of the Total Condylar 2 design from the Hospital for Special Surgery, based on research which showed that the center of the femur displaced posteriorly with flexion. It was used surgically from 1978

developed relationships with surgeons at the Robert Brigham Hospital: Clem Sledge, Fred Ewald, Bill Thomas, and Bob Poss. Within a year, a collaborative effort had produced the Kinematic Knee System. This consisted of a bi-cruciate retaining type, a posterior cruciate retaining type (CR), and an alternate to the Total Condylar where both cruciates were resected called the Kinematic Stabilizer. The starting point for the Stabilizer was the TC2. Rather than a tall central tibial peg in a femoral housing which restrained varus-valgus motion, the peg and housing were reduced in height so that the main function was control of anterior-posterior motion. Throughout the range of flexion, the femur was constrained from anterior displacement on the tibia, and the femur was progressively displaced posteriorly with flexion to increase the range. The design achieved excellent function and durability in long-term follow-up with a 95% survival rate at 10 years (Emmerson et al. 1996).

However, of the different design options in the Kinematic Knee System, the Stabilizer was the least favorite of the Robert Brigham Group, who were more disposed to the cruciate retaining types. This was primarily due to familiarity with previously used designs including the Ewald anatomic design which had been used only a few years previously. Moreover Howmedica themselves did not promote the Stabilizer as much as the other designs in the Kinematic Knee System, mainly because the Total Condylar was still selling well and continued to be supported by John Insall and Chit Ranawat. The Kinematic Knee System however was successful in both the USA and in Europe, especially in the UK and Scandinavia. One of the features of this knee system was that the tibial components were exclusively metal-backed. As described in Chap. 8, as a result of finite element analysis studies, experimental data, and the advantages of being able to switch the tibial inserts at surgery, metal-backing had almost completely replaced all-plastic components by the late 1970s.

In 1976, Albert (Al) Burstein PhD was appointed as the new Director of the Biomechanics Laboratory at the Hospital for Special Surgery. Burstein's interest in biomechanics began in 1963 while he was a mechanical engineering student at Brooklyn Polytechnic Institute. He attended a course on Orthopaedic Biomechanics given by Victor Frankel, a surgeon from the Hospital for Joint Diseases (HJD) in New York (now New York University Langone Orthopedic Hospital). On completing his degree, Burstein accepted a position as Director of the new Biomechanics Lab at the Hospital, established by Victor Frankel. Then in 1966, both Frankel and Burstein left HJD to work at Case Western Reserve University in Cleveland. There they carried out numerous biomechanical studies, mainly on fracture fixation. They created a well-attended annual course on biomechanics, which was targeted mainly for Residents. To go along with this course, they wrote a book entitled *Orthopaedic Biomechanics*, the first book of its type which established the role of biomechanics as an important part of orthopedic surgery. Frankel and Burstein, more than anyone, were responsible for the expansion in activity in orthopedic biomechanics in the ensuing years.

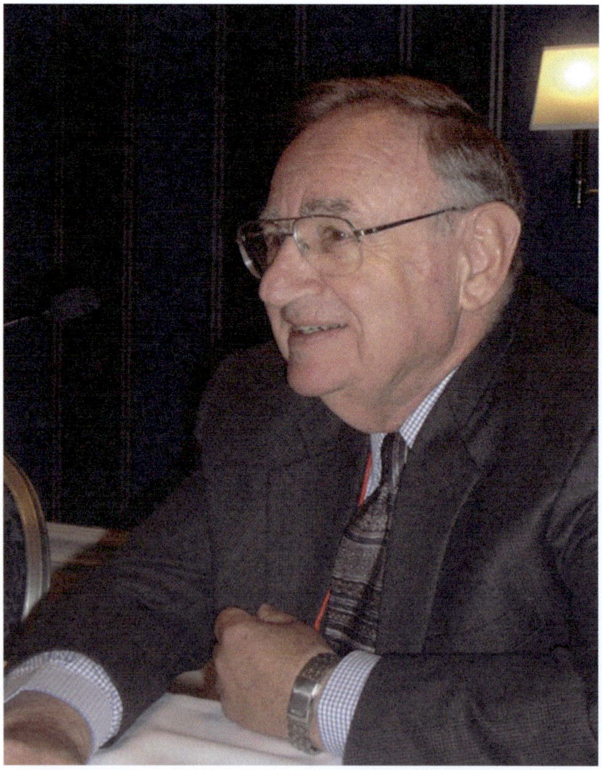

Fig. 10.4 Albert Burstein PhD started his career with Victor Frankel MD at Case Western University in Cleveland and established orthopedic biomechanics as a prominent activity, essential to progress in the field of artificial knee design. One of his significant achievements was the design of the Insall-Burstein knee, with John Insall, at the Hospital for Special Surgery in the late 1970s. Al Burstein was a clear-thinking designer and lecturer who is still involved with the field today. (Photo c 2015) (© Peter S Walker)

Insall-Burstein (IB) PS Knee

Soon after arriving at the Hospital for Special Surgery (HSS) in 1977, Al Burstein appointed several PhDs with expertise in different areas. Among these new staff were Tim Wright PhD and Claire Rimnac PhD who continue to be active in the area of joint replacement and biomaterials today. Very soon Al Burstein was approached by John Insall to make some modifications to the Total Condylar knee. Although the clinical results were successful, there of the Total Condylar knee were successful, there were two deficiencies which needed attention. The first was that the range of flexion was only averaging 90 degrees of flexion, about 10–20 degrees less than was being achieved for the Duo-patella and for other cruciate retaining designs being used at the time. The second limitation was that in some cases, when the knee was flexed and then extended, the femur would slide anteriorly on the tibia. The main reason for this was inadequate soft tissue balancing at surgery where the knee was too loose in flexion. In retrospect, both of the deficiencies may have been ameliorated by making the tibial cut slope posteriorly by five or six degrees, as it is anatomically. However at that time, the prevailing technique was that the tibial resection plane was perpendicular to the long axis of

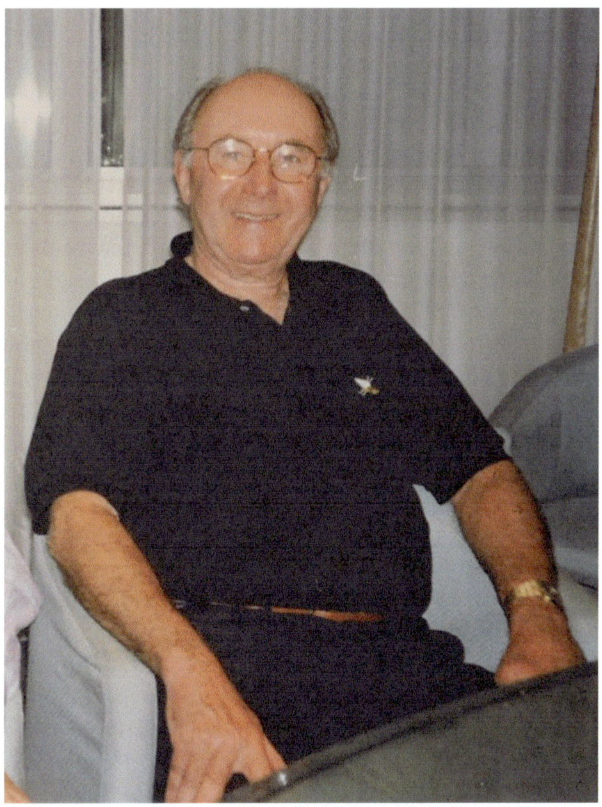

Fig. 10.5 John Insall MD was Chief of the Knee Service at the Hospital for Special Surgery from 1969 to 1996 and was a major contributor the early artificial knee designs, most particularly the Total Condylar and its instrumentation. In the late 1970s, he and Al Burstein designed the Insall-Burstein posterior stabilized knee. Over several decades John Insall was a leading authority on the technique of total knee arthroplasty and trained innumerable Residents and Fellows, who continue his legacy. (Photo mid 1990s) (© Peter S Walker)

the tibia in both the frontal and sagittal planes. Within 2 years, Insall and Burstein had developed the eponymous Insall-Burstein (IB) knee, the type now generically called a posterior stabilized or PS knee (Insall et al. 1982). It was first used in surgery in 1978. The development was simultaneous to that of the Kinematic Stabilizer, but there was no connection between the two projects.

The IB knee used an intercondylar cam-post to produce increased flexion and prevent anterior femoral displacement in high flexion. Burstein analyzed numerous shapes of intercondylar cam-post configurations and arrived at a design where a crossbar within an intercondylar housing in the femoral component interfaced with a short tibial post projecting from the center of the plastic tibial component. As the knee was flexed, contact between the crossbar and the post occurred at about 70 degrees flexion, which subsequently caused femoral rollback up to maximum flexion. Also the bottom of the dish of the tibial component was more posterior than that of the Total Condylar knee, which provided a longer lever arm for the quadriceps. Burstein's design method was impressive in that he analyzed the kinematic motion patterns at quadruple size on sheets of transparent paper of substantial dimensions. Computer-aided design (CAD) was not available at that time; everything had to be designed with paper and pencil. An important mechanical factor was also theorized regarding stability of the tibial component in high flexion. Due to the femoral-tibial contact points being close to the posterior, this might cause excessive compressive stresses on the posterior trabecular bone and uplifting of the anterior of the tibial component. On the other hand, the anterior shear force acting on the plastic post would have the opposite effect. Burstein showed that the resultant of these two forces was a single force close to vertical acting near the center of the component.

Another favorable mechanical feature of the IB was that the tibial component was designed to be at five-degree posterior slope on the tibia with the contact point of the femur on the tibia in early flexion a few millimeters posterior of the center, resembling the normal anatomic position. The height of the lateral and medial bearing surfaces was increased anteriorly to limit the anterior sliding of the femur on the tibia in the flexion arc prior to the engagement of the cam-post. There was also an advancement in materials, namely, molded polyethylene for the tibial component, which was shown to have superior wear properties to the machined components used for most artificial knees on the market at the time.

A US patent was filed for the design in 1980, which was issued in 1981 (Burstein and Insall 1981). The fundamental mechanism was explained in the patent as follows: "The camming action between the cam follower and cam surface forces the zones of contact between the condylar portions of the femoral component and concavities in the tibial component posteriorly as the leg approaches full flexion, thereby increasing the range of flexion without interference between posterior surfaces of the femur and the tibial component and preventing anterior dislocation of the femur. The plateau of the tibial component slopes inferiorly and posteriorly, also to increase the range of flexion without interference." The emphasis was on prevention of anterior displacement in flexion, combined with femoral rollback, to fulfil the main two design criteria.

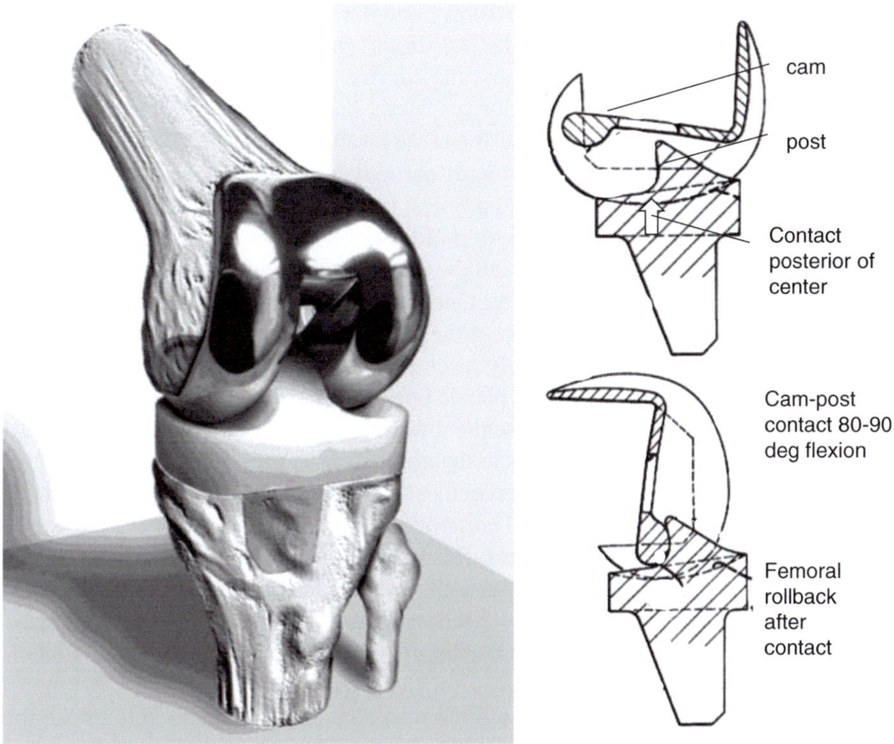

Fig. 10.6 The Insall-Burstein PS total knee was designed at the Hospital for Special Surgery and used surgically from 1978. It was intended as an improvement to the Total Condylar knee, where the cam-post would prevent anterior sliding of the femoral component and cause rollback in high flexion, increasing the range of flexion. (Figure on left courtesy of Fabio Catani MD, University of Modena & Reggio Emilia. Figure on right from US Patent 4,298,992, filed 1980, issued 1981)

Zimmer, who manufactured the knee, immediately recognized the potential of the IB knee design. While the Total Condylar had been very successful for over 5 years, clearly the next development from HSS, and from Insall and Burstein in particular, had a high market potential. Zimmer gave strong promotional support, while Insall and Burstein gave numerous lectures about the knee at prominent conferences. By the late 1970s, there were many courses on total knee replacement run not only by the AAOS and other organizations but by major institutions. Companies often organized special courses featuring their new knee designers. There was considerable demand for attending such courses from surgeons who were motivated to join the fast-growing practice of artificial knee surgery. As a result of the excellent short-term results of the IB design, the credibility of the developers, the prestige of the Hospital for Special Surgery, and the efforts of Zimmer, within a few years, the IB became one of the top selling knees.

The IB knee proved to be relatively easy to insert, yet forgiving due to its inherent stability. It increased the average range of flexion by about 15 degrees and had higher functional scores compared with the Total Condylar. It was modestly described as a "valuable adjunct to the Total Condylar prosthesis" (Insall et al. 1982). In a long-term follow-up of 100 cases at 15–19 years, the survivorship was 92.4% (Abdeen et al. 2010). Most of the revisions were due to patella problems. From the radiographic examination, it was found that there is no observable osteolysis. This would have been expected due to the accumulation of particulate debris, as has been seen with other designs at even shorter follow-up times. In the case of the IB design, the lack of osteolysis was attributed to the use of molded polyethylene and a monoblock construction where the plastic was fused to the metal-backing at manufacture. This prevented backside wear from occurring. One design detail with the IB design which was overlooked was that the posterior of the vertical plastic post was flat. This meant that when the femur rotated internally or externally, the contact with the transverse metal bar was on the corners of the plastic post, causing wear and local fragmentation in some cases, as shown in subsequent retrieval studies. Other studies of the IB design, including subsequent models to the original, have noted "patella clunk." This was explained as mal-tracking of the patella and entrapment of tissue due to the wide intercondylar housing of the femoral component.

Because of the advantages of the Insall-Burstein type of design, from the early 1980s, many surgeons used it for almost all of their cases, while several other companies designed their own versions, circumventing the patents for the Kinematic Stabilizer and the Insall-Burstein. In the larger companies, the PS was usually incorporated into a knee system which also included the still widely used CR type of design. One of the benefits of this was the cost advantage of being able to use the same metal tibial tray for both designs. Much of the popularity of the IB knee was due to Insall's attention to teaching a succession of Residents and Fellows and also his comprehensive book, *Surgery of the Knee*. Production of several editions of this book was greatly facilitated by Norman Scott, who eventually became the main Editor. John Insall also established a travelling fellowship program. Norman Scott maintains the program to this day, which continues to provide so much benefit to its participants.

Since the early 1980s, the IB posterior stabilized design has been redesigned to take advantage of the extensive clinical experience. One example of this is that the "patella clunk" problem was avoided when the PS knee was redesigned into the NexGen Knee System in the late 1990s (Lonner et al. 2007). The kinematics of the PS and its cam-post was studied in detail using fluoroscopic imaging of a loaded lunge activity (Suggs et al. 2008). The patients in this study were Asian with an average passive range of flexion postoperatively of 142 degrees. The cam-post engaged at an average of 91 degrees, after which there was posterior femoral displacement, contributing to the high flexion and fulfilling the design objective. The limited internal-external rotation in the early IB models was later solved by rounding the tibial post. In the NexGen, different dimensional combinations were also added to the femoral component to account for statistical variations between genders and races. This aspect of the ideal dimensions and shape for both the femoral and tibial components was further refined when the Persona Knee System was introduced in 2013. The different versions of the PS design, as well as John Insall's many contributions to artificial knee designs and surgery, have been described in a well-illustrated article (Scuderi et al. 2001).

However, the above lineage of the Insall-Burstein PS knee was not the only development of the cam-post concept. In 1996, John Insall left the Hospital for Special Surgery (HSS) to form the Insall Scott Kelly Clinic. In the same year, Al Burstein also left HSS, but not before starting work on a new posterior stabilized knee. This development involved surgeons affiliated with HSS and was to be called the Optetrak, manufactured by Exactech. The design goals were to minimize the wear and to improve the patella tracking. Wear was considered to be affected by contact stress. Working with Don Bartel PhD at Cornell University, a finite element analysis determined that reducing the frontal plane radii of the bearing surfaces and making the femoral and tibial surfaces almost conforming reduced the contact stresses significantly (Bartel et al. 1995). In addition, Burstein worked with Steve Li PhD, formerly a member of the HSS Biomechanics Laboratory, on a new net-shaped molding methodology for the polyethylene. The Optetrak knee was compared with the IB 2 knee in a study of 68 patients, with bilateral knees implanted, followed for 11 years (Robinson and Green 2011). For both knee designs, survivorship was 98%, and there was no report of any osteolysis which may have been caused by particulate wear. In another study of 171 knees followed for 7 years, the range of flexion averaged 120 degrees, a slight improvement over previous PS versions, while there were no patella "clunk" or other patella problems reported (Ehrhardt et al. 2011). Hence this second PS line of development met with improved results over the previous PS versions of the original Insall-Burstein.

Ultracongruent Knee

As pointed out in Chap. 3, to every design problem, there is usually more than one solution. In this case the relevant design criteria were to provide sufficient anterior-posterior stability and a high range of flexion in the absence of the cruciate ligaments. A different solution to the PS was introduced by Aaron Hofmann in the late 1990s, in the form of the Natural knee (Hofmann et al. 2010). Comparing the basic mechanisms of the two most widely used types of design, the CR and the PS, the sagittal radius of the CR tibial bearing surface is typically larger than that of the PS. In other words, the CR tibial surface is shallower and less constrained in an anterior-posterior direction, while the PS is more constrained. This seems logical based on the absence of both cruciate ligaments in the PS design, where the cam-post substitutes for the function of the posterior cruciate and the elevated anterior bearing surfaces of the tibial component substitutes for the posterior cruciate. In laboratory studies of the stability and laxity of designs with different radii, it was determined that the boundary in the tibial radius values between the CR and the PS had a sound rationale (Luger et al. 1997). For cruciate resection, it was stated by Hofmann that "Relatively shallow posterior tibial curvature and a steep anterior curvature were concluded to provide the most satisfactory combination of laxity and stability." But it was later determined from fluoroscopy studies of patients with CR and PS designs that there was a limit to how shallow the posterior curvature should be (Dennis et al. 2003). When it was too shallow, as in typical CR designs, "paradoxical sliding" occurred. The reason was that due to the absence of the anterior cruciate, the femoral-tibial contact point was often located too posteriorly. On the initiation of function, the anterior shear force component caused the femur to slide anteriorly until it was stabilized by the anterior slope of the tibial surface. But because the anterior slope of the CR was relatively shallow, the sliding distance could be felt by the patient as instability.

These considerations of stability and laxity occurred to Aaron Hofmann after a decade of experience with his Natural knee, which was a CR type (Hofmann et al. 2000; Hofmann 2010). Hofmann reasoned that if the tibial bearing surface was elevated anteriorly, it would effectively substitute for the PCL. The tibial insert was called the Ultracongruent. "The increased anterior build-up prevents the tibia from subluxing posteriorly through the entire arc of knee motion." However there was no mechanism for causing the femur to displace posteriorly during high flexion, and this might cause a reduction in the maximum flexion angle achieved. Surprisingly, clinical results by both Hofmann and an independent group showed that the ranges

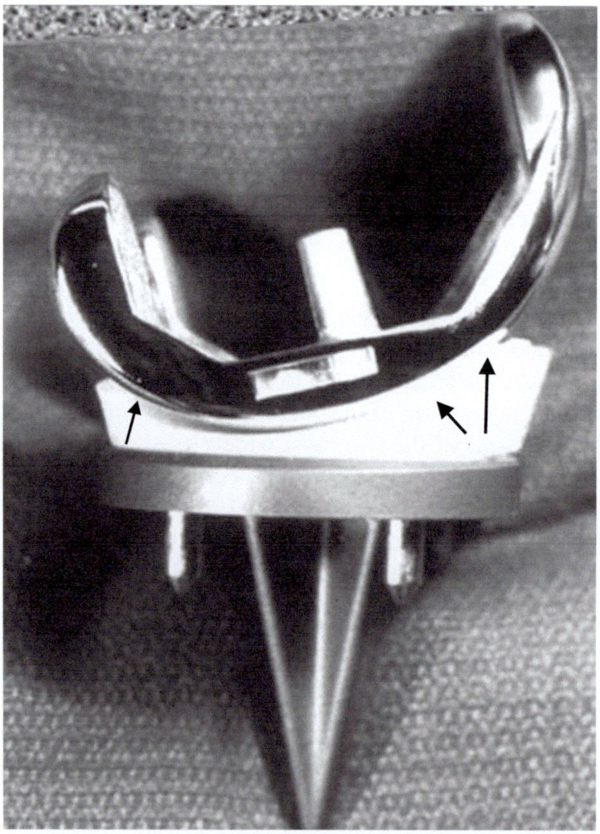

Fig. 10.7 The Natural knee designed by Aaron Hofmann MD with input on fixation aspects from Roy Bloebaum PhD, from the University of Utah, Salt Lake City. The raised anterior surface of the tibial insert (arrows) limits the anterior sliding of the femoral component particularly in early-mid-flexion. The posterior lip on the tibia (arrow) also limits the AP displacements and prevents excessively posterior contact. An advantage of the design is that it can replace both CR and PS types of design (Hofmann 2010). (Reprinted with permission from American Journal of Orthopaedics)

of flexion, or the gains between pre-op and post-op, were similar for the CR and the ultracongruent (Lutzner et al. 2017). The ultracongruent concept has a number of advantages over a PS configuration. There is no need to cut an intercondylar housing in the distal femur, the femoral trochlea can be extended distally giving improved patella tracking, and surgical insertion is easier. The ultracongruent concept is a valid alternate to the cam-post, and the concept may attract increasing attention in the future. It is still not clear however why the lack of femoral rollback does not reduce the flexion angle achieved. It is possibly due to a relatively low posterior lip on the tibial component, so the posterior femoral cortical impingement does not occur too early and block flexion. Further investigation of the geometrical and surgical factors which affect the range of flexion, a very important outcome parameter for an artificial knee, is warranted.

What Was the Design Rationale of the Posterior Stabilized Knee?

The reason that the posterior stabilized knee was designed was the limitations in the Total Condylar knee, a flexion range in patients averaging only about 90 degrees, and flexion instability in some cases. It was thought by John Insall that there should be a solution to these problems, and accordingly he and Al Burstein invented the Insall-Burstein knee. This was termed a posterior stabilized (PS) knee. The first characteristic of the PS was that a cam-post mechanism caused femoral rollback from mid-flexion to full flexion, rollback being thought to be the factor which produced a high flexion. The cam-post would also prevent anterior femoral subluxation in flexion. A further principle was that the resultant of the downward compression force near the posterior of the tibial condyles and the anterior force on the plastic post would be a force which would be more central, so as not to cause rocking of the tibial component. Molded polyethylene in a monoblock tibial component would minimize polyethylene wear.

References

Abdeen AR, Collen SR, Vince KG. Fifteen-year to 19-year follow-up of the Insall-Burstein-1 total knee arthroplasty. J Arthroplast. 2010;25(2):173–8.

Attenborough CG. Total knee replacement using the stabilized gliding prosthesis. Ann R Coll Surg Engl. 1976;58:4–14.

Bartel DL, Rawlinson JJ, Burstein AH, Ranawat CS, Flynn WF. Stresses in polyethylene components of contemporary total knee replacements. Clin Orthop Relat Res. 1995;317:76–82.

Burstein AH, Insall JN. Posterior stabilized total knee joint prosthesis. US Patent number 4,298,992. Filed 1980, issued 1981.

Deane G. New concept in total knee design. Conference on Total Knee Replacement. London: Institution of Mechanical Engineers; 1974. p. 16–8.

Dennis DA, Komistek RD, Mahfouz MR. In vivo fluoroscopic analysis of fixed-bearing total knee replacements. Clin Orthop Relat Res. 2003;410:114–30.

Ehrhardt J, Gadinsky N, Lyman S, Markowicz D, Westrich G. Average 7-year survivorship and clinical results of a newer primary posterior stabilized total knee arthroplasty. HSS J. 2011;7:120–4.

Emmerson KP, Moran CG, Pinder IM. Survivorship analysis of the Kinematic Stabilizer total knee replacement: a 10- to 14-year follow-up. J Bone Joint Surg British volume. 1996;78(3):441–5.

Hofmann AA, Tkach TK, Evanich CJ, Camargo MP. Posterior stabilization in total knee arthroplasty with use of an ultracongruent polyethylene insert. J Arthroplasty. 2000;15(5):576–83.

Hofmann AA. The design principles of the Natural-Knee system. Am J Orthod (Belle Mead, NJ). 2010;39(6 Suppl):2–4.

Insall JN, Lachiewicz PF, Burstein AH. The Posterior Stabilized condylar prosthesis: a modification of the Total Condylar design. Two to four-year clinical experience. J Bone Joint Surg Am. 1982;64(9):1317–23.

Lonner JH, Jasko JG, Bezwada HP, Nazarian DG, Booth RE. Incidence of patellar clunk with a modern posterior-stabilized knee design. Am J Orthop (Belle Mead NJ). 2007;36(10):550–3.

Luger E, Sathasivam S, Walker PS. Inherent differences in the laxity and stability between the intact knee and total knee replacements. The Knee. 1997;4(1):7–14.

Lutzner J, Beyer F, Dexel J, Fritzsche H, Lutzner C, Kirschner S. No difference in range of motion between Ultracongruent and Posterior Stabilized design in total knee arthroplasty: a randomized controlled trial. Knee Surg Sports Traumatol Arthrosc. 2017;25(11):3515–21.

Robinson RP, Green TM. Eleven-year implant survival rates of the all-polyethylene and metal-backed modular Optetrak posterior stabilized knee in bilateral simulataneous cases. J Arthroplast. 2011;8(26):1165–9.

Scuderi GR, Norman W, Scott WN, Tchejeyan GH. The Insall Legacy in Total Knee Arthroplasty. Clin Orthop Rel Res. 2001;392:3–14.

Suggs JF, Hanson GR, Park SE, Moynihan AL, Li G. Patient function after a posterior stabilizing total knee arthroplasty: cam-post engagement and knee kinematics. Knee Surg Sports Traumatol Arthrosc. 2008;16(3):290–6.

Walker PS, Shoji H. Development of a stabilizing knee prosthesis employing physiological principles. Clin Orthop Relat Res. 1973;94:222–33.

Guided Motion Knees

11

Do Guided Motion Designs Have Advantages over the CR and PS?

The two most popular condylar replacement knees today are the CR, where the posterior cruciate ligament is retained, and the PS, where both cruciate ligaments are resected and an intercondylar cam-post provides stability. The starting point of this chapter is the condylar replacement knee, where the femoral condyles resemble those of the anatomic femur, although with simplified geometry, while the tibial surfaces have radii which are larger than those of the femoral surfaces in both the frontal and sagittal planes. The collateral ligaments are retained. In such a knee, the femur can displace anterior-posterior or medial-lateral and rotate internal-external on the tibia, until the femur is constrained by the ligaments or the curvature of the bearing surfaces. This applies to the PS knee, until the femoral cam interfaces with the tibial post, after which the femur is guided to displace posteriorly. In that sense, the PS is a guided motion knee. A rotating platform knee where the displacements between the femur and tibia are prevented or are very limited, but where the rotation is not constrained by the bearing surfaces but by the retained ligaments, will also be considered as a guided motion knee.

Therefore, the definition of a guided motion knee is where mechanical features control or guide the femoral-tibial motion, in a way which is different to the conventional bearing surfaces of a condylar replacement knee; usually, a guided motion knee will be designed to reproduce some motion characteristics of the anatomic knee. Some guided motion knees were invented before 1980 and have been used clinically, while others have emerged only recently and are not yet being used. In this chapter, rotating platform, meniscal bearing, and medial pivot knees will be included. Some guided motion knees which have similar design features to the PS have already been discussed in the previous chapter. One of the questions that will be addressed during this and later chapters is in what way can the kinematics of the artificial knee be changed such that it will result in improved function or offer advantages in other ways.

P. S. Walker, *The Artificial Knee*, https://doi.org/10.1007/978-3-030-38171-4_11

Freedom of Rotation

Allowing freedom of internal-external rotation was originally introduced to address tibial loosening and to allow some freedom of rotation as in the anatomic knee. At Syracuse University, New York, in the early 1970s, David G Murray, MD, an orthopedic surgeon, and James Shaw, PhD, a mechanical engineer, had built a knee simulating machine to study the rotational laxity in the anatomic knee, with a view to applying the research to an artificial knee design (Shaw and Murray 1973, 1974). They invented the Variable Axis knee which had a convex spherical surface in the center of the femoral component, articulating in a concave spherical dish in the center of the plastic tibial component. This design was unconstrained in rotation but was constrained in the anterior-posterior and medial-lateral directions. The main load-bearing surfaces were cylindrically shaped femoral condyles and flat tibial surfaces, which provided a wide base for varus-valgus stability. The knee was strongly constructed in having a metal-backing for the tibial component and a femoral component without an intercondylar cutout. Fixation was augmented with cemented intramedullary stems. In a clinical follow-up (Murray 1982), a problem of the Variable Axis was subluxation and pain in the patella, due to the projecting spherical surface in the center of the femoral component interfering with patella tracking at higher flexion angles. As with the Total Condylar knee, there were also cases of anterior femoral subluxation in flexion if the collaterals were excessively loose. Use of the Variable Axis had tailed off by the end of the 1970s mainly due to these problems, as well as to the over-invasive fixation stems. The design had overcome the loosening problem but had introduced other problems. However, the Variable Axis knee was one of the first designs which allowed complete freedom of internal-external rotation.

An interesting variation of the Variable Axis concept was designed in the late 1980s, called the BiSurface knee (Ueo et al. 2011). As in the Variable Axis, a spherical surface projected from the femoral component and was located in a recess in the tibial insert. In the BiSurface, the sphere was posterior so that it did not interfere with patella tracking. Contact between the sphere and recess only occurred after 90° flexion so that freedom of rotation occurred in high flexion. This addressed the requirements of the eastern lifestyle where high flexion was an everyday requirement. The knee has a strong following in Japan to this day, partly because the manufacturer, Kyocera, is a Japanese company, but also because the femoral component is made from alumina ceramic, which reduces the wear.

Another example where rotation was unconstrained was the UCI knee (University of California, Irvine), designed in the early 1970s by Theodore (Ted) Waugh, MD, working with the Biomechanics Laboratory at the University of California, Irvine (Evanski et al. 1976; Waugh et al. 1973). The UCI was an ingenious arrangement where the femoral condyles were toroidal, while the tibial bearing surface was shaped by the path swept out by the femoral condyles when they were rotated about a central vertical axis. As with the Variable Axis, anterior-posterior and medial-lateral displacements were constrained, but in the UCI, both cruciates were retained. While the femoral component was well fixed due to a triangular prong which was

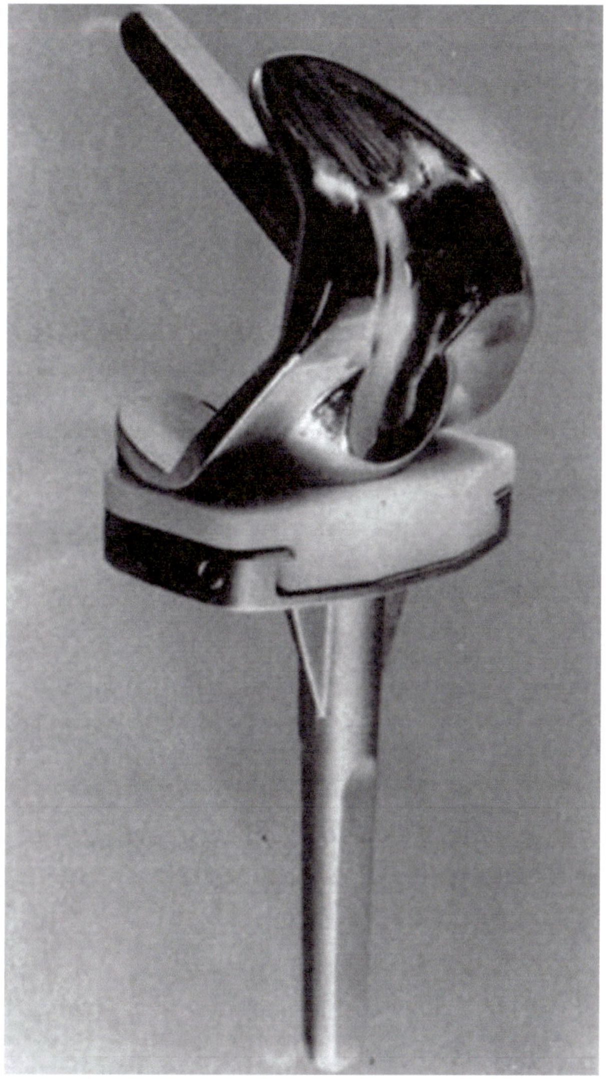

Fig. 11.1 The Variable Axis knee was designed by David G Murray, MD, and James Shaw, PhD, in the early 1970s. The first design criterion was durable fixation, achieved with the intramedullary stems. An additional criterion was stability with freedom of rotation. This was provided by a spherical surface projecting from the distal femur locating in a spherical trough in the center of the tibial surface. The plastic insert was fixed with a transverse metal pin (Murray et al. 1982). (Reprinted with permission from Orthopaedic Clinics of America)

impacted into the distal femur, due to the inadequate stiffness of the all-plastic tibial component, there was a relatively high incidence of loosening and deformation. Nas Eftekhar's Intramedullary Adjustable knee had a similar circular track on the tibial surface, allowing freedom of rotation. Eftekhar's femoral component was a Total Condylar with the addition of a central stem. One-piece plastic tibial inserts were housed in a metal tray, which had a large central stem and two small side pegs. Due to this rugged construction, there was only one revision at an 8-year follow-up of 112 cases (Eftekhar 1983).

Freedom of rotation would result in reduced shear stresses at the cement-bone interface of the tibial component and would allow for errors in the rotational position at surgery. In the anatomic knee, however, the axis of internal-external rotation, while not fixed, is biased to the medial side. Whether a central pivot is a major disadvantage, especially after soft tissue balancing at surgery, is not known.

Reproducing the Menisci

In the early 1970s, evidence was emerging of the importance of the menisci to knee function (Bullough et al. 1970; Walker and Erkman 1975; Krause et al. 1976). An important mechanical property of the menisci was that they allowed the lateral and medial femoral condyles to slide anteriorly and posteriorly on the tibial plateau, while interposition between the femoral-tibial bearing surfaces produced congruity. This was possible because of the deformability of the menisci, their loose peripheral attachments, and their high tensile strength. The mobility of the lateral meniscus was much greater than that of the medial. It was not surprising that artificial menisci would be considered for inclusion in an artificial knee design, because the problem of lack of congruity between the femoral-tibial bearing surfaces would be solved.

Three different types of meniscal bearing knees originated independently at almost the same time. The first of these was at the Nuffield Orthopaedic Centre in Oxford, England. Joseph Trueta, MD, and Peter Bullough, MD, both pathologists, had made fundamental discoveries in the etiology of osteoarthritis of the knee concerning the areas of load transmission. Also involved with this research were John Goodfellow, FRCS, an orthopedic surgeon at the Nuffield Hospital, and John O'Connor, PhD, a Professor of Engineering at Oxford University. There was also collaboration with the research group at Imperial College London, notably Alice Maroudas, PhD, a physiologist; Geoff Kempson, PhD, a mechanical engineer; and Michael Freeman, FRCS, an orthopedic surgeon. Working at Imperial College and the London Hospital, they were studying the properties of articular cartilage and synovial fluid in relation to the mechanical factors which led to cartilage degeneration and osteoarthritis. These collaborations are notable because they provided a stimulating research environment.

Central to all of this work was an understanding of the anatomy of the joint and the mechanisms of load transmission. Areas of cartilage which experienced only small loads were subject to disuse atrophy and degeneration, while areas of excessive loading degenerated due to mechanical failure (Bullough et al. 1968). This theory was investigated for the hip joint by Seth Greenwald who developed an elaborate loading rig and devised novel methods using colored dyes for showing the areas of contact as loads were progressively applied (Greenwald and Haynes 1972). Greenwald had graduated in structural engineering from Massachusetts Institute of Technology and was about to embark on a PhD at Oxford on the design of cooling towers. While waiting to meet his intended supervisor in a public house in Oxford, he fell into conversation with John O'Connor and John Goodfellow, who persuaded him that hip joints were a far more interesting topic than cooling towers. Although Greenwald's work on the hip was never followed up at Oxford by parallel work on the knee, it had a major influence on the understanding of knee mechanics. These studies strongly suggested that in the knee, in order to maintain areas of contact which were sufficiently large to avoid excessive contact stresses, the menisci had to be playing a major role in force transmission.

Goodfellow had observed that osteoarthritis of the knee most frequently initiated anteriorly on the medial side, over an area which contacted in full extension. Hence, the problem was identified as compartmental rather than involving the whole joint. The artificial knees which had been designed at that time, including the Freeman-Swanson, were designed for arthritis involving the entire joint. On the other hand, a unicompartmental knee could be used to treat the osteoarthritis at an early stage. Several unicompartmental designs were already in use, but they had a serious problem according to Goodfellow and O'Connor (1978): the incongruent bearing surfaces produced small contact areas with high contact stresses between the metal and the polyethylene, which would lead to deformation of the plastic and long-term wear. Moreover, they had determined using the Oxford knee rig with a similar dye technique as Greenwald's that the contact points on the tibial surfaces displaced posteriorly during flexion. Hence, a fully conforming unicompartmental knee where the components were fixed to the femur and tibia was not an option.

A solution to this dilemma was elusive until O'Connor and Goodfellow attended a conference at the University of Leeds in late 1973, where Seedhom presented his research on the importance of the menisci in distributing the load but allowing sliding motion to occur (Seedhom 1976). In a sudden insight in the car trip back to Oxford, it was realized that a bearing which included a movable meniscus made from polyethylene was a solution. The femoral component would be a curved metal runner with a spherical outer surface. A polished metal plate would cover the resected

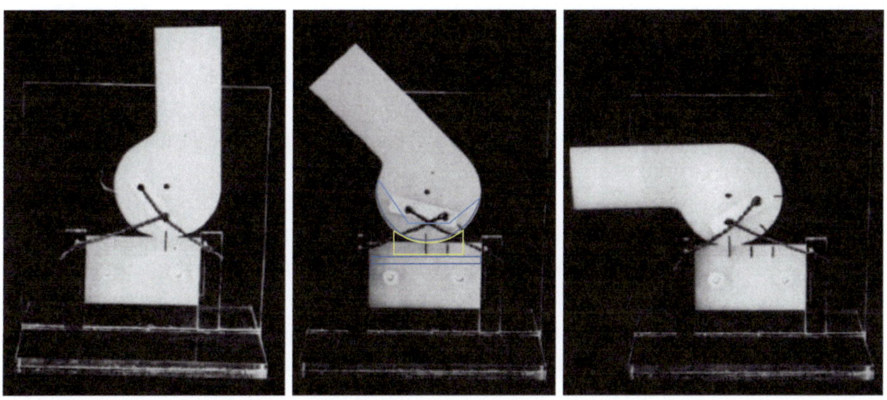

Fig. 11.2 The Oxford unicondylar knee was based on the four-bar linkage model of normal knee mechanics consisting of the cruciates, the femur, and the tibia. The linkage produces posterior rolling of the femur on the tibia while flexing. To maintain full congruency of the femoral-tibial contacts in order to minimize contact stresses, a meniscal-shaped plastic bearing (yellow) was interposed between the metal femoral component (blue), and the metal tibial plate (blue), fixed to the resected tibial surface. The meniscus slides anterior-posterior on the tibial plate during flexion (Goodfellow and O'Connor 1978). (Reprinted with permission from Journal of Bone & Joint Surgery B)

medial tibial plateau. In between would be a plastic meniscus, with a spherical upper surface to match the femoral component and a flat lower surface to match the tibial plate. With this configuration, a full contact area could be achieved for all flexion angles, even if displacements and internal-external rotations occurred. For convenience of manufacture, half of the femoral component of a Geometric knee was used, because of its spherical bearing surface. The tibial plate and the plastic meniscus were relatively easy to manufacture (Goodfellow and O'Connor 1978). The knee was called the Oxford meniscal bearing knee, since shortened to the Oxford Uni.

The design had a possible failure mode in that the meniscus, being unrestrained, could dislocate anteriorly or posteriorly. However, trials on knee specimens showed that if the thickness of the meniscus was made in millimeter increments, selection of the correct thickness at surgery would prevent dislocation from occurring. Nonetheless dislocation did occur occasionally, but this was solved by slightly increasing the lip height of the meniscus and ensuring the correct slope of the tibial metal plate in the sagittal plane. In laboratory wear testing, and in subsequent clinical application, the polyethylene wear was shown to be minimal, attributed to the fully conforming bearing surfaces. The Oxford Uni, which has had a few minor changes to the design and technique over the years, has continued to be widely used and is the largest selling unicompartmental knee (Pandit et al. 2015). The long-term results are similar to those of an artificial knee, as reported by the developing group. However, to achieve such results, David W Murray, FRCS, has emphasized the necessity of frequent use and acquiring expertise in case selection and surgical technique. Carrying out the procedure only occasionally leads to inferior results. A history of the Oxford knee has been documented (Price et al. 2007).

One of the first meniscal bearing artificial knees was designed by Julian Minns, PhD, a medical physicist working at Dryburn Hospital in Durham in northeast England. The major responsibility of Minns was to maintain the technical equipment of the hospital, although being inventive, he found artificial joint design an intriguing outlet. He had also formed a number of contacts in the joint replacement field including the staff at Wrightington Hospital where John Charnley was located. Minns did not want to design just another condylar knee, as he saw the knee as a complex mechanism with many functional parts which he wanted to represent. He recognized the multiple motions which occurred between the femur and the tibia and the role that the cruciate ligaments played in guiding those motions. He also noted that wear in total hips was still a problem even with polyethylene in the conforming Charnley hip. He started initially with a unicompartmental design in 1978 where the anterior-posterior motion of a plastic meniscus was guided in a T-slot (Minns and Campbell 1978). Using a photoelastic technique, he demonstrated the much lower plastic contact stresses in a full conformity bearing surface compared with the stresses in a fixed-bearing shallow polyethylene surface. Minns then moved to a meniscal bearing artificial knee consisting of a condylar femoral component and a metal tibial baseplate with a cutout to preserve the cruciate ligaments. Each tibial condyle had a dovetail slot which housed a polyethylene meniscal bearing with an upper surface in close conformity with the metal femoral condyle. As the knee was flexed and extended, the lateral and medial menisci moved independently in their tracks. Extensive testing was carried out, showing low wear and low torque transmission (Minns 1989). A consequence was no loosening of tibial and femoral components in 450 cases at up to 5 years. Dislocation of the plastic bearings was thought to be avoided because of the dovetail grooves, except in a few cases where there was excessive laxity (Minns 1989). The Minns meniscal knee was used by a few surgeons in England, but it was eventually discontinued for commercial reasons.

Meanwhile, in New Jersey in the USA, Fred Buechel, a surgeon from New Jersey Medical School, and Michael Pappas, PhD, a mechanical engineer at New Jersey Institute of Technology, had been thinking of how artificial joints could be designed which had low contact stresses to minimize wear while still allowing freedom of motion. In 1977 they designed a floating shoulder with an interposed polyethylene bearing and were considering how to apply the design concept to the knee. The main design criteria were low contact stresses but freedom of motion. They had studied the Geometric knee which had low contacts stresses, but the motion was so

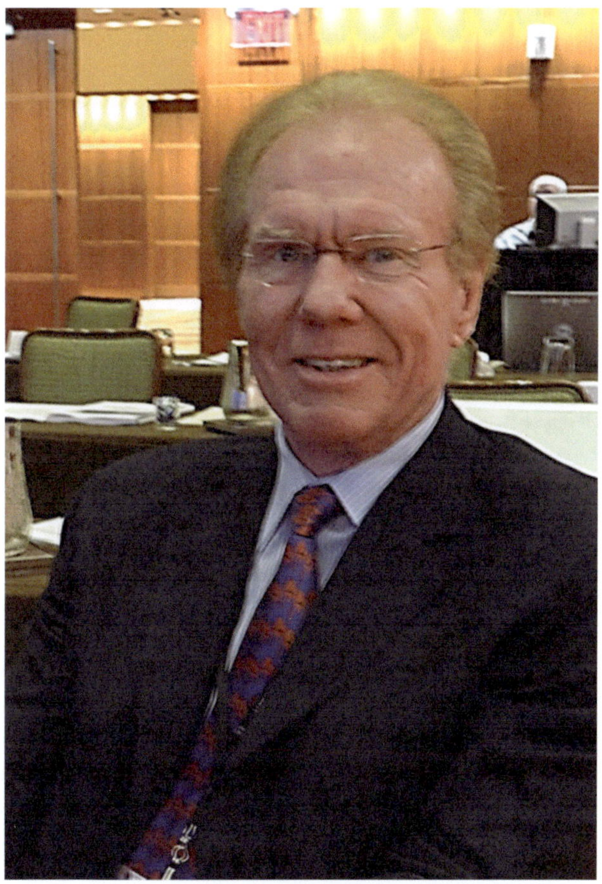

Fig. 11.3 Fred Buechel, MD, from New Jersey Medical School, formed a life-long partnership with Mike Pappas, PhD, a Professor of Mechanical Engineering at New Jersey Institute of Technology. Together, in the late 1970s, they designed the low contact stress (LCS) rotating platform knee. This unique configuration minimized the contact stresses, yet allowed freedom of rotation so that the knee could move more naturally without constraint. The systematic surgical technique and careful follow-up studies have resulted in the continuous clinical success of this design to the present day. (Photo taken at The Knee Society 2018) (© Peter S Walker)

restricted that loosening and limitation of motion were problems. Buechel and Pappas initially designed a meniscal bearing knee very similar to that of Minns, but with curved tracks instead of straight. This was consistent with an axis of rotation close to the center of the knee (Buechel and Pappas 1986). As with the Minns, the design was intended to retain both cruciates, but they also extended the concept to retention of only the posterior cruciate. In both designs, the sagittal radii of the femoral condyles were larger distally and smaller posteriorly, as for the anatomic knee. As a result the contact areas would be slightly reduced in flexion with an increase in contact stresses, although this would only have a small effect on the wear because most weight-bearing activity is carried out with the knee at lower angles of flexion. The short-term clinical results of the meniscal bearing knee reported by Buechel were excellent, with no mechanical failures (Buechel and Pappas 1986).

Soon after, Buechel and Pappas extended their design concepts to a rotating platform design. Using the same femoral component as before, the metal tibial component was a polished flat plate covering the resected surface of the tibia, with a tapered central peg for fixation. An interposed one-piece plastic rotating platform was dished medially and laterally to match the femoral condyles, with a central peg which pivoted in a hole in the central peg of the tibial plate. This configuration allowed for freedom of internal-external rotation about a central axis. The knee was called the LCS, low contact stress. This system successfully combined low constraint forces in rotation with low contact stresses. Initially this was only intended for limited application: "the use of the rotating intermediate bearing element in cases where cruciate function has been lost." Gradually, however, Buechel and other surgeons recognized the easier surgery and the more reliable results with this design.

Previous research studies on anatomic knee kinematics had shown that the rotational axis of internal-external varied with the flexion angle but was biased towards the medial side, consistent with the higher conformity on the medial side and the mobility on the lateral side. In contrast, the axis of rotation of the LCS was central. Despite this apparent mismatch of the kinematics imposed by the rotating platform, the freedom of axial rotation provided advantages. In function, the knee could find its preferred rotational position, so that the knee was unconstrained in turning and twisting actions. In addition, freedom of rotation compensated for any rotational error in placing the tibial component at surgery. This was useful in that there was no general agreement for the optimal rotational position. The absence of the cruciate ligaments with the rotating platform design was an advantage in simplifying the surgery, and in any case, anterior-posterior stability was provided by the conforming bearing surfaces themselves. At 10-year follow-up, the LCS rotating platform design gave 97% survivorship (Buechel et al. 2001).

The LCS rotating platform of Buechel and Pappas built up a strong following. The rotating platform concept was incorporated into most artificial knee systems from several companies. The way this was done was to use the same femoral component as for the CR design, in combination with a rotating platform tibial component. The original purpose of the design was to minimize the wear, and this would be valid at the time the LCS was designed. However, today's polyethylenes are much more wear resistant, so reducing the contact stresses is no longer such an advantage. Even when there is relatively low conformity such as in a typical CR design, the wear measured in tests on simulating machines and observed on retrievals is usually quite small, not sufficient to be a major concern. Another factor is that it has been shown that while the wear on the condylar bearing surfaces of the rotating platform is small, when this wear is added to that between the tibial plate and the lower surface of the plastic component, the total wear is similar to that of a partially conforming artificial knee (Haider and Garvin 2008; Stoner et al. 2013). Wear tracks on the tibial plate have shown circular arcs indicating rotation during function, which has been confirmed in fluoroscopic kinematic studies (Lacour et al. 2014). Consequently the advantage of the rotating platform concept has now become its rotational freedom, an advantage at surgery, and in the reduction in the torque transmitted to the tibial fixation. Particularly when applied to a PS design, the rotational freedom is useful in high flexion where typically a fixed-bearing PS design can be too constrained (Meftah et al. 2012). A positive appraisal of the mobile bearing concept, with a European perspective, was provided by Karol Hamelynck (2006): "Three decades after its introduction, the mobile bearing design remains relevant and important."

Different Medial and Lateral Laxity and Stability

In the 1970s and 1980s, many studies were carried out on the laxity of the knee, under both unloaded and loaded conditions (see Chap. 4), but there was little attention given to the relative laxities between the lateral and medial sides. For example, in measuring rotational laxity, the center of rotation in the transverse plane was not identified. In one study of knee motion controlled by the quadriceps during flexion, there was an average of 8.6 mm posterior displacement of the center of the femur accompanied by 15° external rotation of the femur (Rovick et al. 1991). That could only mean an axis of internal-external rotation on the medial side of the knee, but this was not highlighted. Nevertheless, such motion and laxity studies provided the guidelines for a number of artificial knee designs of the CR and PS types. The understanding of knee motion had been influenced by the four-bar linkage model in the sagittal plane, where the femoral-tibial contact points displaced posteriorly with flexion, guided by the cruciate ligaments (O'Connor et al. 1989). Hence, there were two perspectives of knee mechanics, one focusing on the ligaments being elastic and extensible allowing laxity, the other on their stiffness and in defining the motion.

In the mid-1990s, in a teaching session on knee motion at the London Hospital, successive lectures by Michael Freeman and Peter Walker confused the audience. Walker described rigid body motion of the femur relative to the tibia, with fixed axes being defined in the femur and tibia. The external rotation and the posterior displacement of the femur with flexion were shown separately. The posterior displacement of the origin of the distal femur was referred to as "rollback," giving the impression that the femur displaced posteriorly on the tibia as the knee was flexed from extension to flexion. Freeman on the other hand insisted that there was no posterior displacement of the femur on the tibia and no rollback. Instead, he claimed that as the femur was flexed, there were two simultaneous rotations, flexion and axial rotation, but no displacements. However, Walker's posterior displacement was defined with respect to the origin of the femur relative to the origin of the tibia, which would also occur in Freeman's model. Both explanations of knee motion were consistent, but it was not appreciated at the time. Nevertheless, Freeman's model was easier to visualize.

In subsequent studies, Freeman and other researchers further demonstrated the medial pivot action as the knee was flexed using MRI studies of loaded and unloaded knees for knee specimens and for living subjects (Freeman and Pinskerova 2005; Pinskerova et al. 2004; Williams and Logan 2004). Prominent co-authors of this work were Freeman himself; Vera Pinskerova, MD, a pathologist from Prague; and Andy Williams, FRCS, an orthopedic resident from Saint Mary's Hospital in London. Their data was consistent with the anatomy of the knee whereby the medial tibial plateau was dished and the meniscus relatively immobile, while on the lateral side, the tibial plateau was convex, sloped downwards posteriorly, and with a mobile meniscus. It seemed logical to apply this important finding to the design of an artificial knee. This idea was developed in England and in the USA at about the same time, in the mid- to the late 1990s.

In England, Michael Freeman worked with Michael Tuke, PhD, a faculty member at Imperial College, London, who later founded Finsbury Instruments. A US patent was issued in 1993 describing a spherical conforming bearing medially and a curved track laterally to allow internal-external rotation pivoting about the medial

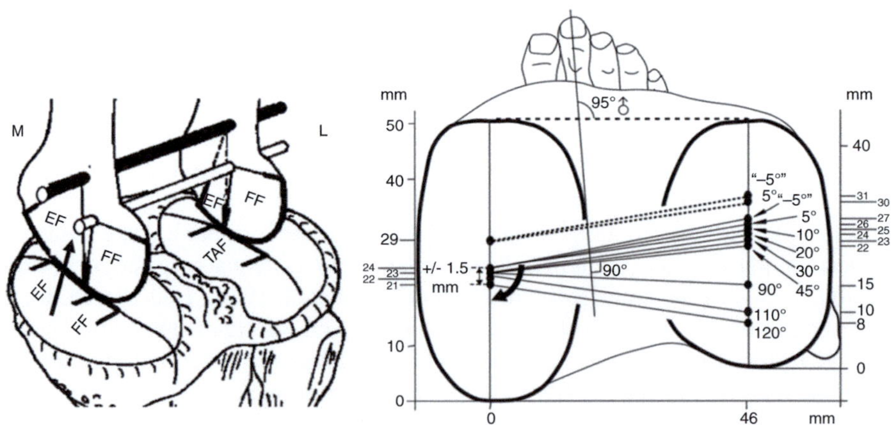

Fig. 11.4 A basis for a medial pivot type of artificial knee. Knee specimens were flexed to different angles and MRI scans taken. The succession of transverse flexion axes (white axis at left, arrow) through the femoral condyles were projected on to the tibial surface. The femur appears to pivot on the medial side as it flexes. The anterior positions near extension are due to femoral rolling up the anterior facet on the tibial plateau (Iwaki et al. 2000). Subsequent MRI studies on subjects showed that the axial rotation depended on different positions and muscle actions of the subjects, but still with relatively small medial displacements. (Reprinted with permission from Journal of Bone & Joint Surgery B)

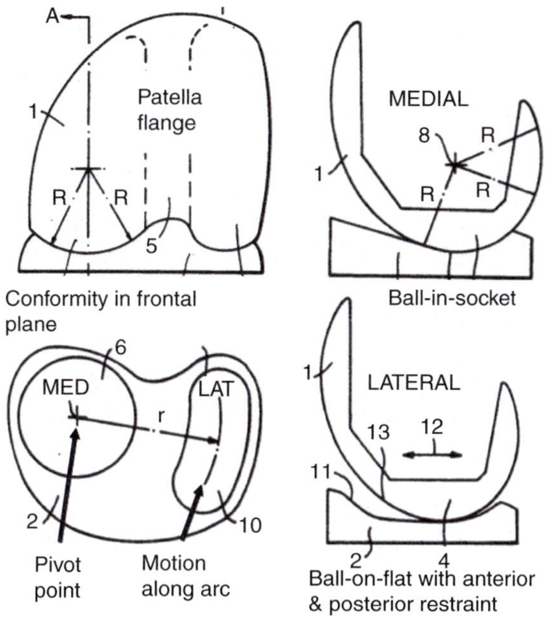

Fig. 11.5 The first US patent for a medial pivot knee, filed in February 1992 by Michael Tuke and Michael Freeman, of the University of London, England. The design was modified from the original Freeman-Swanson knee by making a spherical bearing medially and by flattening the lateral tibial surface. (US Patent 5,219,362. Filed 1992, issued 1993. Tuke and Freeman 1993)

side (Tuke and Freeman 1993). Tuke and Freeman described the invention as follows: "The present invention accordingly seeks to provide an improved knee prosthesis which will allow the patient to move his knee substantially in the same manner as though he had not had to undergo implantation of a knee prosthesis". The recently introduced "Forgotten Joint Score" expresses a similar way of evaluating a patient's artificial knee.

Finsbury Instruments was already manufacturing the Freeman-Samuelson knee, a further development of the original Freeman-Swanson. This design was then modified to produce the Medial Rotation Knee based on the patent. In a mean 6-year follow-up (Mannan and Scott 2009), the loosening was not increased, and there was an improved survivorship of 98% compared with the Freeman-Samuelson knee, while the "deep medial dish provided enhanced stability without recourse to an intercondylar cam and post." This last phrase refers to a posterior stabilized (PS) type of knee. Anterior-posterior stability of the knee has been noted by patients in subsequent evaluations of the medial pivot knee, which represents an important positive feature of this type of design.

The Medial Rotation Knee was used clinically until Finsbury Instruments was purchased by DePuy in 2009. The knee was then redesigned by Mike Tuke who formed a new company in 2011 called MatOrtho. The new design was called the SAIPH Knee. Freeman and Pinskerova pursued the medial pivot concept separately

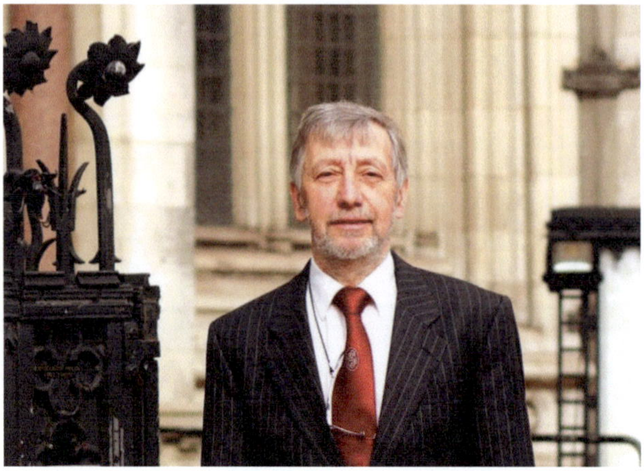

Fig. 11.6 Michael Tuke worked in Alan Swanson's Biomechanics Laboratory in the late 1960s and played a major role in early knee designs of Freeman and Swanson. Mike Tuke founded his own company, Finsbury Orthopaedics in 1978, with a successful record of innovative designs for the knee and hip. Among these designs was the Medial Rotation Knee, used now for 25 years. Later, after the formation of a new company MatOrtho, based in Leatherhead, England, Mike Tuke upgraded the knee, calling it the SAIFF knee. This knee continues to increase in popularity worldwide. (Photo courtesy Michael Tuke)

through the Swiss company Medacta, calling their design the GMK Sphere (Scott et al. 2016). Pinskerova's explanation of the rationale was "The concept of the GMK Sphere TKA is based on medial antero-posterior stability combined with lateral freedom of motion, resulting in a medial center of longitudinal rotation as exhibited by the normal knee… This movement is possible because the lateral collateral ligament is loose in flexion. The combination of a fully congruent medial compartment and an unconstrained lateral tibial surface together with tight medial collateral ligament and loose lateral collateral ligament enables flexion accompanied by femoral external rotation around the stable medial condyle" (Pinskerova 2016). This motion was demonstrated in a computer model (Morra et al. 2012).

While the development of the medial pivot knee was proceeding in England, a separate but related development took place in the USA, also from the mid-1990s. The main driver of this work was David Blaha MD, from Ann Arbor, Michigan, who had taken an interest in knee mechanics and total knee design since his residency in the mid-1970s. At that time, Larry Matthews, MD; David Sonstegard, PhD; and Herb Kaufer, MD, from the University of Michigan Medical Center in Ann Arbor, were designing the Spherocentric knee (Matthews et al. 1975). As reported in a paper to the Orthopedic Research Society (ORS) in 1975, this knee was conceived as a combination of a hinge and a condylar replacement where a centrally embedded ball-in-socket allowed rotational laxity such that the implant absorbed far less energy when torque or bending were applied, compared with a fixed hinge, and hence would move more naturally and experience less loosening. In principle the Spherocentric had some similarity to the Attenborough, but the latter had more

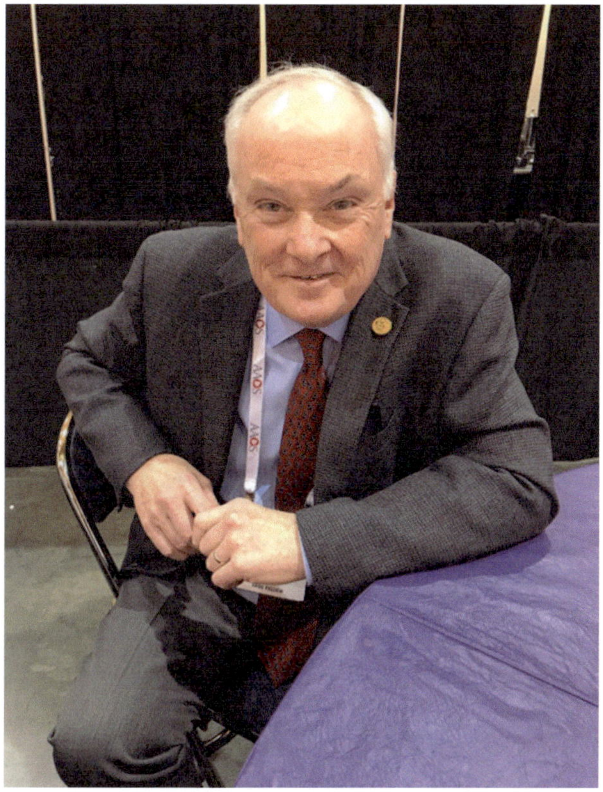

Fig. 11.7 David Blaha was one of the early originators of the medial pivot knee concept. His early interest in biomechanics was sparked by working with Herb Kaufer, MD, and Larry Matthews, MD, at the University of Michigan, Ann Arbor in the USA. Following a fellowship with Mike Freeman, he returned to Ann Arbor to continue experiments on knee motion, which he applied to a medial pivot knee design. Working with Steve White, this was accomplished in the Advance Medial Pivot knee made by Wright Medical. (Photo taken at AAOS meeting, 2018) (© Peter S Walker)

substantial fixation stems than the Spherocentric. David Blaha found an ideal environment in the area of knee mechanics during a fellowship with Michael Freeman at the London Hospital in the late 1970s. They were both skeptical that the knee motion was guided by the cruciate ligaments in a four-bar link mechanism as first proposed by Zuppinger and Strasser in the nineteenth century and later embellished by O'Connor and others at Oxford (O'Connor et al. 1989). However, Freeman and Blaha did not formulate any systematic experiments on which to base a more advanced theory, other than making empirical observations that as the knee was flexed, the medial femoral condyle appeared to be in a nearly constant position on the tibia while the lateral condyle displaced posteriorly. On returning to the Ann Arbor in the early 1980s, Blaha initiated a knee motion study on specimens using Vicon equipment, which suggested that during flexion, the axis of rotation moved in three dimensions and was not restricted to planar motion. Subsequent experiments on knee specimens confirmed this, by using an "open chain" model where the femur was fixed horizontally and the tibia was initially fully flexed (Blaha et al. 2003). The tibia was then extended by pulling on the quadriceps tendon. Gradual external rotation of the tibia was observed. A remarkable finding was that the motion changed very little when the cruciates were excised, from which Blaha concluded that the four-bar linkage model for guiding knee motion was inconsistent with the

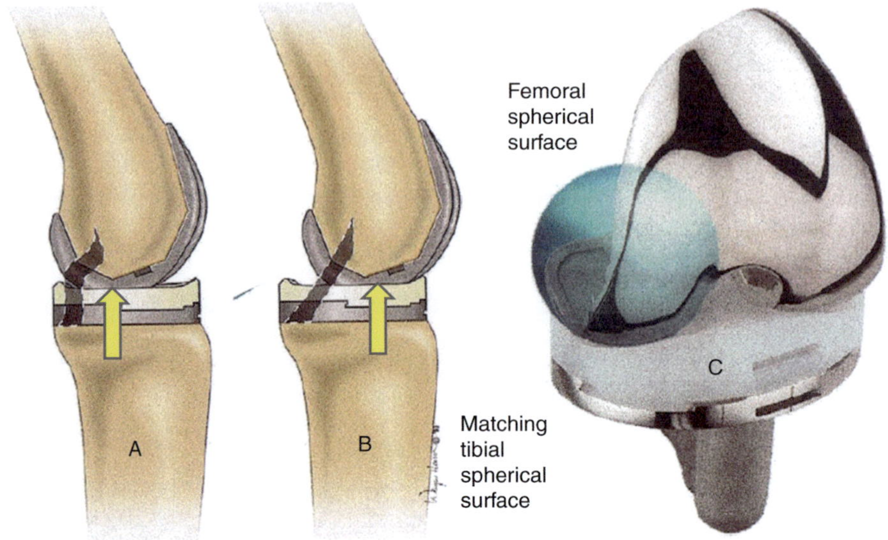

Fig. 11.8 David Blaha was one of the main proponents of the medial pivot concept in the USA. This figure shows the main concepts. The basic principle was anterior-posterior stabilization using a ball-in-socket on the medial side. (**a**) In a CR posterior cruciate retaining knee, just before load acceptance. (**b**) On load acceptance, anterior sliding of the femur occurs. (**c**) In a medial pivot knee the conforming medial side prevents the anterior sliding (Blaha 2004). (Reprinted with permission from Journal of Arthroplasty)

experimental data. By 1991 a total knee design based on a more stable medial side and an unconstrained lateral side had emerged. It took a long time to find interest from a company, but the idea was eventually taken up by Wright Manufacturing in Memphis, who were then making the 913 PS type design from the Hospital for Special Surgery. The new concept became the Advance Medial Pivot due mainly to the efforts of David Blaha and Steve White, but it was not until 1998 that the first knees were used in patients. Other surgeons involved with the project were Murale Jasty, Brad Penenberg, and Bill Maloney.

In the first few years of clinical application, there was uncertainty about how to align the femoral component on the distal femur to produce the best balance of collateral tightness in extension and flexion, and whether the posterior cruciate should be retained or resected. Lack of high flexion in many cases was largely solved by sloping the tibial cut posteriorly to the anatomic 5–7°. The idea of a medial pivot knee was not as widely accepted as anticipated. There were several likely reasons. The MRI studies by Freeman, Pinskerova, and others, showing the medial pivot motion of the anatomic knee, had not yet been published, while the same applied to Blaha's own studies with open and closed chain experiments (Blaha et al. 2003). Wright Manufacturing had limited marketing capabilities compared with Zimmer, Stryker, DePuy, and Biomet. But probably the main factor was that the larger companies had their flagship CR and PS designs well represented by prominent surgeons from renowned institutions. A further factor was that there was an absence of a sufficient body of evidence from follow-up studies that the medial pivot was performing any better in patients than the CR and PS knees that dominated the market. Even by 2002 (Blaha 2002), there was only one study of the Advance Medial Pivot, in which it was stated: "In the author's series, knees at two years follow-up had an average Knee Society score of 91 and average 116° range of motion. In a multicenter study of four hundred and one patients, the average range of motion was 118°. In a comparison study of forty-three patients with a medial pivot in one knee and a CR or PS design in the other knee, a majority of patients rated the medial pivot knee superior in ease of rehabilitation, motion, stability, and overall satisfaction."

This latter study of bilateral cases was reported separately in a publication in 2004 (Pritchett 2004). In the same study, Pritchett also found that an ACL + PCL retaining design was preferred over a CR or PS, while there was equal preference for an ACL + PCL and medial pivot designs. In a further paper by Blaha (2004), where the biomechanical principles of the medial pivot concept were expounded, he emphasized the anterior-posterior stability throughout flexion as being the key characteristic. In a later clinical paper, Pritchett considered different reasons for the patient preferences (Pritchett 2011). In his view, the most important was the AP stability provided, as well as an enhanced quadriceps lever arm. Other factors were the paradoxical sliding of the CR and patella problems with the PS. A strength of the studies by Pritchett was that these were bilateral cases, with different knee designs in opposite sides. Hence, there is a consistency between these two authors, although in the actual clinical trials, it was difficult to specifically identify anterior-posterior stability from the standard clinical evaluation schemes used at the time. The overall picture was that the medial pivot knee performed at least as well as standard CR and PS knees and may have been superior in certain aspects. Recently a 15-year average follow-up study was reported of 347 medial pivot knees (Macheras et al. 2017). The average range of flexion was 120°, and the survivorship at 17 years was 98.8%. On the important aspect of anterior-posterior stability, a major benefit proposed for this design was "No post-operative instability was observed in our study. All knees were objectively stable throughout the range 0–90°... The patients in our study noted a great sense of stability, particularly in single-leg weight-bearing positions, they felt strong on stairs and they judged their knees comfort during walking stable and natural overall... Undoubtedly the medial pivot design gives an inherent stability to the TKA." On the question of whether the posterior cruciate ligament (PCL) should be retained, a difficult question when the design was introduced, these authors found no difference in clinical results, but somewhat more difficulty balancing the knee when the PCL was intact.

A different type of tibial insert where the medial side was more dished than the lateral to provide more constraint was introduced in 2015. The medial side was not fully conforming, in contrast to the medial pivot designs. Called the Medial Congruent Bearing, this insert was to be used with the existing cruciate retaining (CR) femoral component in the Persona Knee System. Designed by Steve White and Bill Maloney, MD, this insert was a modification of Aaron Hofmann's ultracongruent insert. The Medial Congruent Bearing can be described as a "loose medial pivot" in that there was still some anterior-posterior laxity, especially in flexion due to the reducing radius of the femoral component. This design can be claimed to be more anatomic than a fixed medial pivot, as the medial side of the anatomic knee does have some anterior-posterior laxity, but much less than on the lateral side.

Guided Motion Knees with Biomimetic Motion or Geometry

In the past, the design of most standard condylar replacement knees has been based on geometrical parameters, with ease of manufacture as an important design criterion. In the sagittal plane of the femoral component, a larger distal radius has blended into a smaller radius posteriorly. In the frontal plane, the radii have ranged from anatomic at about 20 mm to being close to flat. The radii of the tibial surfaces in the frontal and sagittal planes have been larger than those of the femoral component to provide laxity in anterior-posterior and rotation. The depth and V-angle of the patella flange has usually been based on anatomic values. Intercondylar cam-posts have further constrained the relative motion, mainly in the anterior-posterior direction. At surgery, ligament balancing has been carried out so that the ligaments still perform their primary functions, particularly in providing varus-valgus stability. Such condylar knees, even with symmetric condyle shapes, can move asymmetrically, but not in the same way as an anatomic knee.

The design goal of Guided Motion knees is to go one step further than a standard condylar knee in guiding or controlling the femoral-tibial motion, to more resemble the motion of the normal anatomic knee. That said, it is not easy to define what "normal anatomic knee motion" is, because there are many activities an individual can perform, and every individual's knee moves differently. There are even differences in performing the same function repetitively. Using knee specimens, the motion has been measured in passive flexion, in flexion under quadriceps action, and where forces act in both the quadriceps and hamstrings. In the living subject, fluoroscopy has been used to measure motion in squatting, in leg raising, lunging, and step and chair rise. Now that mobile fluoroscopy units are available, motion has been measured in regular walking and in other activities. In an attempt to summarize, there are certain motion characteristics that are common to everybody. For level walking studied on a mobile fluoroscopy unit, Gray et al. (2019) stated: "Anterior-posterior translations of the tibio-femoral contact centers were significantly greater in the lateral compartment than the medial compartment. Posterior translations… were associated with increasing knee flexion. The center of rotation of the knee in the transverse plane was located predominantly on the medial side…" In walking, however, the flexion angles during the loaded stance phase are limited to about 20°. In a lunge activity up to 115° flexion, again using fluoroscopy, Feng et al. (2015) found that the medial femoral condyle translated first anteriorly and then posteriorly up to maximum flexion. The lateral side moved continuously posteriorly, but with much larger displacements than on the medial side. The internal rotation of the tibia was 27°. At maximum flexion, the lateral condyle was at the very posterior of the tibia (risky for an artificial knee). Another important measure of knee motion is the laxity. At a given flexion angle on the neutral path of motion, the magnitudes of the anterior-posterior laxity and internal-external laxity are an important parameter in defining motion. Nobody designing an artificial knee with anatomic motion would rigidly constrain the motion to the average. The values of laxity depend on the compressive load acting, but in all conditions, the medial side has much less anterior-posterior laxity compared with the lateral side (Reynolds et al. 2017). It can be concluded that if a Guided Motion knee is to mimic anatomic motions in function, the displacements and rotations as they are known at this time should be reproduced.

There have been several attempts to achieve anatomic knee motion. The first was to use a "tibial surface generation" method. This was first described by Ewald and by Seedhom in the 1970s (see Chap. 9). An anatomically shaped femoral component was moved in a flexion path, including some laxity, to generate the tibial surface. This process was later carried out by Walker and Ewald (1988) using computer graphics, where motion data from knee specimens was input. The tibial surfaces generated from the above were all similar, a relatively shallow lateral side and a more concave medial side. This "tibial surface generation" method (Walker 2001) was later expanded upon by starting with different femoral component surfaces (Walker 2014). This included a converging condyle version, which had been patented in 2001 by Takei. In addition, intercondylar surfaces and housings on the femur produced ramps or projecting posts on the central tibia.

Yet further application of the "tibial surface generation" method was by a group at Massachusetts General Hospital, including Harry Rubash, MD; Guaon Li, PhD; and Varadarajan, PhD (Varadarajan et al. 2015; Zumbrunn et al. 2015). Starting with a femoral component, they input motion data obtained from Guaon Li, PhD, using fluoroscopy of normal subjects. What was unique about their method was that the motion comprised all 6 degrees of freedom, including vertical displacements and varus-valgus rotations. The resulting tibial surfaces were "biomimetic" in that the medial tibial surface was moderately dished but the lateral surface was convex in the sagittal plane. At the anterior and posterior of each surface were lips representing the spaces that would be occupied by the menisci at the extremes of motion. The design was called the biomimetic knee. In the version of the knee designed by Varadarajan, the anterior cruciate ligament was resected. Nevertheless, using KneeSim software for motion analysis, it was found that "the biomimetic knee showed an overall medial pivot and greater rollback of the lateral femoral condyle than the medial condyle." In the version analyzed by Zumbrunn, the anterior cruciate was retained with the proposition that there would be even further reproduction of anatomic motion. In this version, certain nuances of the motion were found be even closer to normal. A computer modelling approach to a similar concept was described by Liu et al. (2012).

In about 2004, a different approach was taken to designing a guided motion knee. It was recognized by Jan Victor, MD; Johan Bellemans, MD; Michael Ries, MD; and others that the limited range of flexion achieved by artificial knees was inhibiting a number of functional activities where higher flexion was required. It was proposed that if normal kinematics could be achieved, together with other factors such as

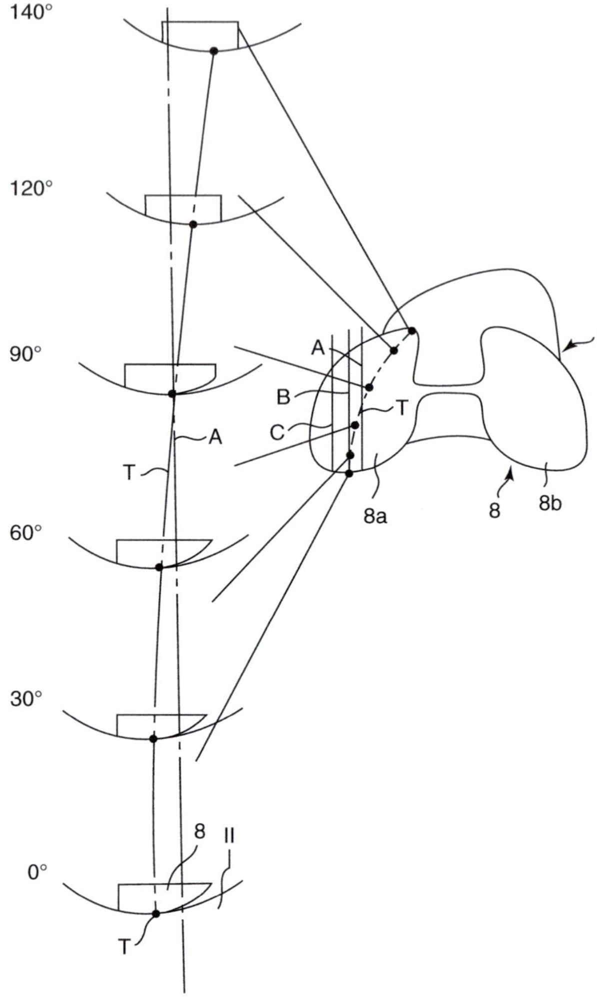

Fig. 11.9 Tsunenori Takei designed a total knee in 2001 where the lateral femoral condyle converged towards high flexion. This facilitated posterior rollback of the lateral femoral condyle with axial rotation, increasing the range of flexion. (US Patent 6,406,497 B2. Filed 2001, issued 2002)

condylar offset, flexion could be increased (Victor and Bellemans 2006). The design group decided to use the PS concept but to make the lateral tibial surface almost flat: "Preserving the anterior and posterior cruciate ligament has been attempted and resulted in more normal kinematics and better flexion. Surgical feasibility limits the potential of this solution. The other solution is to provide kinematic guidance and stabilization by the prosthetic design through surface geometry and the cam-post mechanism." This arrangement produced posterior displacement with flexion, but substantially more laterally than medially. The name of the device was the Journey BCS knee introduced in 2005. In several clinical follow-up studies, the knee did achieve a high range of flexion, but there were some complications of instability, possibly due to excessively posterior contacts and rotation. Accordingly, a redesign was made by moving contacts anteriorly, the modified design being evaluated by fluoroscopy (Zambianchi et al. 2018). The results were "The design adjustments performed onto the second-generation prosthesis to limit excessive posterior displacement of the femoral condyles, as well as femoral component rotation in weight-bearing conditions, contributed to modify replaced knee's kinematics during daily living activities, as confirmed by fluoroscopy data." This Journey design is biomimetic in certain ways, but relying on the mechanics of a cam-post to provide much of the motion guidance reproducibly, rather than relying on ligaments which vary with the individual.

In 2008, a biomimetic type of guided motion knee was conceived, based on a kinematic analysis (Floerkemeier et al. 2011; Frosch et al. 2009). The originality was that the bearing surfaces of the tibial component were asymmetric, convex for the lateral side and concave for the medial, together with a sagittal offset between the lateral and medial profiles. The preference for rolling rather than sliding would reduce the wear of the polyethylene. The idea was the basis of an artificial knee design called the Aequos knee. After clinical application, fluoroscopic studies were carried out which showed that the patella tendon angle resembled that of normal knees (Wachowski et al. 2011). This was due to the femoral rollback which reduced the angle with flexion, reducing the force between the patella and the anterior femur.

A further approach was to introduce a third bearing between the lateral and medial tibial bearing surfaces, which would replace the function of the anterior cruciate in early flexion, by limiting the anterior-posterior displacements and maintaining an anterior position of the femur (Walker and Borukhov 2017). The work

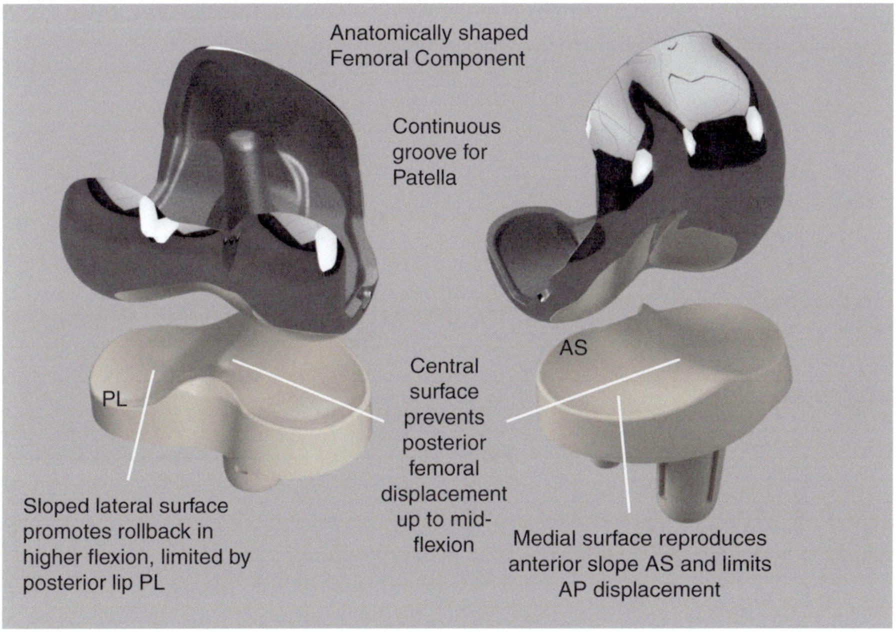

Fig. 11.10 A guided motion knee based on reproducing the stabilizing mechanisms of the natural structures and on reproducing the normal motion patterns. There are three bearing surfaces each performing different functions, with the medial side being more conforming than the lateral, to produce anatomic motion, laxity, and stability characteristics (Walker and Borukhov 2017). (CAD models by Stephen Chan)

was carried out in Walker's Laboratory for Orthopaedic Implant Design at the NYU Langone Orthopedic Hospital. The design was called the Replica Anatomic knee. This guided motion design was based on replicating the laxity and stability normally provided by the cruciate ligaments and the menisci, which had been determined in previous biomechanical studies (Walker et al. 2015; Reynolds et al. 2017). The testing method for the design was to impose a sequence of anterior-posterior and internal-external forces on the knee, over a full flexion range and measure the laxities. The laxity values were then compared with those from an average of 23 anatomic knees (Walker et al. 2015). It was shown that the laxity values, and the lateral and medial displacement paths, were closer to normal than a typical PS knee. For the latter there was much higher rotational constraint in early and late flexion, compared with that of the anatomic knee.

Another example of a knee where the intercondylar space was used to provide extra guidance was a Third Condyle knee designed by Bytgyqi et al. (2017). The concept was similar to that above, but this design had already been subject to clinical evaluation. It was found that while the motion was still not similar to anatomic, the approach had further possibilities.

A refined way to address guided motion knee design was later devised by Amiri et al. (2011) where specific kinematic functions were assigned to each region of the bearing surfaces. The potential problem of overconstraining the knee was addressed as follows: "the ultimate shape of the tibial component… can be defined by tuning the shapes and clearances until an optimal compromise between guiding and laxities is formed." The aim of this idea was to minimize the wear of the polyethylene.

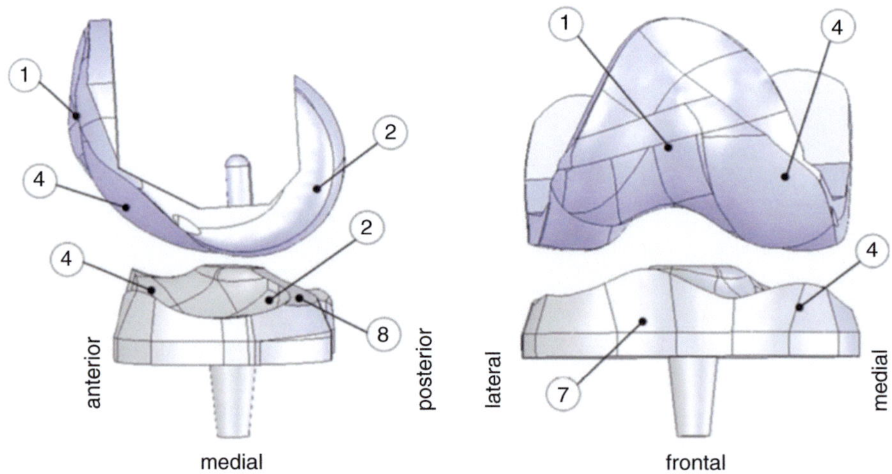

Fig. 11.11 A Guided Motion knee where the surfaces of the femoral and tibial bearing surfaces are shaped in different regions (numerals on figure) to provide the required guidance to motion, together with optimizing the surfaces for wear. The target motion is close to a medial pivoting action. Cruciate preservation is not essential, but can provide anatomic fine-tuning to the motion (Amiri et al. 2011). (Reprinted with permission from Journal of Medical Devices ASME)

Do Guided Motion Designs Have Advantages Over the CR and PS?

Rotating platform and medial pivot designs have shown clinical results equivalent to those of standard CR and PS knees. There is evidence that they provide a feeling of anterior-posterior stability. This effect may be more apparent in a medial pivot knee due to the medial location of internal-external rotation, whereas in a rotating platform, the line of anterior-posterior stability is central. However, the anatomic knee does not have absolutely fixed axes for axial rotation. Guided Motion designs which closely replicate the shapes of the normal anatomic knee have the advantages of a more accurate fit and correct "flow" of the soft tissues around the components. Guidance of the motion from the bearing surfaces, without requiring the cruciate ligaments, has the advantage of greater reproducibility and ease of surgery. Producing more anatomic motion and laxity will provide more accurate lever arms for the muscles. Evaluation of guided motion designs can conceivably be carried out by a computer modeling method (Rullkoetter et al. 2017). These authors point out the complexity of a modeling system but are optimistic that "future TKA designs will be optimized using preclinical computational modelling." This approach can evaluate guided motion knees without the considerable expense of a company financing physical production and clinical trials. It is likely that future knee systems will include Guided Motion knees based on the evidence so far that these type of designs more closely simulate normal kinematics in different functions, as well as embodying normal laxity and stability. The most practical guided motion design will be one which relies on the mechanical features to provide the anatomic motion, laxity, and stability, without having to rely on the cruciate ligaments which require a high accuracy of surgery which cannot always be achieved. A key question is, however, to what extent such normal kinematics will be felt by the patient and what type of evaluation method should be used.

References

Amiri S, Cooke TDV, Wyss UP. Conceptual design for condylar guiding features of a total knee replacement. J Med Devices. 2011;5(2):025001.

Blaha JD. A medial pivot geometry. Orthopedics. 2002;25(9):963–4.

Blaha JD. The rationale for a total knee implant that confers anteroposterior stability throughout range of motion. J Arthroplast. 2004;19(4 Suppl 1):22–6.

Blaha JD, Mancinelli CA, Simons WH, Kish VL, Thyagarajan G. Kinematics of the human knee using an open chain cadaver model. Clin Orthop Relat Res. 2003;410:25–34.

Buechel FF, Pappas MJ. The New Jersey low-contact-stress knee replacement system: biomechanical rationale and review of the first 123 cemented cases. Arch Orthop Trauma Surg. 1986;105(4):197–204.

Buechel FF Sr, Buechel FF Jr, Pappas MJ, D'Alessio J. Twenty-year evaluation of meniscal bearing and rotating platform knee replacements. Clin Orthop Relat Res. 2001;388:41–50.

Bullough P, Goodfellow J, Greenwald AS, O'Connor J. Incongruent surfaces in the human hip joint. Nature. 1968;217(5135):1290.

Bullough PG, Munuera L, Murphy J, Weinstein AM. The strength of the menisci of the knee as it relates to their fine structure. J Bone Joint Surg. 1970;52(3):564–7.

Bytgyqi D, Shabani B, Cheze L, Neyret P, Lustig S. Dores a third condyle TKA restore normal gait kinematics in varus knes? In vivo kinematic analysis. Arch Orthop Trauma Surg. 2017;137(3):409–16.

Eftekhar NS. Total knee-replacement arthroplasty. Results with the intramedullary adjustable total knee prosthesis. J Bone Joint Surg Am. 1983;65(3):293–309.

Evanski PM, Waugh TR, Orofino CF, Anzel SH. UCI knee replacement. Clin Orthop Relat Res. 1976;120:33–8.

Feng Y, Tsai T-Y, Li J-S, Wang S, Hu H, Zhang C, Rubash H, Li G. Motion of the femoral condyles in flexion and extension during a continuous lunge. J Orthop Res. 2015;33:591–7.

Floerkemeier T, Frosch KH, Wachowski M, et al. Physiologically shaped knee arthroplasty induces natural roll-back. Technol Health Care. 2011;19(2):91–102.

Freeman MAR, Pinskerova V. The movement of the normal tibio-femoral joint. J Biomech. 2005;39:197–208.

Frosch KH, Floerkemeier T, Abisht C, Adam P, Dathe H, Fanghanel J, Srurme KL, Kubein-Meesenburg D, Nagerl H. A novel knee endoprosthesis with a physiological joint shape. Part 1: biomechanical basics and tribological study. Unfallchirurg. 2009;112(2):1687–175.

Goodfellow J, O'Connor J. The mechanics of the knee and prosthesis design. J Bone Joint Surg. 1978;60-b(3):358–69.

Gray HA, Guan S, Thomeer LT, Schache AG, Stieger R, Pandy MG. Three-dimensional motion of the knee-joint complex during normal walking revealed by mobile biplane x-ray imaging. J Orthop Res. 2019;37:615–30.

Greenwald AS, Haynes DW. Weight-bearing areas in the human hip joint. J Bone Joint Surg. 1972;54(1):157–63.

Haider H, Garvin K. Rotating platform versus fixed-bearing total knees: an in vitro study of wear. Clin Orthop Relat Res. 2008;466(11):2677–85.

Hamelynck KJ. The history of mobile-bearing total knee replacement systems. Orthopedics. 2006;29(9 Suppl):S7–12.

Iwaki H, Pinskerova V, Freeman MAR. Tibiofemoral movement 1: the shapes and relative movements of the femur and tibia in the unloaded cadaver knee. J Bone Joint Surg Br. 2000;82(8):1190–5.

Krause WR, Pope MH, Johnson RJ, Wilder DG. Mechanical changes in the knee after meniscectomy. J Bone Joint Surg Am. 1976;58(5):599–604.

LaCour MT, Sharma A, Carr CB, Komistek RD, Dennis DA. Confirmation of long-term in vivo bearing mobility in eight rotating-platform TKAs. Clin Orthop Relat Res. 2014;472(9):2766–73.

Liu YL, Chen WC, Yeh WL, et al. Mimicking anatomical condylar configuration into knee prosthesis could improve knee kinematics after TKA – a computational simulation. Clin Biomech (Bristol, Avon). 2012;27(2):176–81.

Macheras GA, Galanakos SP, Lepetsos P, Anastasopoulos PP, Papadakis SA. A long term clinical outcome of the Medial Pivot Knee Arthroplasty System. Knee. 2017;24(2):447–53.

Mannan K, Scott G. The Medial Rotation total knee replacement: a clinical and radiological review at a mean follow-up of six years. J Bone Joint Surg. 2009;91(6):750–6.

Matthews LS, Sonstegard D, Kaufer H. Impact considerations in prosthetic loosening. In: Proceedings Orthopaedic Research Society, San Fransisco, 27 February–1 March, 1975.

Meftah M, Ranawat AS, Ranawat CS. Ten-year follow-up of a rotating-platform, posterior-stabilized total knee arthroplasty. J Bone Joint Surg Am. 2012;94(5):426–32.

Minns RJ. The Minns meniscal knee prosthesis: biomechanical aspects of the surgical procedure and a review of the first 165 cases. Arch Orthop Trauma Surg. 1989;108(4):231–5.

Minns RJ, Campbell J. The mechanical testing of a sliding meniscus knee prosthesis. Clin Orthop Relat Res. 1978;137:268–75.

Morra EA, Heim CS, Greenwald AS. Preclinical computational models: predictors of tibial insert damage patterns in total knee arthroplasty: AAOS exhibit selection. J Bone Joint Surg Am. 2012;94(18):e137(131–5).

Murray DG. Total knee replacement with a variable axis knee prosthesis. Orthop Clin North Am. 1982;13(1):155–72.

O'Connor JJ, Shercliff TL, Biden E, Goodfellow JW. The geometry of the knee in the sagittal plane. Proc Inst Mech Eng H J Eng Med. 1989;203(4):223–33.

Pandit H, Hamilton TW, Jenkins C, Mellon SJ, Dodd CA, Murray DW. The clinical outcome of minimally invasive Phase 3 Oxford unicompartmental knee arthroplasty: a 15-year follow-up of 1000 UKAs. Bone Joint J. 2015;97-b(11):1493–500.

Pinskerova V. GKM sphere medially stabilized knee. 2016. https://media.medacta.com/media/gmk-sphere-publication-review-99-26sphere-pubus-rev00.pdf

Pinskerova V, Johal P, Nakagawa S, Sosna A, Williams A, Gedroyc W, Freeman MAR. Does the femur roll-back with flexion? J Bone Joint Surg. 2004;86(6):925–31.

Price AJ, O'Connor JJ, Murray DW, Dodd CA. Goodfellow JW. A history of Oxford unicompartmental knee arthroplasty. Orthopedics. 2007;30(5 Suppl):7–10.

Pritchett JW. Patient preferences in knee prostheses. J Bone Joint Surg. 2004;86(7):979–82.

Pritchett JW. Patients prefer a bicruciate-retaining or the medial pivot total knee prosthesis. J Arthroplast. 2011;26(2):224–8.

Reynolds RJ, Walker PS, Buza J. Mechanisms of anterior-posterior stability of the knee joint under load-bearing. J Biomech. 2017;57:39–45.

Rovick JS, Reuben JD, Schrager RJ, Walker PS. Relation between knee motion and ligament length patterns. Clin Biomech (Bristol, Avon). 1991;6(4):213–20.

Rullkoetter PJ, Fitzpatrick CK, Clary CW. How can we use computational modeling to improve total knee arthroplasty? Modeling stability and mobility in the implanted knee. J Am Acad Orthop Surg. 2017;25(Suppl 1):S33–s39.

Scott G, Imam MA, Eifert A, et al. Can a total knee arthroplasty be both rotationally unconstrained and anteroposteriorly stabilised? A pulsed fluoroscopic investigation. Bone Joint Res. 2016;5(3):80–6.

Seedhom BB. Loadbearing function of the menisci. Physiotherapy. 1976;62(7):223.

Shaw J, Murray DG. Knee joint simulator. Clin Orthop Rel Res. 1973;94:15–23.

Shaw JA, Murray DG. The longitudinal axis of the knee and the role of the cruciate ligaments in controlling transverse rotation. J Bone Joint Surg Am. 1974;56(8):1603–9.

Stoner K, Jerabek SA, Tow S, Wright TM, Padgett DE. Rotating-platform has no surface damage advantage over fixed-bearing TKA. Clin Orthop Relat Res. 2013;471(1):76–85.

Takei T. Artificial knee joint. US Patent 6,406,497. Filed July 2001, issued June 2002.

Tuke MA, MAR Freeman. Knee prosthesis. US Patent 5,219,362. Filed Feb 1992, issued June 1993.

Ueo T, Kihara Y, Ikeda N, Kawai J, Nakamura K, Hirokawa S. Deep flexion-oriented bisurface-type knee joint and its tibial rotation that attributes its high performance of flexion. J Arthroplast. 2011;26(3):476–82.

Varadarajan KM, Zumbrunn T, Rubash HE, Malchau H, Li G, Muratoglu OK. Cruciate retaining implant with biomimetic articular surface to reproduce activity dependent kinematics of the normal knee. J Arthroplast. 2015;30(12):2149–53.

Victor J, Bellemans J. Physiologic kinematics as a concept for better flexion in TKA. Clin Orthop Rel Res. 2006;452:53–8.

Wachowski MM, Fiedler C, Walde TA, Balcarek P, Schüttrumpf JP, Frosch S, Frosch KH, Fanghänel J, Gezzi G, Kubein-Meesenburg D, Nägerl H. Construction-conditioned rollback in total knee replacement: fluoroscopic results. Acta Bioeng Biomech. 2011;13(3):35–42.

Walker PS. A new concept in guided motion total knee arthroplasty. J Arthroplast. 2001;16(8 Suppl 1):157–63.

Walker PS. Application of a novel design method for knee replacements to achieve normal mechanics. Knee. 2014;21(2):353–8.

Walker PS, Borukhov I. Replication and substitution of anatomic stabilizing mechanisms in a total knee design. J Med Devices. 2017;11(4):041005.

Walker PS, Erkman MJ. The role of the menisci in force transmission across the knee. Clin Orthop Relat Res. 1975;109:184–92.

Walker PS, Ewald FC. Bearing surface design in total knee replacement. Eng Med. 1988;17(4):149–56.

Walker PS, Arno S, Borukhov I, Bell CP. Characterizing knee motion and laxity in a testing machine for application to total knee evaluation. J Biomech. 2015;48(13):3551–8.
Waugh TR, Smith RC, Orofino CF, Anzel SM. Total knee replacement: operative technic and preliminary results. Clin Orthop Relat Res. 1973;94:196–201.
Williams A, Logan M. Understanding tibio-femoral motion. Knee. 2004;11(2):81–8.
Zambianchi F, Fiacchi F, Lombari V, Venturelli L, Marcovigi A, Giorgini A, Catani F. Changes in total knee arthroplasty design affect in-vivo kinematics in a redesigned total knee system: a fluoroscopy study. Clin Biomech. 2018;54:92–102.
Zumbrunn T, Varadarajan KM, Rubash HE, Malchau H, Li G, Muratoglu OK. Regaining native knee kinematics following joint arthroplasty: a novel biomimetic design with ACL and PCL preservation. J Arthroplast. 2015;30(12):2143–8.

Instrumentation and Technique

12

Are Mechanical Instruments Accurate Enough?

The early devices for the treatment of osteoarthritis, tibial spacers and fixed hinges, required little in the way of instrumentation for their insertion. For the spacers, the tibial resection was achieved using an osteotome, with the local bone geometry as the guide for the direction and depth of the cut. For the hinges, a saw was used to resect the distal femur and proximal tibia with a T-shaped rod and plate for aligning the cuts relative to the canals. The overall alignment of the component was defined by the long intramedullary stems. Once the condylar replacement type was introduced however, two problems were highlighted: how to prepare the bones for accurate fitting of the component and how to achieve the required overall alignment of the femur relative to the tibia.

Principles of Alignment and Force Transmission

To achieve these goals, the instrumentation and technique were based on a combination of anatomic and biomechanical considerations. Key reference points on the bones were identified as the basis for reference lines or axes. In the frontal plane, the points included the center of the femoral head, the centers of the distal femur and proximal tibia, the extreme lateral and medial points of the distal femur and proximal tibia, the center of the ankle level with the malleoli, and the centers of the diaphysis of the femur and tibia. These points were then used to define the anatomic axes of the femur and the tibia, the mechanical axis of the limb (as distinct from the mechanical axis of the femur and tibia separately), and the joint line. In the sagittal plane, the anatomic axis of the femur and the tibia and the tibial slope were defined. The angle between the femoral and tibial anatomic axes in the sagittal plane denoted the flexion angle although there is some uncertainty due to the anterior bowing of the femur.

In his book on kinesiology, first published in 1955, Arthur Steindler MD showed the frontal plane axes as described above and concluded that "because of the obliquity of the anatomic axis of the femur the greater amount of pressure is borne by the

P. S. Walker, *The Artificial Knee*, https://doi.org/10.1007/978-3-030-38171-4_12

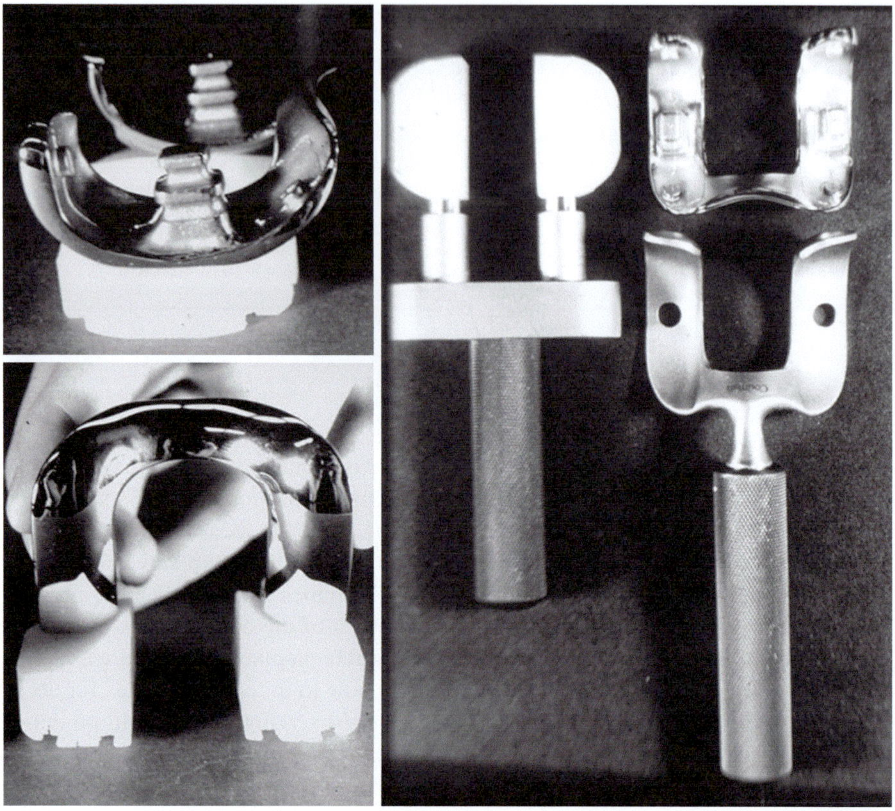

Fig. 12.1 In the early 1970s, the instrumentation for inserting the Duo-condylar knee consisted only of two tools, one for shaping the femur and one for positioning the tibial components. The surgeon held the femoral tool over the distal femur and marked the area which was to be recessed about 3 mm so the component would just project from the surrounding surface. It was not easy to match the shape of the anterior bridge. The tibial tool did position correctly spaced and parallel tibial bearing surfaces. Very soon afterwards, alignment guides were designed to check alignment of the components to the long axes of the femur and tibia

lateral condyle, and a greater tension is sustained by the soft structures of the medial condyles." (Steindler 1955). This perception was based on the assumption that a vertical force would be applied from the top of the femoral shaft, the line of action passing outside of the lateral condyle and hence applying the highest load on that side of the knee. This misconception was due to the lack of biomechanical knowledge at that time. By the mid-1960s however, based on radiographic observations of arthritic knees with varus deformity, it was clear that cartilage loss and densification of the trabecular bone were due to medial overloading, a state that became worse as the deformity progressed. This was the basis for tibial osteotomy described by Mark Coventry MD and others at the Mayo Clinic (Coventry 1965). By 1969, James Morrison PhD and John Paul PhD from the University of Strathclyde, Glasgow, Scotland, had concluded from their in vivo biomechanical studies that the larger proportion of the force on the knee passed through the medial side of the joint, even in normal subjects (Morrison 1970). Later, Ed Chao PhD, Mark Coventry MD, and Frank Sim MD developed software to calculate the lines of action of the resultant force across the knee in varus deformity and calculated the ideal alignment for an osteotomy in order to centralize the forces. In their analysis they defined the major force of the femur on the tibia being applied along a line from the center of the femoral head to the center of the tibial plateau.

Nevertheless, in some designs of hinged knees, the femoral and tibial stems were co-axial, not reproducing the 5 degrees of valgus between the femur and tibia as in the normal knee. Hence it is not surprising that in the early 1970s, when new designs of condylar replacement knees were being introduced, there was inadequate understanding of the correct frontal plane alignment to apply to the surgical procedure. Indeed at the conference on Total Knee Replacement organized by the Institution of Mechanical Engineers and the British Orthopaedic Association in 1974, the brief instructions for the Freeman-Swanson total knee included "The bone ends are resected at right angles to their long axes to leave two flat cancellous surfaces parallel to each other." (Freeman et al. 1974). This would leave the knee joint in about 5 degrees of varus deformity on average. Other prominent participants at the conference, who had also developed new artificial knees, omitted to emphasize the importance of frontal plane alignment or describe how it was achieved at surgery. This was at odds with a statement made by Ian Harrington PhD from Strathclyde University at the same conference: "....joint load tending to increase with increasing joint angular deformity. This is more apparent with varus and flexion deformities of the knee than for valgus....the normal pattern is to unload the lateral component." This was however recognized by Mark Coventry and Richard Bryan from the Mayo Clinic in relating their experience with the Polycentric and Geometric devices: "If the limb is in varus it must be overcorrected to 5 degrees of valgus...." (Coventry and Bryan 1974). The development of an axial guide had made it possible to estimate the axial alignment accurately. The consequence of too little attention being given to frontal alignment was tibial component loosening, mostly due to excessive varus alignment. It was this, rather than applying the earlier experience with osteotomies or the biomechanical data, that led to the recognition of the problem and the development of reliable alignment guides.

Even so, designers of the early condylar knees seem to have relied on their own unpublished studies of the normal alignments of the lower extremity, as there did not appear to be any published study on the topic. As evidence of this, in the papers of the First Scientific Meeting of the Knee Society in 1984 edited by Larry Dorr MD, in a paper on Axial Alignment, Moreland and Hanker wrote: "Since some authors have reported that the alignment of the lower extremity and component positioning are important for durability....and since we were unable to find a radiological study of normal alignment....". Their study was republished a few years later in the *Journal of Bone and Joint Surgery* (Moreland et al. 1987). The frontal plane alignment does have an effect on the force distribution between the lateral and medial sides of the knee, as implied by Moreland et al. It might be assumed that on average, there would be equal forces through the lateral and medial sides of the

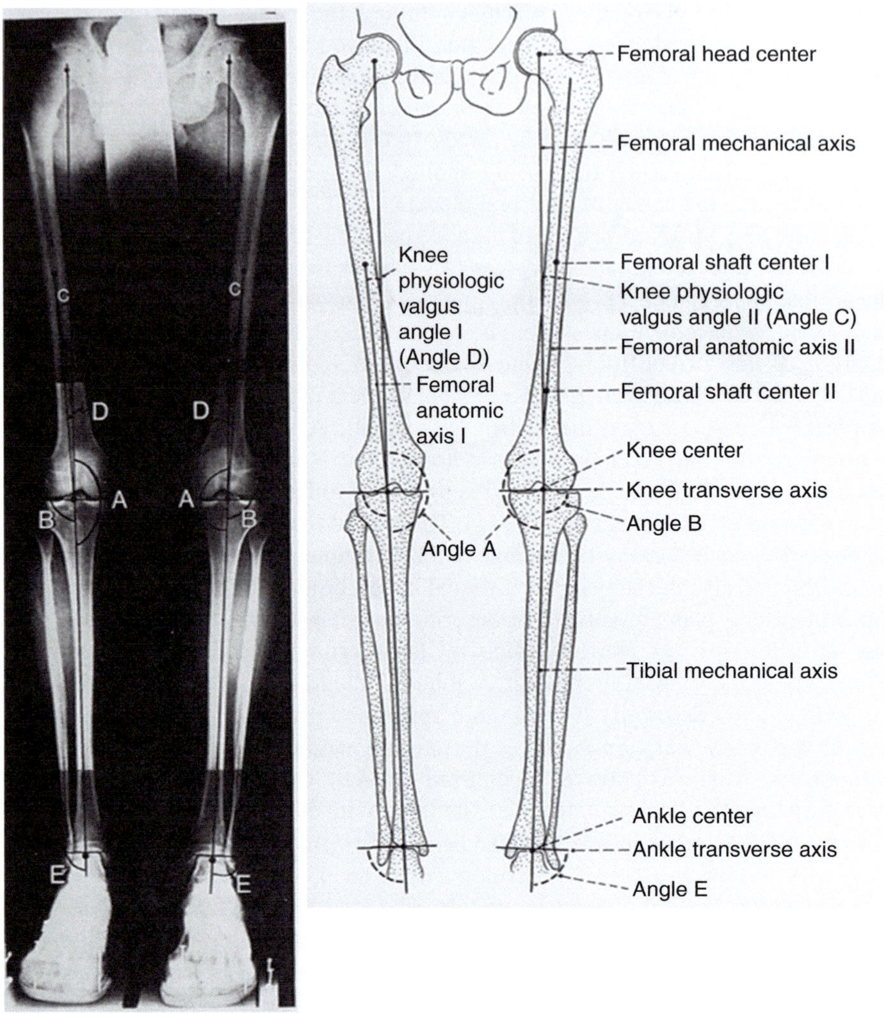

Fig. 12.2 One of the first studies where reference axes and angles were defined in the frontal plane and average values measured. It was found that the mechanical axes of the femur and tibia were not collinear, with an angulation of about 1.5 degrees, implying that the mechanical axis of the limb (center of hip to center of ankle, not shown in figure) passed medial to the center of the knee. The joint line, called the knee transverse axis, was angled at 2–3 degrees to the mechanical axis of the tibia, a slight varus slope (Moreland et al. 1987). (Reprinted with permission from Journal of Bone & Joint Surgery A)

knee. This was found to not be the case in a monumental study carried out by Georg Bergmann PhD and associates at the Charite Hospital in Berlin. Total knee implants were instrumented and the force data extracted wirelessly. The results from five patients, carrying out activities including walking, going up and down the stairs, and sit-to-stand, were published (Kutzner et al. 2010; Halder et al. 2012). The peak forces were in the range of 2.2–3.5 times body weight, the highest values being for stair ascend and descend. For an alignment between the anatomic axes of the femur and tibia of 5 degrees, a normal mean value, 65–73% of the force passed through the medial side. Every 1 degree more varus, the medial share value increased by 5%. This might imply that an excess of varus would be detrimental for component wear and loosening and the possibility of lateral lift-off. The resultant force on the tibia was found to be predominantly in a direction in-line with the long axis. However there were deviations from vertical in certain phases of activity, especially stair activities, where there were shear force components. These could act in an anterior or posterior direction on the tibia, of magnitude about 15–20% body weight. There were even medial-lateral shear force components, somewhat less at about 10% body weight. This data is relevant to the posterior slope of the tibial component, which will affect the anterior shear forces as well as the femoral-tibial position. In general, alignments of the components will affect the force distributions and hence the stability and kinematics of both the femoral-tibial joint and the patella-femoral joint.

Development of Mechanical Instruments

Applying principles of alignment to instrument design was illustrated by the work of Charles O. Townley, a surgeon in Port Huron, Michigan, who started this work in the late 1940s (Pritchett 1988). Before entering medical school, Townley graduated with a degree in physical education, after which he spent a year studying mechanical engineering. During his residency he formulated solutions for treating the arthritic knee and actually made drawings of a design of total knee consisting of metallic shells which accurately reproduced the femoral and tibial surfaces (Townley 1988). He did not implement this, however, because of the likely problems with wear and friction, but he saw that there was utility in using only the tibial component. His stainless steel articular-plate replacement as it was called was used from 1953 to 1972. In cases of varus or valgus deformity with wear and bone compression on one side of the tibia, Townley used different methods for correction. With the leg straightened, the defect was filled with bone chips or by an osteotomy and elevation of the bone near the plateau surface: "This results in a tightening of the collateral ligament on the involved side and correction of the disturbance in the weight-bearing line at the knee joint. It is suspected that the increased stability.... plays a major role in the postoperative relief of pain." However by the late 1960s, with the availability of the materials being used for the total hip and the early knees of Freeman-Swanson and Gunston, Townley was once again able to turn his attention to his own total knee design, to which his principles on knee arthroplasty in the articular-plate replacement could be applied. These principles were "to provide an articular replacement procedure that would simulate the normal anatomic and functional modalities of the knee joint." To achieve this required a combination of implant design and technique including accurate bearing surface shapes and placement, in synchrony with preservation of all of the ligaments, as well as correct alignment of the long axes of the femur and tibia and inclination of the joint line:

"Significant abnormalities in either the size, contour or placement of the femoral component will distort or misplace the condylar articular outline and will place it out of tune with the holding patterns of motion sustained by the ligaments." Townley emphasized the inclination of the mechanical axis of the leg in the frontal plane in a standing or functional position and the disposition of the joint line. This meant that in a standing position, the joint lines of the right and left legs were parallel to the ground. Consequently, the joint line was inclined at 2 degrees to the mechanical axis and to the anatomic axis of the tibia itself. In the sagittal plane, the tibial cut should be at the patient's natural angle, in the range of 6–10 degrees posterior slope. It is notable that Townley was the first to emphasize the approach of achieving normal anatomic alignments for each patient.

Townley designed special cutting guides to achieve these various goals. To accurately identify the center of the femoral head, the proximal reference point of the mechanical axis, radiopaque markers were placed at the level of the femoral head and a radiograph taken at the start of the operation. A length of thick cord, regarded as an "instrument," held taut between the centers of the femoral head and ankle, should pass through the medial condyle of the knee. This strict anatomic approach of Townley was intended to restore the normal ligament length patterns and, in turn, the normal stability and laxity of the knee being operated on. It is consistent with the data on the mechanical properties of ligaments, obtained subsequent to Townley's work, showing the sensitivity of knee motion to even small changes in ligament lengths of only 1–2 millimeters. This puts into perspective the difficult task of the implant designer and the surgeon in achieving such accuracy. One aspect that Townley did not emphasize during the description of his technique was how to handle deformities where normal ligament lengths could have changed, for example, elongation of the lateral collateral and contraction of the medial collateral in varus deformity.

The problem of implanting total knees in cases with deformity was a particular focus of John Insall and Chit Ranawat, from the Hospital for Special Surgery: ".... the problems of accurate placement increases with the preoperative deformity and contracture...." (Insall et al. 1976). Starting in about 1972, a surgical technique and a set of instruments were developed for dealing with these situations. The Total Condylar knee was designed to treat a full range of cases from mild to severe arthritis, a strategy which had the advantage of a standard implant and technique which could be readily learned and provide consistent results. The resection of the cruciate ligaments made the technique easier, and because the anterior-posterior stability of the joint was now provided by the dishing of the tibial bearing surfaces, cruciate resection was not seen as a disadvantage. The essence of the technique was to make the bone cuts so that the soft tissue sleeve around the knee was balanced in both flexion and extension, rather than implanting the components to reproduce the original bearing surfaces, as with Townley's technique. The first step was to flex the knee to 90 degrees; insert the rod of the first instrument, the tibial cutter, into the femoral intramedullary canal; and then pull the tibia downwards so that the joint capsule was tightened. The tibial cutter had a choice of horizontal slots through which to cut the proximal tibia using an oscillating saw. The second instrument was the femoral shaper which also had an intramedullary rod and which had slots for cutting the anterior and posterior surfaces of the femur. The third instrument was the distal femoral cutter that had a plate locating on the already-cut proximal tibial surface and which was pulled down to tighten the soft tissue capsule with the knee at 0 degrees flexion. The slot in the femoral cutter was then used to make the distal femoral cut.

It was, however, realized that when the capsule was tightened on the lateral and medial sides, the frontal plane alignment of 5 degrees valgus between the femur and tibia may not have been achieved: "In the more common varus deformity, the medial ligament shortens and the lateral ligament stretches: unless corrected, this imbalance will persist after replacement." A few degrees of bone misalignment were accepted, but for large varus deformities, the medial structures were partially released from the tibia prior to making the femoral cuts. Valgus releases were not recommended however. In the above procedure for making the bone cuts, in cases of varus deformity, it usually occurred that the posterior femoral cut on the medial condyle was a few millimeters more in thickness than the cut on the lateral condyle. The anterior femoral cut would be parallel to the posterior cut. The result was an external axial rotation of the femoral component on the distal end of the femur, of a few degrees. While this rotation would reduce the steepness of the lateral face of the patella groove at the anterior aspect of the femoral component, where the patella articulates in early flexion, in practice this did not produce any serious consequences.

The above two approaches to surgical technique, focusing either on anatomic alignment of the femur to the tibia and the components to each bone or producing equal soft tissue tensions and gaps in extension and flexion, have been the fundamental starting points for subsequent technique development. It was evident that both alignment and soft tissue balancing were necessary which subsequently led to a fusion of both concepts. This was emphasized by David Hungerford and Ken Krackow (1984) at the first Scientific Meeting of the Knee Society: "In order for non-constrained total knee systems to work properly, the retained ligaments must function at normal lengths….To achieve nearly normal function each component must be positioned not only in the correct varus-valgus, flexion-extension, and rotational attitude, but also in the correct proximal-distal and anterior-posterior attitude." The mention of "non-constrained" has significance in that it was not necessarily implying that the same rules applied to the more constrained cruciate resecting total knee designs, which were popular at the time. In the area of alignment, techniques have included redefining the angles of the bone cuts as well as attempting to improve accuracy. Hungerford and Krackow focused on the overall alignment from full-leg standing x-rays to confirm what Townley had already pointed out that the joint line in the frontal plane sloped medially by an average of 2–3 degrees, such that the joint line was parallel to the ground in a standing position. Reproducing this at surgery was an important element in placement of the femoral component on the distal femur, where the bone resected laterally and medially in both flexion and extension was exactly the same as the thickness of the femoral component. This was considered to be crucial because any deviation in component

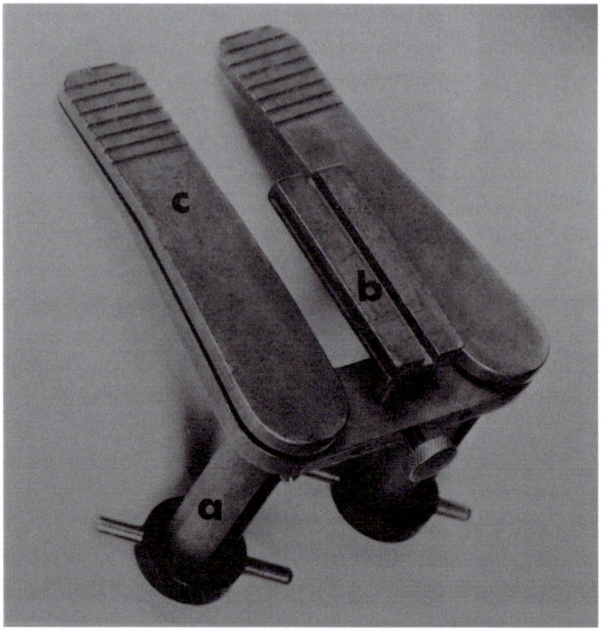

Fig. 12.3 A mechanical distractor where the gaps on the lateral and medial sides were measured, was designed in the mid-1980s by Chit Ranawat and Larry Dorr as part of their Precision knee instruments. The aim was to achieve accuracy at every step of the procedure through well-designed instruments and steps in the technique. (Reprinted with permission from Springer Nature)

position would change the center of rotation of the femur producing an incorrect ligament length pattern during flexion. Hence the instrumentation was designed to key off the distal and posterior femoral condyles, but allowing for any cartilage wear or bone collapse that had occurred.

There was one compromise that the distal femoral cut needed to be at the anatomic angle to the femoral shaft, as indicated by both intramedullary and extramedullary rods, and hence the distal cut was keyed off the most prominent condyle. This frontal plane angle was individual to each patient, based on their long-leg radiographs (Hungerford and Kenna 1983), which was an original idea at the time when most knee systems recommended a standard angle. This aspect was addressed later by Johan Bellemans et al. (2012), noted below. Having now positioned the femoral and tibial components correctly, balancing was carried out in two steps. Firstly, to achieve stability in both flexion and extension, either extra bone could be resected from the distal femur, or a thicker tibial component could be used. Secondly, varus-valgus instability was solved by releasing the tight side or tightening the loose side. While the major goals of this technique were similar to those of Townley, the steps were more systematic and the instruments more accurate. Attention was given to avoiding an excess of varus or valgus, while the ligament balancing steps were clearly spelled out. A limitation was that the balancing was carried out by "feel" rather than with any instrument such as a tensor.

This deficiency was addressed by Chit Ranawat and Larry Dorr (1985), in their "Precision Cut Instrumentation" which was applicable to mechanical alignment, an advancement of the instruments used for the Total Condylar. By this time, several posterior stabilized (PS) designs had emerged, for which mechanical alignment was

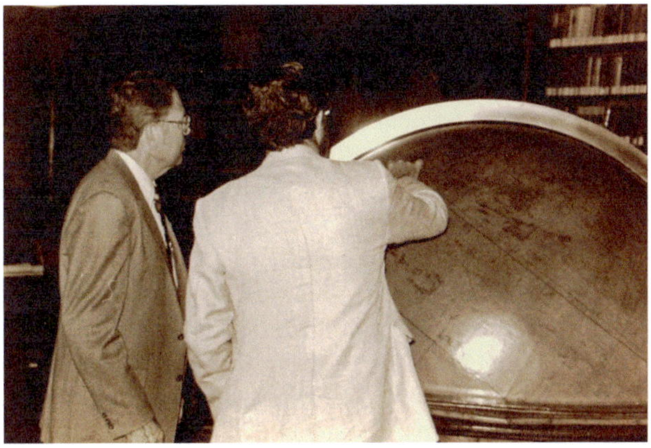

Fig. 12.4 Richard Bryan (left) from the Mayo Clinic and David Hungerford from Baltimore appreciate the ancient globe at the Umberto Library in the Rizzoli Institute in Bologna, Italy. The globe was made in 1762 by Father Rosini, based on maps and descriptions from numerous explorers. Fabio Catani points out that Australia is not shown on the globe, a destination not known at the time. The occasion was a conference on artificial knees, organized by Mario Marchetti in the early 1980s. (© Peter S Walker)

also recommended: "These instruments allow for precision bone cutting and restoration of the mechanical axis. The tensor allows balancing of the ligaments both in flexion and extension". The tensor was first used with the knee at 90 degrees flexion after cutting the proximal tibia and the anterior and posterior femur. The lateral and medial arms of the tensor were expanded, and if the gaps on the medial or lateral side were unequal, the ligament on the tight side was released in small steps until the gaps were equal. The knee was then extended with the femur at 5 degrees valgus to the tibia and the tensor inserted. Distraction again determined any medial or lateral tightness to be corrected, after which the level of the distal cut was marked on the anterior femur. Hence, this technique achieved both the required alignments and ligament balancing. The latter was achieved in both flexion-extension and in varus-valgus by use of the tensor. This method of balancing was far more accurate than using simple spacer blocks inserted between the cut surfaces, where the surgeon assessed the relative tightness of the block in flexion and extension, and the varus and valgus equality by applying side-to-side movements. Nevertheless, this particular tensor still relied on the surgeon assessing the tightness of the distractor wheel to come to a "hard stop" when the ligaments were tight.

Different Alignment Goals and Techniques

The literature shows that the various alignments affect outcomes, although considerably more research is needed to gain more insights. The issue is complicated because of the wide range of conditions of the arthritic knee and the different mechanics of the implant designs used for treatment. This means that there may not be a "best" technique for all circumstances. The different techniques have been thoroughly summarized in a recent article by Bill Jaffe MD from NYU Langone Orthopedic Hospital (Jaffe et al. 2018). Following a Fellowship with John Charnley in 1970, Bill Jaffe joined the surgical staff at NYU and maintained a strong interest in biomechanics and biomaterials, working with scientists such as Jim Pugh PhD, Harry Alexander PhD, and Fred Kummer PhD. The most common fundamental tenet of surgical techniques today is to align the limb in some relation to the mechanical axis: "The goal of mechanical alignment in TKA is to create a joint line that is perpendicular to the mechanical axis of the limb, theoretically resulting in even distribution of loads across the medial and lateral surfaces of the components." This differs from anatomic in that normally the joint line is at 2–3 degrees of varus to the mechanical axis, such that the joint line is parallel to the ground in the standing position. Making the bone cuts on the distal end of the femur and the proximal tibia, using mechanical instruments, usually relies on an intramedullary rod in the femur and an external alignment rod in front of the tibia. Most often, average, or close to average, values are used for the cut angles. Cutting the tibia perpendicular to its anatomic axis rather than at 2–3 degrees varus simplifies the surgery and avoids an excess varus cut in case of an inaccuracy. However it is a compromise.

Jaffe then describes the different methods used for producing the bone cuts, assuming a perpendicular tibial cut. In "measured resection" landmarks are used on the distal femur to make the distal femoral cut and the anterior and posterior cuts. The latter produce some internal rotation of the femoral component on the distal femur, partly in compensation for the joint line being perpendicular to the mechanical axis. A choice is made between anterior or posterior referencing, and while posterior referencing is better for controlling the flexion angle and flexion tightness, with multi-sized knee systems of today, it makes little difference.

Regarding the resection technique, the first was "measured resection" where the anterior and posterior femoral cuts were made with reference to the line across the posterior condyles (posterior condylar axis PCA), the line through the epicondyles (epicondylar axis TEA), and the line through the base of the patella groove (Whiteside's line). In mechanical alignment, the anterior and posterior cuts are rotated by about 3 degrees to compensate for the distal cut being perpendicular to the mechanical axis. In the "gap balancing" resection technique, obtaining equal lateral and medial soft tissue tensions is the guide for the resections.

Kinematic Alignment

Kinematic alignment requires special mention because of the increasing interest in recent years (Howell 2019). Steve Howell MD is an orthopedic surgeon who has collaborated on knee mechanics with Maury Hull PhD and others at the University of California, Davis. The goal is to restore the joint lines in extension and flexion to the normal anatomic condition. The technique has some similarity to that advocated by Townley, and by Hungerford and Krackow, called anatomic alignment, but there are some important differences. The method also has connections to the study by

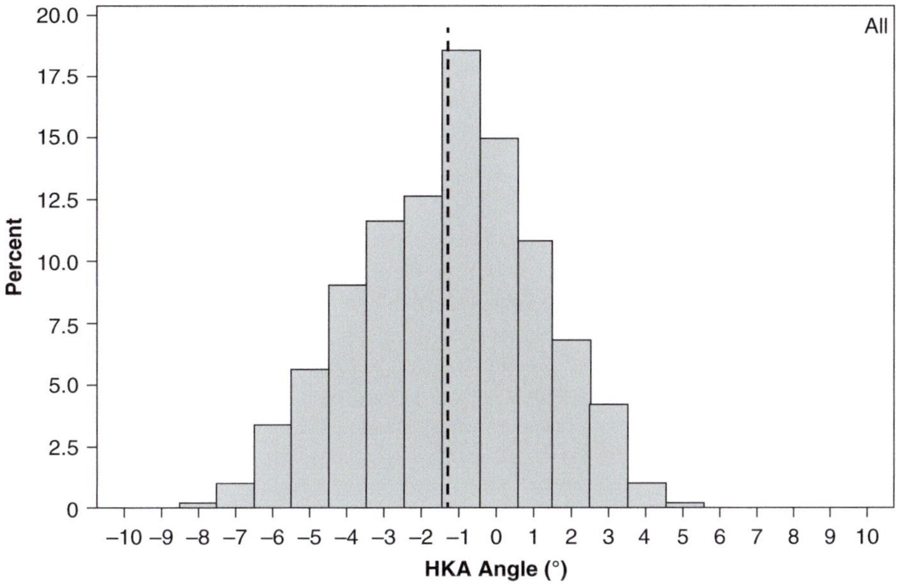

Fig. 12.5 In a study of 250 young males and females (500 knees), Johann Bellemans and Jan Victor from Ghent University, Belgium, measured the angle between the mechanical axis of the femur and tibia (angle A in diagram by Moreland and Hanker). The mean value was about 1 degree. However there were 32% of males and 17% of females where there was a deviation greater than 3 degrees. In positioning an artificial knee, it was questioned whether the best alignment would take account of the angle in the particular patient or still be at the standard alignment perpendicular to the mechanical axis (Bellemans et al. 2012). (Reprinted with permission from Clinical Orthopaedics & Related Research)

Bellemans et al. (2012) where it was shown that many knees have a constitutional varus relative to the mechanical axis. The origin of kinematic alignment was the laboratory study by Anne Hollister et al. (1993) depicting an average transverse axis in the femur about which the tibia flexed and extended and a vertical axis through the medial tibia about which the femur rotated internal-external. This concept can also be connected with that of Freeman and Pinskerova (see Chap. 11). Steven Howell MD added a third axis, transverse in the femur, about which the patella flexes and extends (Howell 2019). These three axes are shown to be parallel and perpendicular to the distal femoral and posterior femoral joint lines. At surgery, distal femoral cuts are made, resecting exactly the thickness of the components, allowing for any cartilage or bone loss. The same process is carried out for the posterior femoral condyles. The tibia is cut, again restoring the line of the transverse axis and the posterior slope. All cuts are measured and checked, adjusting if necessary. It is noted that the anatomic axes in the femur and tibia, the mechanical axis, as well as the epicondylar axis and Whiteside's line, are not referred to. The rotational positional of the tibial component is based on correct fitting of an anatomically shape component, but can also be referred to bony landmarks, the object being to preserve the anatomic Q-angle. Having made the cuts, the balancing steps are

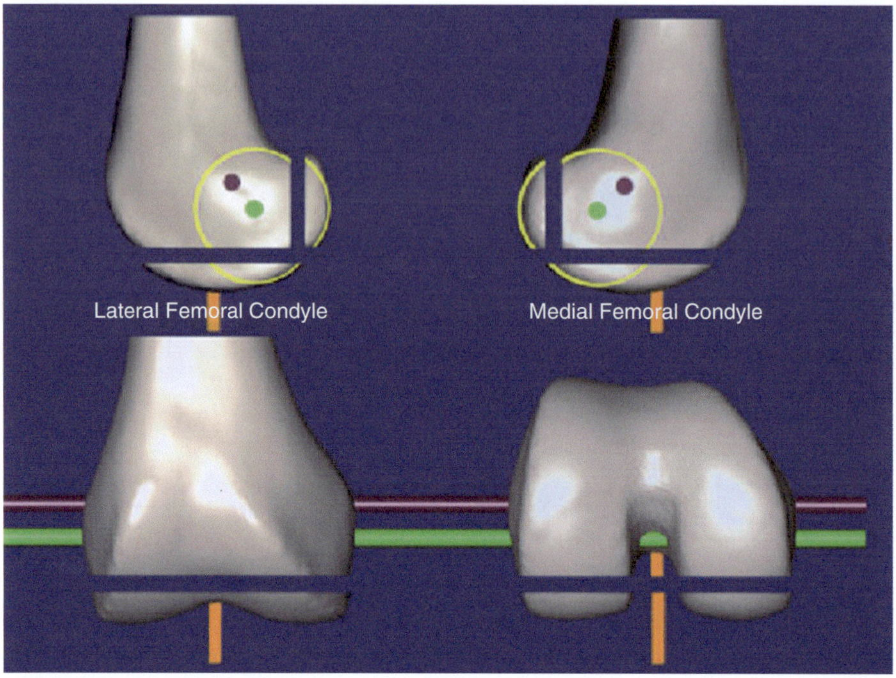

Fig. 12.6 Steve Howell MD from Methodist Hospital, Sacramento, and Maury Hull PhD, from University of California Davis, developed a system of bone cuts called kinematic alignment. A right femur (left) shows the relationships of the three kinematic axes of the knee with respect to the joint lines of the distal and posterior femur and the position of the components. The transverse axis in the femur about which the tibia flexes and extends is the green line. The transverse axis in the femur about which the patella flexes and extends is the magenta line. The longitudinal axis about which the tibia internally and externally rotates on the femur is the orange line. All three axes are either parallel or perpendicular to the joint lines. Resecting bone, after correcting for wear, from the distal and posterior femur equal in thickness to the condyles of the femoral component, kinematically aligns the femoral component. Resecting bone, after correcting for wear, from the tibia equal in thickness to the tibial component, kinematically aligns the tibial component. The resulting frontal plane alignment of the joint line is usually 2–3 degrees varus to the mechanical axis, as for the anatomic knee, but varies with each individual (Howell et al. 2013). (Reproduced with permission from Knee Surgery Sports Traumatology Arthroscopy)

carried out based on a decision tree for corrective measures. For example, a knee which was tight in extension and loose in flexion would be adjusted by a small additional resection from the distal femur. Tightness on the medial or lateral sides would be corrected with a small wedge cut from the proximal tibia. This is consistent with experimental and surgical data where most imbalances could be dealt with by corrections of only 2 mm or 2 degrees (Walker et al. 2014). Verasense devices were used at surgery to measure the actual compartmental forces. Anatomic values are targeted, such as a looser lateral side than medial side in flexion. The relative medial and lateral forces were measured as a function of overall alignment measured postoperatively from long-leg radiographs (Shelton et al. 2017). The idea of the study was that knees that had larger deviations from the mechanical axis, either in varus or valgus, would show large inequalities in the contact forces at surgery. The "take-home message" from the study was "Kinematic alignment has a high proportion of varus and valgus outliers according to mechanical alignment criteria - Medial and lateral tibial compartment forces of subjects with varus or valgus outlier alignment were comparable with those with in-range alignment." In terms of clinical results, a 10-year follow-up of 222 knees showed 98.4% survivorship, despite a high proportion aligned outside of recommended limits (Howell et al. 2018). For example there were 27% outside of +/− 3 degrees from the mechanical axis (mostly in varus) and an almost uniform distribution of varus tibial tilt up to 6 degrees from horizontal. Even so, a knee with a large deviation from the mechanical axis should be treated with some caution according to Rivière et al. (2018) in which case there should be a hybrid approach where that knee is aligned less than the deviation. This does have a rationale for high varus deformities, where there would be substantial increase in medial force (Halder et al. 2012), which in an artificial knee could cause excessive wear or loosening.

Accuracy of Mechanical Instrumentation

Mechanical instrumentation has steadily evolved up to the present time, with more precise alignment for the various angles, provision for modifying bone cuts, and options for different levels of cut. There are two issues with any instrumentation system: what is the accuracy which can be achieved, as measured by the deviations from the target alignment values, and how much inaccuracy can be tolerated without having an adverse effect on survivorship or function. The latter is a difficult question because there is no compelling evidence as to what should be the correct target, components perpendicular to the mechanical axis, or a more patient-specific alignment.

The accuracy of the bone cuts was measured for a typical instrument system in the 1990s (Mahaluxmivala et al. 2001). While the mean values of the frontal plane angles were close to target, the standard deviations for the femoral and tibial component alignments were 2.2–3.9 degrees, the least value being for the tibial frontal plane. Only 75% of overall alignment angles were within 3 degrees of target. The looseness of the IM rod in the femoral canal was identified as large source of error. In a more recent and often-quoted paper, 398 consecutive cases of 3 types of total knees were carried out by a single surgeon at the Mayo Clinic in a 5-year time period (Parratte et al. 2010). Full-length radiographs were used to measure the frontal plane angles. Although the mean deviation from the mechanical axis was zero degrees, the standard deviation was 2.8 degrees with a range from 8 degrees varus to 9 degrees valgus. However the survivorship was no different between cases within 3 degrees and all outliers of more than 3 degrees. The authors concluded nevertheless that "a neutral mechanical axis remains a reasonable target…." In a recent revisit of the same cohort of patients followed for a further 5 years, there were no changes in the conclusions (Abdel et al. 2018). The effect of alignment was of great interest to Merrill Ritter MD and colleagues in Mooresville, Indiana, using the AGC knee implant. By constantly evaluating their results as a basis for yet further improvements in treatment modalities, Ritter and a group of expert knee and hip surgeons made numerous contributions to the advancement of the field. In their study of no less than 6070 knees, failures were tested for a correlation with the femoral-tibial angles. Remarkably there were only 54 failures (0.89%) at an average of 5 years (Ritter et al. 2011). Their angles were measured on short radiographs. The mean femoral-tibial angle was 4.7 degrees of valgus, with a standard deviation of 2.5 degrees. (The mean femoral-tibial angle in normal knees is 5.7 degrees). The range however was from −12 degrees to +20 degrees. The overall conclusion was "a surgeon should aim to place the tibial component at an angle of 90 degrees from the tibial axis and the femoral component in <8.0 degrees of valgus in order to yield an overall anatomic alignment (tibiofemoral coronal alignment) between 2.5 degrees and 7.4 degrees of valgus, which should be achievable with conventional instruments." This range is similar to that of the Mayo Clinic study, although in Ritter's study, the failures occurred at higher deviations.

Based mainly on observations of individual cases, many authors have suggested that alignment errors can result in problems other than component loosening. These problems have included patella mal-tracking, excessive polyethylene wear, instability, and reduced flexion angle, as well as cosmetic effects. While mechanical instrumentation has been associated with high survivorship values, it may be that inaccuracies have resulted in some patients not reaching their optimal functional performance, although it has been difficult to reach definite conclusions when there is such granularity.

Up till now the most common method for performing an artificial knee has been the use of traditional mechanical instrumentation. It cannot be assumed that all systems are similar in their accuracy and precision or ease of use. However, overall, it is recognized that there are certain inherent errors in the use of such instruments. There are only a few papers to be found on the magnitude and causes of errors, so the following list is compiled from observations made in papers, conference lectures, and anecdotal discussions.

- The intramedullary rod for defining the frontal plane angle of the distal femoral cut. In larger canals, the error can be around +/− 2 degrees. This can be even larger if the entry point of the rod is not lined up with the center of the femoral canal, which is about 6 mm medial to the center of the intercondylar notch.
- Angular deflection of the saw blade when passing through the slot due to clearance or offset forces applied.
- Error in pinning the slotted cutting block to the bone.
- Distance of the cutting block from the starting point of the bone cut.
- Bending of the saw blade as it encounters hard bone more on one side of the blade than the other.
- Error in placement of the distal clamp of a tibial cutting guide at the ankle.
- Lack of parallelism of the vertical rod of the tibial cutting guide to the anatomic axis of the tibia, in the sagittal plane.
- Looseness in the modular parts of the instruments or even a misunderstanding of the method of assembly or attachment to the bone.

- Loosening of the pins holding the slotted cutting guides, as the bone cut is being made.
- Cutting blocks which have flat surfaces over which the blade is passed, allowing for some tilting of the blade (although visualization may be better).

A number of these factors have been addressed in some systems, but in general, there is still room for improvement. Hence it can be concluded that while there are inherent errors in the use of mechanical instruments, the errors could likely be reduced by improvements in the design and use of the cutting guides and saw blades. The final word in this section is given by a study from the Rothman Institute in Philadelphia (Küçükdurmaz et al. 2015). They attempted to match the flexion and extension gaps. There were three groups of 25 patients, each group having a different instrumentation system from a major company. Their results were that only 44 percent of cases had all three bone cuts within 2 millimeters of target. This is not ideal considering the sensitivity to ligaments to length changes of only 1–2 mm.

Range of Flexion

One outcome measure, the maximum range of flexion achieved, has still not reached anatomic levels. This could be partly explained by the fact that an artificial knee does not sufficiently mimic the anatomic structures which it is replacing. In the anatomic knee, flexion beyond about 120 degrees involves complex movements of the femoral condyles on the tibial plateaus and displacement of the menisci, such that impaction between the posterior femoral cortex and the posterior tibial plateau, which would block flexion, is avoided (Pinskerova et al. 2009). These authors concluded that "The anatomical and functional features of the arc from 120 to 160 degrees suggest that it would be difficult to design a total knee replacement giving physiological movement." Nevertheless there are design features of an artificial knee which do have an effect.

Impingement of the posterior femoral cortex on the posterior edge of the tibial insert was highlighted as a limitation to flexion in one study (Bellemans et al. 2005). They focused on the posterior slope of the tibial cut as affecting the height of the posterior edge of the tibial bearing surface and concluded that every 1 degree of slope changed the flexion angle by 1.7 degrees. However simply cutting a large slope angle beyond what is normal for the particular knee is not advisable because the contact points between the femoral and tibial condyles displace posteriorly, which can cause instability or extension lag (Cantin et al. 2015; Weinberg et al. 2017). Bellemans also showed how the posterior offset of the femoral condyles relative to the posterior cortex was another factor in determining when impingement occurred, with a high offset giving the most flexion. A further possibility in limiting flexion is abnormal tensions in the soft tissues around the implant components, in regions where a component projects beyond the boundaries of the original femur or tibia. Around the anterior patella flange is one area where this might occur, but there is little literature on this aspect. Nevertheless if the preoperative flexion angle is already limited due to changes in the soft tissue properties around the knee, it may not be possible to regain a high flexion angle after the artificial knee.

Patient-Specific Instrumentation (PSI)

Due to the complexity and number of the mechanical instruments and the attention needed for cleaning, sterilizing, and storing, it is not surprising that alternate methods for making the bone cuts were explored. One method for simplifying the system was to use imaging to design and manufacture patient-specific cutting guides for making the primary cuts of the distal femur and proximal tibia (Lombardi & Frye 2012). The idea was to generate computer models of the femur and tibia using MRI or CT scans. From those models, the bone cuts were defined to produce the required alignments in the frontal and sagittal planes. Cutting guides were then designed to fit precisely on to the distal femur and proximal tibia, matching the surfaces of the patient's bones. To manufacture such guides with their complex geometry was a challenge, the answer being 3D printing using rigid polymeric materials. At surgery, the cutting guides were positioned in their unique positions on the bones and pinned in place. This greatly simplified the surgical procedure. The method became known as patient-specific instrumentation (PSI). As pointed out by Lombardi and Frye, an important advantage is the ability to customize the bone cuts for each individual patient.

The first PSI system, the Visionaire, was approved by the FDA in 2008. Since then seven other systems have been designed and introduced. However, overall, the

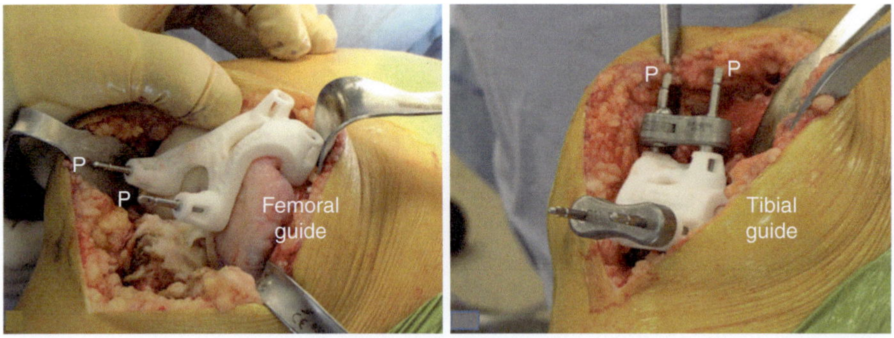

Fig. 12.7 Patient-specific instrumentation (PSI) made by 3D printing for each individual patient. CT or MRI scans are taken of the hip, knee, and ankle and reference axes determined, together with the cutting planes of the femur and tibia. The guides are designed to be a precise fit on the distal femur and proximal tibia (best seen on the left picture). After pinning the guides (P), holes are drilled into the bone through the other two guide holes which define the position of a standard slotted cutting guide. The number of outliers, cuts more than 3 degrees from target, was approximately 25%, at least as good as that of conventional instruments. (Ng et al. 2012). (Reproduced with permission from Clinical Orthopaedics & Related Research)

method has not shown any striking advantages over the traditional mechanical instrumentation, based on a number of studies. The verdict from one author Bill Mihalko (2015) was "but until more definitive functional and patient-perceived outcome data, along with cost effectiveness data, are obtained, we do not have adequate evidence to recommend for or against the use of PSI for total knee arthroplasty." Subsequent publications provided further information. Based on a meta-analysis of 44 studies comparing almost 3000 each of PSI cases and mechanical cases (Thienpont et al. 2017), the conclusion was "The present meta-analysis revealed an increased risk of malalignment of the tibial component for PSI, and its impact on implant longevity remains to be seen. This study showed that PSI only has a minor impact on the risk of malalignment of the mechanical axis. Moreover, there is still a lack of evidence of clinical effect associated with use of PSI." A multicenter study found no differences between PSI and mechanical instrumentation for alignment, operative time, blood loss, and Knee Society Function Score (Abane et al. 2018). In a recent meta-analysis where 38 studies were analyzed including almost 350 cases, it was concluded that PSI does not improve patient-reported outcome measures, surgery time, and complication rates as compared to standard techniques. While there is much overlap in the above studies, the conclusions are the same. A cautionary note is that all systems do not necessarily produce the same results, some systems may be measurably superior to others in certain ways, but this is difficult to discern from the literature.

Hence while there were no striking advantages cited, there were no major disadvantages in using PSI in terms of alignment accuracy and functional performance. In that case it might be thought that the simplicity of the surgical procedure would be a positive factor. The drawback however was that the patient had to be scheduled for imaging a few weeks prior to surgery, and the surgeon had to study the design of cutting guides proposed by the manufacturer, all adding time and cost. A further point is that many surgeons were somewhat nervous about relying on the fit of the cutting guides to the distal femur and proximal tibia to produce the correct alignments, without having a secondary check. It is unlikely that PSI will be abandoned, because of its elegance, and it represents the point of view that while mechanical instruments may produce similar accuracy, simplification would be an advantage. Possibly modifications of PSI may be put forward to address the disadvantages.

Computer-Assisted Instrumentation

In the late 1990s, efforts were underway to develop a computer-assisted surgical technique which could improve both accuracy and precision of the bone cuts and the alignment. Electronic digitizers were already widely used in engineering whereby the coordinates of a point on an object could be determined by touching the point with a probe. This technology was applied to a surgical navigation system where various reference points on the femur and tibia were exposed and the coordinates determined with reference to a global axis system. The positions of the femur and tibia in space were also determined in this axis system by fixing trackers into the middle of the diaphyses of the femur and tibia which were optically tracked. All points were then tracked in real time even when the femur and tibia moved. The location of the center of the femoral head, impossible to access directly but necessary for defining the mechanical axis of the leg, was determined by an ingenious method. The femur was rotated in different directions about the hip joint, while points on the femur were continuously tracked. The coordinates of the center of the hip could then be calculated.

Using such a system, it was immediately evident that the alignments of the bone cuts were more accurate and outliers were greatly reduced (Jenny and Boeri 2001). Since the first system, several others were developed and used extensively around the world. A recent meta-analysis from 21 studies comparing 844 knees performed by mechanical instrumentation with 869 knees using navigation (Clayton et al. 2014) showed that "These results demonstrate that the use of computer navigation in TKA achieves both superior mechanical alignment and an increase in functional scores. This increase requires the investment of additional time and financial resources."

While navigation still has a dedicated following today, the increased surgical time has been the main reason why the method has not become widely popular, coupled with some skepticism as to whether the more accurate alignment makes a significant difference in longevity and function. A positive step in recent years has been the refinement to navigation systems in measuring the varus and valgus laxities as the knee is put through a range of flexion. This enables the surgeon to balance the knee in a more quantitative way than before. However if the laxities are still measured by the surgeon applying the forces by hand, there is still a subjective element to the readings obtained.

It was inevitable that robotics would enter the arena in total knee surgery (Bargar 2007). This was initiated by an orthopedic surgeon working with a veterinary surgeon. The orthopedist, Bill Barger, had a background in mechanical engineering before entering the medical field. The veterinarian, Howard "Hap" Paul, was a creative and adventurous individual who is still recognized today by the HAP Paul Award for innovation, given by the International Society for Technology in Arthroplasty (ISTA) at its annual meetings. Based on initial funding from IBM, Bargar and Paul were able to perform their first robot hip surgery on a dog in 1990. The name they gave to their equipment was Robodoc. Part of the driving force for choosing the hip was the enthusiastic movement between many surgeons around the world for uncemented customized artificial hip joints, for which a perfect fit between the implant and the canal of the bone was required. The milling tool on the robot arm could prepare such a cavity. During the 1990s, clinical hip trials proceeded on humans, but then in 2000, the first total knee surgery was performed, the company making the equipment being called Think Surgical. Concurrent with this development, Professor Brian Davies at Imperial College, London, began development of a medical robot in 1991 called the Probot, for prostate surgery. By 1999 Davies had developed an active constraint system called the Acrobot for minimally invasive orthopaedic applications including total knees. After a number of iterations of the robot, the Acrobot company was acquired by Stryker where patent problems prevented its further application. Brian Davies is still active in the field of medical robotics.

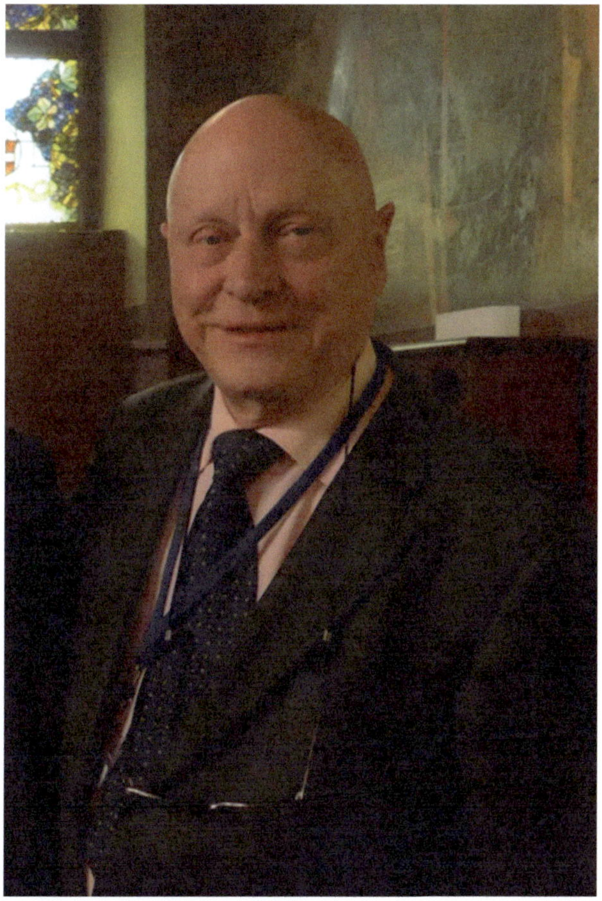

Fig. 12.8 Brian Davies PhD, from the Mechanical Engineering Department at Imperial College London, developed the first active constrained robot systems for performing artificial knee procedures, first performed on patients in 2002. This work set the stage for other robotic developments which are gradually gaining recognition for their capabilities in accuracy in effecting the optimal surgical plan. (Photo taken in London c 2015). (© Peter S Walker)

There are currently several robotic systems available, described in a review by Jacofsky and Allen (2016). Some systems were developed by enterprising individuals, either in a university setting or in a startup company. For example, Rony Abovitz, a visionary, connected with Maurice Ferre MD in 2004 to form MAKO Surgical, to develop the first haptic robot system, applied initially to unicompartmental knees. The company has since been acquired by Stryker which is concentrating primarily on the application of the robot for total knee replacement. Rony is presently involved with virtual reality but not in the world of orthopedics. Dr. Tony DiGioia, a surgeon in Pittsburgh, collaborated with faculty members in robotics at Carnegie Mellon University, to develop a handheld robotic tool called Navio for performing a minimally invasive knee replacement procedure. As with Bill Bargar, DiGioia held an engineering degree before entering the medical field. A company was formed in 2013, Blue Belt Technologies, which was acquired by Smith & Nephew in 2015. The Navio is a handheld tool with cutting implements such as burrs and is used in conjunction with a navigation system to shape the bone without

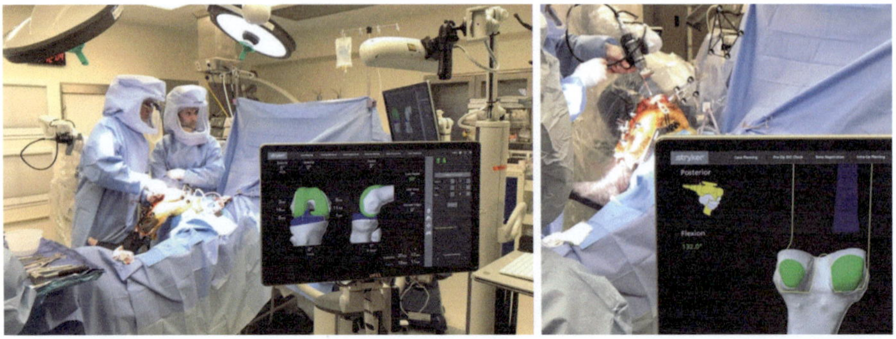

Fig. 12.9 An artificial knee procedure using the Mako robot (Stryker). Left, the surgeon has planned the procedure by placing the femoral and tibial components on the images of the bones, shown on the computer screen. The key reference points are being digitized. Right, the robot arm with an oscillating saw mounted on the end, is being deployed to resect the posterior femoral condyles. The progress of the cuts is shown on the computer screen. (Photos courtesy of Patrick Meere MD, NYU Langone Orthopedic Hospital, New York)

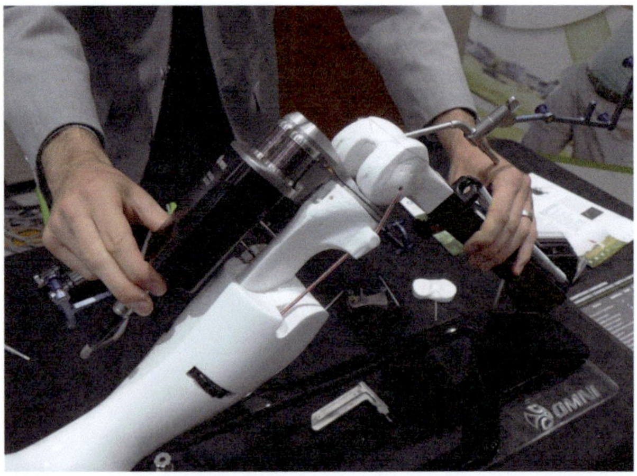

Fig. 12.10 A device for distracting the lateral and medial condyles separately at surgery as a guide to the balancing required. This is part of the Omnibot system for carrying out an artificial knee surgery. Designed by Christopher Plaskos. (Photo taken at CAOS International Conference, New York, April 2019)

needing any adjunct cutting guides. Chris Plaskos PhD developed a small bone-mounted robot which moved a cutting guide into prescribed positions, without requiring any prior imaging. Chris was a PhD in the area of medical robotics and co-founded OMNILife Science in 1999 to further develop this invention. A new addition to the system has been a distractor system for balancing ligaments. The company was acquired in 2019 by Corin Group in England. Zimmer entered the computer-assisted surgery area in 2007 with the acquisition of ORTHOsoft Inc., based in Montreal. The concentration has been on smart tools such as the iAssist. Zimmer recently acquired the ROSA robotic arm system from French-based medtech. Rosa was originally developed for brain and spine surgery, but within a short period of time, Zimmer developed software for artificial knee surgery. The accuracy of the system was tested in knee specimens by eight surgeons on different knee designs (Parratte et al. 2019). The accuracy was within about 1 degree and 1 mm. DePuy Synthes (J&J) recently acquired a Paris-based robot company Orthotaxy. This is a compact robot, at a relatively low price, which will be easy to operate and speed up the surgery. It is currently being developed for knee surgery.

Hence robotics for total knee surgery is an active and expanding field, currently being evaluated in many centers. Jacofsky and Allen (2016) summarized the current status as follows: "Regardless of what target a surgeon may desire for limb alignment or component position, it is clear that robotics will enable surgeons to carry out more precise and accurate procedures on a more consistent basis with a more patient-specific plan. In the future, robotics is moving toward becoming a valuable adjunct to the surgeon in optimizing patient-specific arthroplasty." The authors also point out that there is a very high price tag for a hospital to enter this field, which limits the level of acceptance at this time.

Another area of computer-assisted surgery which has gained support is the use of "smart tools" incorporating inertial measurement units (IMUs) and other sensors. While not receiving the same amount of attention as robotics, such devices offer the advantages of simplicity, utility, and low cost, without adding time to the procedure. They are intended to be used seamlessly in a system of mechanical instruments. The smart tools fit in the palm of the hand and are designed to place cutting guides in a location on the femur and tibia to make precise cuts relative to the reference axes such as the mechanical axis. The tools are initially registered to bony landmarks and then the cutting guides are pinned in place. Two of the most widely used devices have received positive appraisals. In a follow-up of the KneeAlign system, Nam et al. (2012) concluded: "This study demonstrates that accelerometer-based navigation can obtain the same degree of accuracy as previously reported with large console CAS systems, while avoiding the use of additional pin sites, arrays, or large console platforms." For the iAssist, Kinney et al. (2018) reached a similar conclusion: "we have demonstrated that the use of a handheld guidance system in TKA results in decreased mechanical axis variability and a decreased rate of unacceptable postoperative alignment compared to conventional instruments, without resulting in significant increases in operative time or blood loss."

On the subject of computer-assisted surgery, brief mention will be made of computer-assisted training of the surgical technique. In 2003, Noble and Conditt devised a method whereby the surgeon was provided with a computer model of the arthritic knee and then positioned artificial components on to the bones in the correct alignments (Noble and Conditt 2008). The surgeon then performed the procedure physically on sawbones and attempted to implement the computer model. A scoring system was devised for how accurately the dimensional parameters were achieved. A similar method was carried further (Gunther et al. 2002) in that the entire set of instruments and implants was modelled in the computer. The surgeon performed the procedure in the computer, learning the sequential steps. The alternative was to study the manufacturer's manual. Surgeons in the computer group and the manual group then performed the procedure on saw bones. The computer-trained surgeons performed in a shorter time and with fewer errors. This type of approach has potential and is clearly more convenient and less expensive than

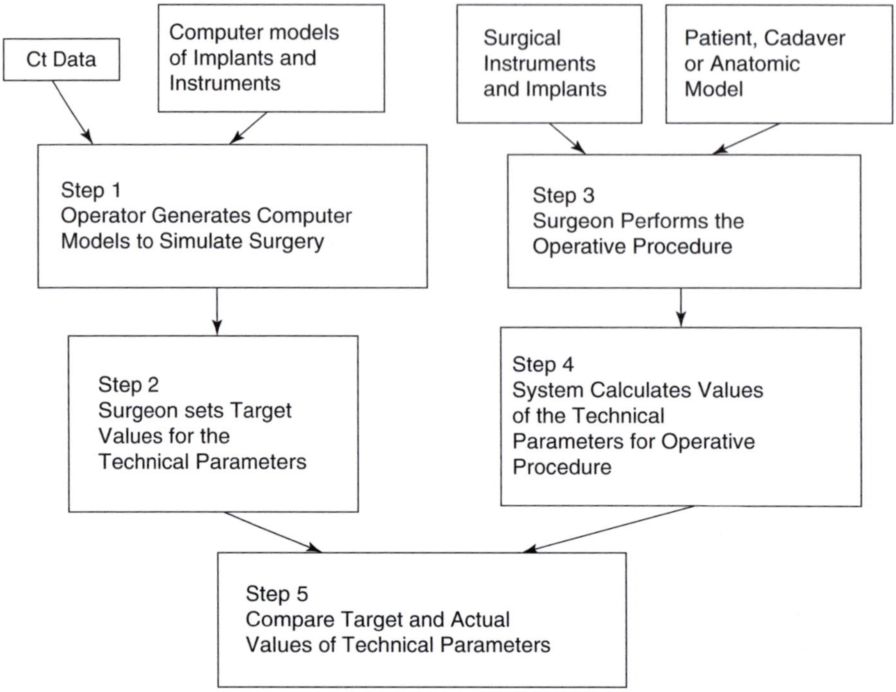

Fig. 12.11 A method devised by Philip Noble and Michael Conditt while at Baylor College of Medicine and Methodist Hospital, Houston. The figure shows the strategy for evaluating a total knee surgical procedure for accuracy, comparing the end result to the target values. The method was demonstrated to be applicable to actual surgical cases or in a training environment where surgeons work with sawbones or with leg specimens. (US patent 7,427,200 B2, filed 2003, issued 2008)

using cadaveric specimens. At the same time, there is the limitation that a computer simulation is unlikely, in the short term at least, to simulate the anatomy and properties of the actual tissues of the knee, the methods being most applicable to the bones themselves. Recently, the American Academy of Orthopaedic Surgeons has initiated a study of virtual reality as a modality for surgical training. This possibility is a subject of extensive research at Imperial College, London.

Soft Tissue Balancing

One facet of surgical technique that deserves special attention is soft tissue balancing, also called ligament balancing, or simply "balancing". Balancing is carried out at surgery, where loads which occur during function cannot be safely applied. Hence balancing needs to be carried out with the knee in a passive condition. Even then, because of the weights of the thigh and shank, there are forces and moments between the femur and tibia. In this passive condition, it was discovered in experiments at the NYU Langone Orthopedic Hospital that there are forces acting across the lateral and medial condyles due to "pre-tensions" in the soft tissues (Verstraete et al. 2017). The forces were highest in extension, averaging 114 Newtons (25 pounds) on the medial side and 63 Newtons on the lateral side. The forces reduced quickly in early flexion and then more gradually for the remaining flexion range. The purpose of the soft tissue tensions, it can be proposed, is to maintain the femoral and tibial condyles in a defined relative position during a passive range of flexion. If the tensions are too high, it would cause stiffness; if too low, there would be excessive laxity and incorrect positions. When an artificial knee is placed, the objective is to place the components on the bones so that there are normal soft tissue tensions throughout the flexion range, to maintain the correct femoral-tibial positions. For simplicity it can be proposed that the tensions should be equal at about 100 Newtons per condyle, throughout flexion. This is not easy to accomplish because when a collateral ligament is just tense, every millimeter of extra length causes about 50 Newtons of force. Hence to balance the knee requires that the femoral shape and size are close to the normal anatomy of that knee and the tibial thickness is correct. Imbalances need to be identified at surgery and corrected by various means such as osteophyte removal, soft tissue releases, or modifications to bone cuts (Meere et al. 2016).

While the methods of the early 1970s using simple spacer blocks served well at that time, they may not have achieved the most consistent results. One of the individuals who recognized the complexity of balancing was Leo Whiteside MD, who founded a bioengineering unit near his hospital in St. Louis, Whiteside Biomechanics. Steve White PhD, Darryl Haynes PhD, and other biomechanical engineers carried out pioneering and influential studies at this unit. In 1987 the group published a study (Whiteside et al. 1987) showing the importance of balancing the collateral ligaments correctly to limit varus-varus laxity, but with the effect of also controlling rotational laxity, a phenomenon which had also been noted by John O'Connor from Oxford in relation to unicondylar knees (Goodfellow and O'Connor 1978). Whiteside also explained the importance of placing a femoral component precisely matching the condyles so that the collateral ligament attachment points were correctly lined up with the sagittal contours, otherwise the ligaments will be too tight or too loose in a part of the flexion range. This must be considered in relation to techniques where the femoral component is positioned in relation to the mechanical axis or some other landmarks. Whiteside (2005) emphasized the multiple soft tissue structures across the knee, many with broad attachments, such that different fiber bundles would become loose and tense at different flexion angles. However, insertion of artificial knee components would often lead to abnormalities in these tension patterns. This led to his concept of balancing which was to selectively release the tightest parts of the structures (Whiteside et al. 2000 ch.26): "...release only the ligaments that are excessively tight, leaving those that are performing normally." This approach to balancing, where the tightness of small groups of fibers at different flexion angles is accounted for, has recently been supported by Ranawat after many years of experience with different techniques. Nevertheless, quantifying the balancing in some way during the procedure was an unsolved problem, except for the introduction of distractor devices which could not readily be used with trial components in place.

A different way of thinking about balancing was proposed by Asano et al. (2004). Rather than focusing on gaps or on selective releasing, they hypothesized that the important measure was soft tissue tensions. They devised a special instrument which could measure tensions, the surgical goal being to achieve equal tensions on the lateral and medial sides, as well as in flexion and extension. The tensions in the soft tissues transferred directly to the condylar contacts between the femoral and tibial components. This concept was translated into electronic instrumentation developed recently, an instrumented trial tibial component, called the Verasense. The device was conceived by Martin Roche MD, an orthopedic surgeon from Holy Cross Hospital in Fort Lauderdale, and Marc Stein PhD, an electronics engineer. A company was formed by Jay Pierce, and by 2010, clinical application was initiated. Rather than measuring ligament tensions or distraction gaps, the forces on the cut surfaces of the lateral and medial condyles were measured by an instrumented tibial trial, the forces being generated by the tensions in the soft tissues (Gustke et al.

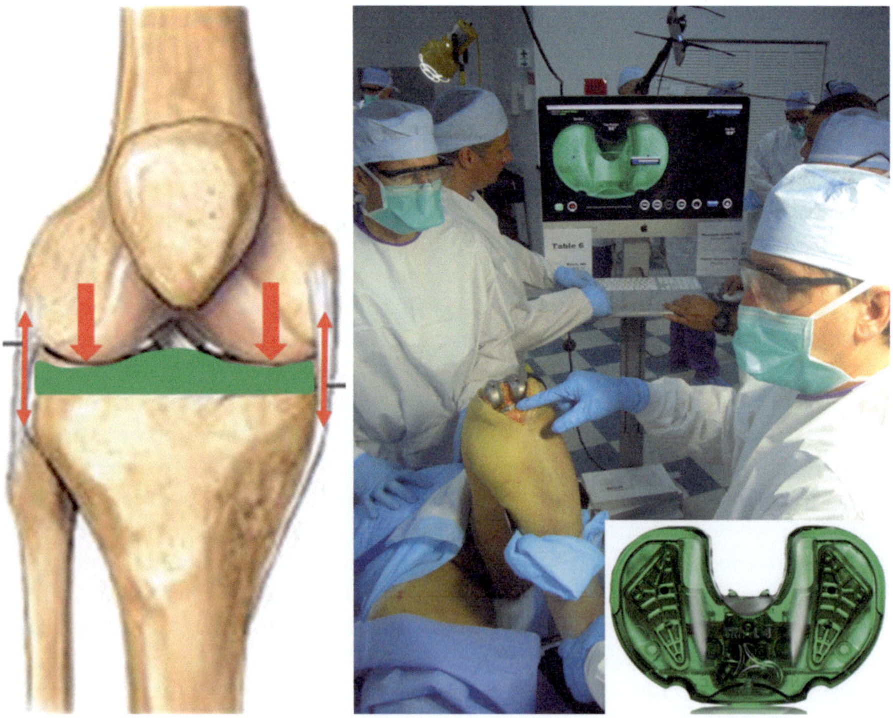

Fig. 12.12 In a normal intact knee, there are forces in the collateral ligaments of about 100 N (22.5 lbf) which apply these forces to the lateral and medial condyles (left figure). The forces reduce with flexion, and the medial force is higher than the lateral. At surgery the surgeon can insert an Orthosensor instrumented tibial trial which measures the condyle forces during flexion-extension (displayed on computer screen). If the knee is unbalanced, the surgeon can make small angular changes to the bone cuts or release tight regions of ligaments

2017). Hence by studying the lateral and medial force patterns as the knee was flexed and extended, the surgeon could determine corrective bone cuts, changes in component thicknesses, or soft tissue releases, in order to obtain the correct balancing. The sensitivity of the balancing process was determined in experiments by Walker et al. (2014) where only 2 mm or 2 degree corrections were usually the maximum needed. This was confirmed in a series of 101 surgical cases (Meere et al. 2016). This also reinforced the importance of accurate condylar shapes of the artificial knee components as well as accurate placement (Zapata et al. 2019). Such small corrections could be carried out by a "systematic selective soft tissue release" technique, although in some cases, bony cut corrections could be made also (Peters et al. 2013).

There are now several technique options for total knee surgery. In the majority of cases, traditional mechanical instruments are used. The main reasons are availability, familiarity, reliability, and acceptable results. However the disadvantages include high initial cost (usually borne by the suppliers of the artificial knees), storage and cleaning requirements, and lack of sufficient accuracy and precision such that surgery to close tolerances is not possible at present. An interesting recent alternate for mechanical instruments is to make the instruments disposable using 3D printing (Hooper et al. 2019). While disposable plastics have a negative environmental impact, there are certain advantages such as elegance of pre-assembled designs and ease of inventory handling. For accuracy and optimization at surgery, robotic systems have a clear advantage. Adoption is so far limited due to high up-front cost, the need for a high level of technical skill, even including a technician in the operating environment, and so far, increased operating time. In the upcoming years, studies on costs, outcome measures, and other aspects, are needed to provide answers to the most appropriate ways forward.

Are Mechanical Instruments Accurate Enough?

In terms of survivorship, where the components do not loosen, the Mayo Clinic and the Mooresville studies concluded that deviations from target limb alignments of at least up to 3 degrees were well tolerated. It is possible that cement technique, design of the implant, and condition of the tibial trabecular bone have more effect than alignment. But assuming that 3 degrees was the maximum error allowed, mechanical instruments are borderline for producing this accuracy routinely. Hence some improvement in the design of the instruments is needed. An improved intramedullary guide, and the smart tools navigation devices, may fill this need. In terms of function, a limitation is that the target alignment and component positions to achieve the optimal results in each patient, and the effect of deviation from the target, are not known with any certainty. However for achieving a target value, computer-assisted methods, such as navigation and robotic surgery, are more accurate. They also offer the opportunity for testing component placements and measurement of ligament laxity at surgery. Ongoing clinical studies will determine whether functional outcome measures can be elevated by the use of the newer computer-assisted techniques.

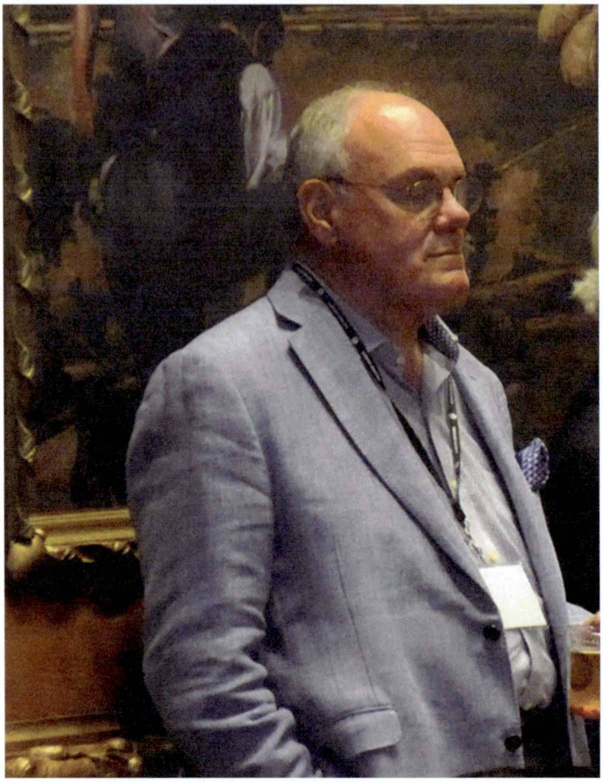

Fig. 12.13 Robert Booth from Jefferson Health, Philadelphia, has performed more total knee surgeries than any other surgeon. His surgical expertise and efficiency is widely known from his numerous lectures at conferences around the world. He is also an authority on American cultural history. (Photo at Knee Society 2018 © Peter Walker.)

References

Abane L, Zaoui A, Anract P, Lefevre N, Herman S, Hamadouche M. Can a single-use and patient-specific instrumentation be reliably used in primary total knee arthroplasty? A multicenter controlled study. J Arthroplast. 2018;33(7):2111–8.

Abdel MP, Ollivier M, Parratte S, Trousdale RT, Berry DJ, Pagnano MW, et al. J Bone Joint Surg Am. 2018;100(6):472–8.

Asano H, Hoshino A, Wilton TJ. Soft-tissue tension total knee arthroplasty. J Arthroplast. 2004;19(5):558–61.

Bargar W. Robots in orthopaedic surgery: past, present, and future. Clin Orthop Rel Res. 2007;463:31–6.

Bellemans J, Colyn W, Vandenneucker H, Victor J. The Chitranjan Ranawat award: is neutral mechanical alignment normal for all patients? The concept of constitutional varus. Clin Orthop Relat Res. 2012;470(1):45–53.

Bellemans J, Robijns F, Duerinckx J, Banks S, Vandenneucker H. The influence of tibial slope on maximal flexion after total knee arthroplasty. Knee Surg Sports Traumatol Arthrosc. 2005;13(3):193–6.

Cantin O, Magnussen RA, Corbi F, Servien E, Neyret P, Lustig S. The role of high tibial osteotomy in the treatment of knee laxity: a comprehensive review. Knee Surg Sports Traumatol Arthrosc. 2015;23(10):3026–37.

Clayton AW, Cherian JJ, Banerjee S, et al. Does the use of navigation in total knee arthroplasty affect outcomes? J Knee Surg. 2014;27(03):171–6.

Coventry MB. Osteotomy of the upper portion of the tibia for degenerative arthritis of the knee. J Bone Joint Surg Am. 1965;47:984–90.

Coventry MB, Bryan RS. Technical pitfalls in the polycentric and geometric total knee arthroplasties. Conference on Total knee replacement. London: Institution of Mechanical Engineers; 1974. p. 16–8.
Freeman MAR, Swanson SAV, Todd RC. Replacement of the knee with the Freeman-Swanson prosthesis. Conference on Total knee replacement. London: Institution of Mechanical Engineers; 1974. p. 16–8.
Goodfellow J, O'Connor J. The mechanics of the knee and prosthesis design. J Bone Joint Surg. 1978;60-b(3):358–69.
Gunther SB, Soto GE, Colman WW. Interactive computer simulations of knee-replacement surgery. Acad Med. 2002;77(7):753–4.
Gustke KA, Golladay GJ, Roche MW, Elson LC, Anderson CR. A targeted approach to ligament balancing using kinetic sensors. J Arthroplast. 2017;32(7):2127–32.
Halder A, Kutzner I, Graichen F, Heinlein B, Beier A, Bergmann G. Influence of limb alignment on mediolateral loading in total knee replacement: in vivo measurements in five patients. J Bone Joint Surg Am. 2012;94(11):1023–9.
Hollister AM, Jatana S, Singh AK, Sullivan WW, Lupichuk AG. The axes of rotation of the knee. Clin Orthop Relat Res. 1993;290:259–68.
Hooper J, Schwarzkopf R, Fernandez E, et al. Feasibility of single-use 3D-printed instruments for total knee arthroplasty. Bone Joint J. 2019;101(7_Supple_C):115–20.
Howell SM. Calipered kinematically aligned total knee arthroplasty: an accurate technique that improves patient outcomes and implant survival. Orthopaedics. 2019;42(3):126–35.
Howell SM, Papadopoulos S, Kyle T, Kuznik KT, Maury L, Hull ML. Accurate alignment and high function after kinematically aligned TKA performed with generic instruments. Knee Surg Sports Traumatol Arthrosc. 2013;21:2271–80.
Howell SM, Shelton TJ, Hull ML. Implant survival and function ten years after kinematically aligned total knee arthroplasty. J Arthroplast. 2018;33(12):3678–84.
Hungerford DS, Kenna RV. Preliminary experience with a total knee prosthesis with porous coating used without cement. Clin Orthop Relat Res. 1983;176:95–107.
Hungerford DS, Krackow KA. In: Dorr LD, editor. Porous coated knee replacement. Papers of the First Scientific Meeting of the Knee Society. Baltimore, MD: Publ University Park Press; 1984.
Insall J, Ranawat CS, Scott WN, Walker PS. Total condylar knee replacement: preliminary report. Clin Orthop Relat Res. 1976;120:149–54.
Küçükdurmaz F, Levicoff EA, Good RP, Sharkey PF. Do standard surgical guides produce accurate and precise femoral bone resections during total knee arthroplasty? Surg Technol Int. 2015;27:225–32.
Jacofsky DJ, Allen M. Robotics in arthroplasty: a comprehensive review. J Arthroplast. 2016;31(10):2353–63.
Jaffe WL, Dundon JM, Camus T. Alignment and balance methods in total knee arthroplasty. J Am Acad Orthop Surg. 2018;26(20):709–16.
Jenny JY, Boeri C. Computer-assisted implantation of total knee prostheses: a case-control comparative study with classical instrumentation. Comput Aided Surg. 2001;6(4):217–20.
Kinney MC, Cidambi KR, Severns DL, Gonzales FB. Comparison of the iAssist handheld guidance system to conventional instruments for mechanical Axis restoration in total knee arthroplasty. J Arthroplast. 2018;33(1):61–6.
Kutzner I, Heinlein B, Graichen F, Bender A, Rohlmann HA, Beier A, Bergmann G. Loading of the knee joint during activities of daily living measured in vivo in five subjects. J Biomech. 2010;43:2164–73.
Lombardi AV, Frye BM. Customization of cutting blocks: can this address the problem? Curr Rev Musculoskelet Med. 2012;5(4):309–14.
Mahaluxmivala J, Bankes M, Nicolai P, Aldam C, Allen P. The effect of surgeon experience on component positioning in 673 Press Fit Condylar posterior cruciate-sacrificing total knee arthroplasties. J Arthroplast. 2001;16(5):635–40.
Meere PA, Schneider SM, Walker PS. Accuracy of balancing at total knee surgery using an instrumented tibial trial. J Arthroplast. 2016;31(9):1938–42.
Mihalko WM. Patient-specific cutting guides were not better than conventional instrumentation for total knee arthroplasty. J Bone Joint Surg Am. 2015;97(22):1891.

Moreland JR, Bassett LW, Hanker GJ. Radiographic analysis of the axial alignment of the lower extremity. J Bone Joint Surg Am. 1987;69(5):745–9.
Morrison JB. The mechanics of the knee joint in relation to normal walking. J Biomech. 1970;3(1):51–61.
Nam D, Nawabi DH, Cross MB, Heyse TJ, Mayman DJ. Accelerometer-based computer navigation for performing the distal femoral resection in total knee arthroplasty. J Arthroplast. 2012;27(9):1717–22.
Ng VY, DeClaire JH, Berend KR, Gulick BC, Lombardi AV Jr. Improved accuracy of alignment with patient-specific positioning guides compared with manual instrumentation in TKA. Clin Orthop Relat Res. 2012;470(1):99–107.
Noble PC & Conditt M. Computer-based training methods for surgical procedures. US Patent no. 7,427,200B2. Filed 2003, issues 2008.
Parratte S, Pagnano MW, Trousdale RT, Berry DJ. Effect of postoperative mechanical axis alignment on the fifteen-year survival of modern, cemented total knee replacements. J Bone Joint Surg Am. 2010;92:2143–9.
Parratte S, Price AJ, Jeys LM, Jackson WF, Clarke HD. Accuracy of a new robotically assisted technique for total knee arthroplasty: a cadaveric study. J Arthroplast. 2019;34(11):2799–803.
Peters CL, Jimenez C, Erickson J, Anderson MB, Pelt CE. Lessons learned from selective soft-tissue release for gap balancing in primary total knee arthroplasty: an analysis of 1216 consecutive total knee arthroplasties: AAOS exhibit selection. J Bone Joint Surg (Am Vol). 2013;95(20):e152.
Pinskerova V, Samuelson KM, Stammers J, Maruthainar K, Sosna A, Freeman MA. The knee in full flexion: an anatomical study. J Bone Joint Surg. 2009;91(6):830–4.
Pritchett JW. Charles O Townley: Design by Reason. 1988. www.seattlejointsurgeon.com.
Ranawat CS, Dorr LD. Technique of Total knee arthroplasty with precision cut instruments. In: Total-condylar knee arthroplasty. Berlin: Springer; 1985. p. 69–83.
Ritter MA, Davis KE, Meding JB, Pierson JL, Berend ME, Malinzak RA. The effect of alignment and BMI on failure of total knee replacement. J Bone Joint Surg Am. 2011;93(17):1588–96.
Rivière C, Lazic S, Boughton O, Wiart Y, Vïllet L, Cobb J. Current concepts for aligning knee implants: patient-specific or systematic? EFORT Open Rev. 2018;3(1):1–6.
Shelton TJ, Nedopil AJ, Howell SM, Hull ML. Do varus or valgus outliers have higher forces in the medial or lateral compartments than those which are in-range after a kinematically aligned total knee arthroplasty? Bone Joint J. 2017;99-B:1319–28.
Steindler A. Kinesiology of the human body under normal and pathological conditions. Springfield: Publ Charles C Thomas; 1955.
Thienpont E, Schwab PE, Fennema P. Efficacy of patient-specific instruments in total knee arthroplasty: a systematic review and meta-analysis. J Bone Joint Surg Am. 2017;99(6):521–30.
Townley CO. Total knee arthroplasty. A personal retrospective and prospective review. Clin Orthop Relat Res. 1988;236:8–22.
Verstraete MA, Meere PA, Salvadore G, Victor J, Walker PS. Contact forces in the tibiofemoral joint from soft tissue tensions: implications to soft tissue balancing in total knee arthroplasty. J Biomech. 2017;58:195–202.
Walker PS, Meere PA, Bell CP. Effects of surgical variables in balancing of total knee replacements using an instrumented tibial trial. Knee. 2014;21(1):156–61.
Weinberg DS, Gebhart JJ, Wera GD. An Anatomic Investigation Into the Relationship Between Posterior Condylar Offset and Posterior Tibial Slope of One Thousand One Hundred Thirty-Eight Cadaveric Knees. J Arthroplasty. 2017;32(5):1659–1664.e1651.
Whiteside LA, Kasselt MR, Haynes DW. Varus-valgus and rotational stability in rotationally unconstrained total knee arthroplasty. Clin Orthop Relat Res. 1987;219:147–57.
Whiteside L. Assess and release the tight ligament. In: Total knee arthroplasty: Springer; 2005. p. 170–6.
Whiteside LA, Saeki K, Mihalko WM. Functional medical ligament balancing in total knee arthroplasty. Clin Orthop Relat Res. 2000;380:45–57.
Zapata G, Sanz-Pena I, Verstraete M, Walker PS. Effects of femoral component placement on the balancing of a total knee at surgery. J Biomech. 2019;86:117–24.

Testing and Tribology

13

How Were Designs Tested for Wear, Strength, and Kinematics?

Any new mechanical device needs to be thoroughly tested before it is put into general use, especially if there would be serious consequences in the event of a failure. Testing requires standard test methods which have been validated as representing service conditions. Yet, in the 1960s when total hips had been used in patients for only a few years, and artificial knees were just being introduced, standard tests for artificial joints did not exist, even though the American Society for Testing and Materials (ASTM) F4 Committee for Medical Devices was initiated in 1962. That is not to say that tests were not carried out or were considered unnecessary. Some of the early designs were indeed subjected to tests devised by their inventors, but many other designs were introduced without any testing at all. The following describes the rationale behind some of the earliest tests and how the test methods gradually became more sophisticated and expanded in scope.

Tribology (Friction, Lubrication, and Wear)

The methodologies for testing the friction and wear in artificial hips and knees originated from studies of the mechanics of the anatomic joint, such as the sliding behavior between the cartilage bearing surfaces. Researchers such as Charles McCutcheon PhD (1962) built machines where specimens of cartilage were loaded on to glass surfaces, reciprocating motion applied, and the frictional shear force measured. The friction was measured under various loading conditions and lubricants, to enable hypotheses to be tested regarding the lubrication mechanisms. The friction coefficients were extremely small, less than 0.01, far less than was possible using metals and plastics. Obtaining the lowest possible friction was a major goal of John Charnley for his artificial hip, which is one reason why the femoral head was only 22 mm in diameter. High torque from a large-diameter metal femoral head would transmit directly to the cement-bone interface of the acetabular component, predicted to cause premature loosening. In an anatomic hip, the average femoral head diameter is 50 mm, but if applied to an artificial hip, this would have left inadequate

P. S. Walker, *The Artificial Knee*, https://doi.org/10.1007/978-3-030-38171-4_13

thickness of the plastic acetabular component and also produced a large frictional torque during flexion-extension.

In the early 1960s a metal-on-metal design of total hip, the McKee-Farrar hip, was widely used, which did use anatomic dimensions for the femoral head, because the acetabular component was made as thin metal shell. However, Charnley considered that the large head diameter as well as the higher-friction coefficient of metal-on-metal compared with metal-on-plastic would be major disadvantages. To demonstrate this, Charnley designed a two-channel pendulum friction machine which is on display at the Wrightington Hospital in England. The hip joints were loaded, and then an arc of flexion was applied and released. The number of swings before a hip finally came to a stop was an indicator of the friction. As expected, the small-diameter metal-on-plastic hip kept swinging for much longer than the large-diameter metal-on-metal hip. This demonstration was a deciding factor for many visiting hip surgeons. Another characteristic of metal-on-metal hips was that high torques could be caused by inadequate ball-socket clearance or by socket distortion when it was inserted into the acetabulum. Metal-on-plastic hips on the other hand were not sensitive to such factors.

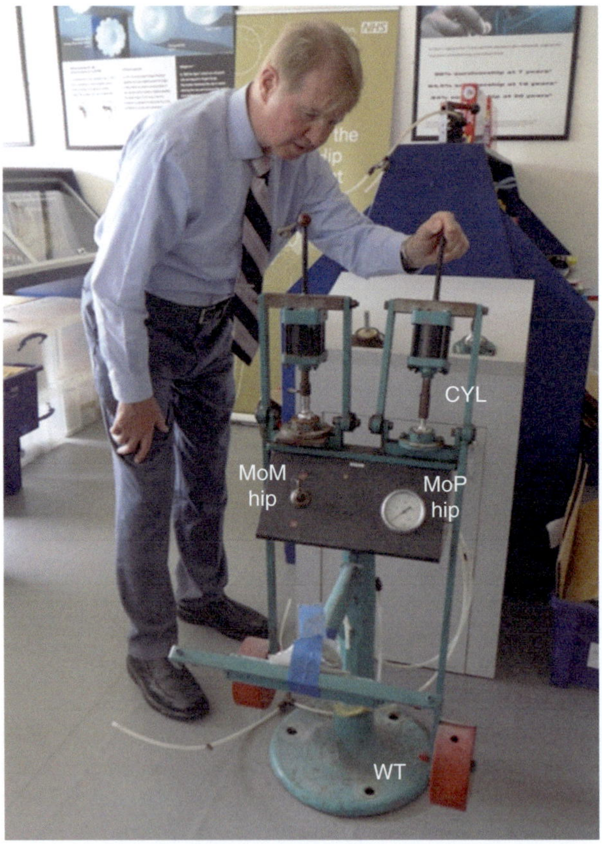

Fig. 13.1 Peter Walker studying the pendulum rig designed by John Charnley for demonstrating the relative frictional torque between two different artificial hip designs. MoM = metal-on-metal hip, McKee-Farrar hip, 36 mm dia. MoP = metal-on-plastic hip, Charnley, 22 mm dia. The center of the ball-in-socket was the pivot for the pendulum. Red weights WT are below. The cylinders CYL at the top apply loads to the hips. Both pendulums were given the same initial displacement. The pendulum which stopped swinging first had the highest frictional torque. The Charnley hip had lower friction than the McKee-Farrar due to the lower friction coefficient of the materials and the smaller diameter. (Photo taken at the Hip Museum, Wrightington Hospital, England, 2017)

Another important requirement for total hips was to minimize the wear of the plastic component. In the Charnley hip design of the late 1950s, the use of polytetrafluoroethylene (PTFE) for the socket had led to excessive wear, even though the friction was small. It is often assumed that low friction equates to low wear, but this is not necessarily true for metal-on-plastic bearings. Charnley realized that a wear test machine was needed which realistically simulated hip function. Rather than just testing samples of the materials themselves, Charnley designed a four-channel machine which tested the actual hip joints, where the machine flexed and extended the joints under a constant load. This test led Charnley to choose high-density polyethylene for the acetabular component, first implanted in 1962. Despite this background in testing of the friction and wear of hip joints, similar testing was not recorded for Gunston's knee, designed in the late 1960s at the same center at Wrightington Hospital. The only reference to testing the knee was: "A program of cadaveric trials and load tests was completed before use of the prosthesis in a patient" (Gunston 1971). There are few records available at Wrightington on the development of Gunston's Polycentric knee, and it is likely that the major attention at that time was still on the Charnley hip.

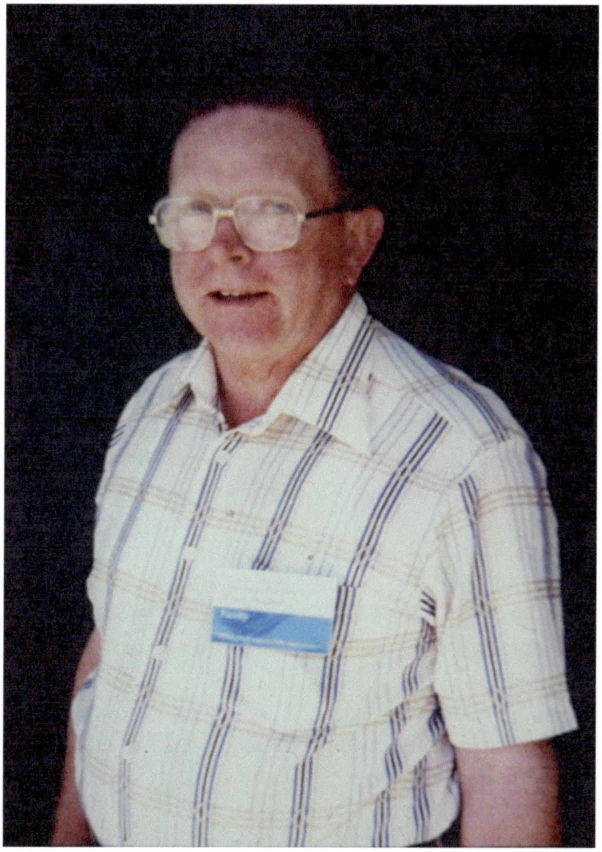

Fig. 13.2 Sir John Charnley FRCS developed the first successful total hip replacement in the early 1960s, which led directly to the development of the artificial knee. It is impossible to overestimate the influence which Charnley had on the field of artificial joints, whether in research, design, technique, or teaching. His continuous critical appraisal and his striving for further improvements moved the entire field forwards. And all this was accomplished in Wrightington Hospital, a small country hospital in North West England, without the benefit of a major University center. (Photo taken at an AAOS conference c 1990) (© Peter S Walker)

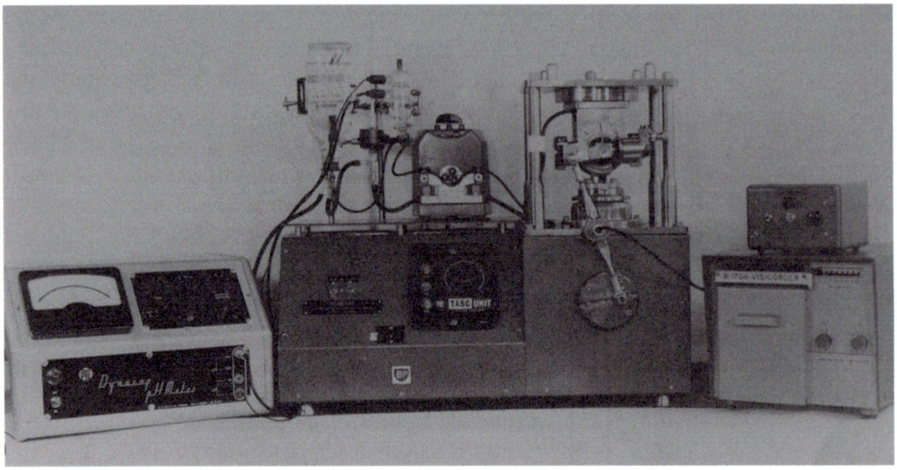

Fig. 13.3 One of the first joint simulating machines designed to test the wear of artificial hip joints. In the early 1960s, there were questions concerning the most efficacious materials for the socket, polyethylene being but one possibility. The machine was designed in John Scales's laboratory at the Royal National Orthopaedic Hospital, Stanmore, England, in collaboration with British Petroleum Research laboratories. (Photo from Conference Proceedings, Lubrication & Wear in Human Joints, Leeds, England, 1970)

Another center in the UK where there was an interest in testing artificial hip joints in the 1960s, was the Royal National Orthopaedic Hospital at Stanmore, located in north London and affiliated with University College London. The Professor of Bioengineering, John Scales MD PhD, collaborated with engineers at the British Petroleum Research Center to develop an elaborate hip simulating machine for friction and wear testing. This machine applied cyclic loads and motions applied along three axes to the hip joint being tested. Tests were carried out on metal-on-metal and metal-on-polyethylene hips, including the Charnley, McKee-Farrar, and Stanmore designs. While Scales agreed that metal-on-polyethylene produced lower friction than metal-on-metal, the volumetric wear of the latter was less, such that Scales concluded: "We believe that it is essential to continue with studies of all-metal bearings, particularly for those prostheses which might have to last for upwards of forty years." This applied mainly to bone tumor implants used in younger patients, which had been developed.

From the 1950s, John Scales working with JT "Ginger" Wilson and other surgeons had developed an expertise in the design and manufacture of prostheses for replacing large segments of bone in cases of bone tumors. The distal femoral and proximal tibial implants included an all-metal fixed-axis knee hinge. By the 1960s, the hinged knee joint had been developed into a stand-alone hinged joint, with plastic bushings in the bearings, used for cases of advanced knee deformity and instability. Some basic wear tests of the bushings were carried out comparing metal and polymeric materials. It was surprising that a metal-polyethylene condylar type of total knee was not developed at Stanmore by 1970 considering that such a design was already being designed by Freeman and Swanson in London and by Gunston at Wrightington. After all, considering the increasing demand for hip replacement, surely the same would apply to the knee. The answer was the skepticism regarding the viability of the condylar replacement type of total knee, because by the 1960s, all-metal hinges had already become well established in England and in other European countries with designs including the Walldius, Shiers, Stanmore, GSB, and St. George. These hinges were thought to be a reliable solution for the typical severe knee problems at the time. Mild to moderate arthritis was still treated with osteotomy or conservative treatments such as debridement. However, by the early 1970s the situation started to change with condylar knees rapidly gaining ground.

At another London location, Imperial College London, laboratory tests were developed in the mid-1960s for wear and fixation testing of the Freeman-Swanson total knee (Swanson et al. 1973; Freeman et al. 1982). The resources of the newly established bioengineering unit housed in the Mechanical Engineering Department were well suited for designing and constructing the equipment and for carrying out the tests. Nevertheless, the wear test machine was relatively simple in construction, in that it oscillated the femoral component through a flexion arc of 90 degrees with a constant load of 210 pounds. The tests were only run to one million cycles, which represents less than a year of usage even for typical patients requiring a total knee. Furthermore, the loading did not include shear or torque which would most likely have increased the wear and deformation of the polyethylene. The rationale was: "Flexion-extension movements….can be applied cyclically….under load. This is the only movement essential to a knee joint." As well as measuring the wear, tibial fixation tests were also considered important. The reason was that the long cemented intramedullary stems of the hinged knee joints being used at the time provided secure fixation, whereas there was the possibility that plastic components cemented only to the surface of the tibia could loosen. The test devised was to cement the components into tibial specimens and then to apply an axial torque until failure of the fixation.

To put these tests in context, while data of the forces in the hip joint during function was obtained at the Bioengineering Department, Strathclyde University, Glasgow, Scotland, in the mid-1960s, parallel data on the knee was not published until 1968, after the testing of the initial Freeman-Swanson knee. The knee force studies carried out as a PhD thesis by James Morrison, under the supervision of John Paul, significantly advanced the understanding of how the knee functioned in real-life conditions and provided invaluable data for the design and testing of artificial knees (Morrison 1968, 1970).

The most well-known center in the field of tribology at the time was the Mechanical Engineering Department at the University of Leeds in England. Professor Duncan Dowson had built up a research activity in tribology and was recognized as one of the leaders in the field with his concepts of elastohydrodynamic lubrication. When Bahaa Seedhom PhD from Leeds University designed his cruciate retaining anatomically shaped total knee in the early 1970s, it was the wear of the polyethylene which was his major concern. The main reason why Seedhom focused on wear was because he had developed a heat-forming method to shape the

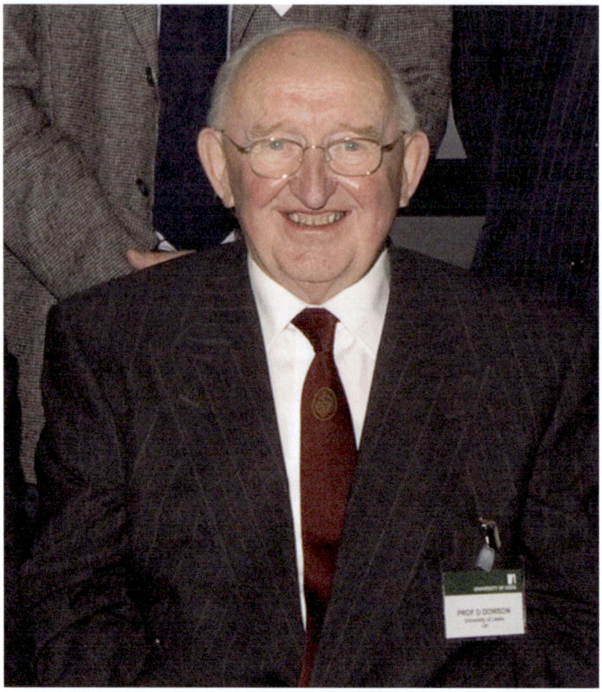

Fig. 13.4 Duncan Dowson PhD at age 80. Dowson was a major pioneer in the area of tribology at the University of Leeds, England. He motivated many researchers to study the tribology of human joints and develop artificial joints with low friction and wear. He was a co-organizer of the first major Conference on Total Knee Replacement held at the Institution of Mechanical Engineers in London, in September 1974. In his later years, he produced the authoritative book on the history of tribology while continuing to participate in committee activities of the Institution of Mechanical Engineers. (Photo taken at celebration event 'Dowson at 80')

tibial bearing surfaces. The shapes of these surfaces were generated by moving the metal femoral condyles through a succession of motion paths which included combinations of flexion-extension, internal-external rotation, and anterior-posterior displacement. The resulting surfaces could not be described by circular arcs and hence were not amenable to machining using the technologies available at that time. Instead, hand-formed metal molds were pressed against polyethylene preforms to produce the final surface.

Seedhom considered designing a wear testing machine for the components themselves, but this would have been time-consuming and expensive. Instead, he used a tri-pin-on-disc apparatus to measure the wear of cylindrical pins made from the heat-formed polyethylene, equipment which was already available (Seedhom et al. 1973). This test method was a standard procedure in the field of tribology where a plastic pin was loaded onto a polished metal disc with a constant load and sliding speed and the wear measured at time intervals. Based on the volumetric wear, the wear coefficient for the material could be calculated.

However, the test did not embody the complex cyclic loading patterns combined with sliding in different directions, as in the anatomic knee joint. Seedhom circumvented these limitations by using the wear data to predict the wear depth of the plastic socket of a Charnley hip joint and comparing his prediction with that measured in clinical studies in which the wear was measured radiographically. On finding close agreement with the actual value of 0.1 mm per year, Seedhom felt confident enough to predict that his knee design would only wear by 1 mm depth in 20 years:

"This is thought to be an acceptable wear rate." To provide credibility for this prediction, Seedhom measured the number of steps a typical patient would take per year. The test subjects were fitted with a pedometer which they used each day over a period of time. Averaging the data from several subjects in each group, the steps per year were housewives 8000, old people on vacation 6000, and university staff 11,000. By combining this data with Morrison's force data, Seedhom was able to calculate the force and distance terms in Archard's wear equation: Wear volume = wear factor x load x sliding distance. (There has recently been a renewed interest in obtaining the activity data of patients with artificial knees, by using electronic wearable sensors.)

Laxity and Stability

While Seedhom's work on an artificial knee was proceeding, Peter Walker was working in the Bioengineering Department at Leeds University, completing his PhD project on the lubrication of anatomic joints. In November 1969, Walker moved to the Hospital for Special Surgery in New York. In the design of the Total Condylar knee in the early 1970s, Walker and colleagues took a different approach to testing, concentrating more on the laxity and stability of the joint, rather than on the wear. The former was regarded as a higher priority given that the designs up to that time

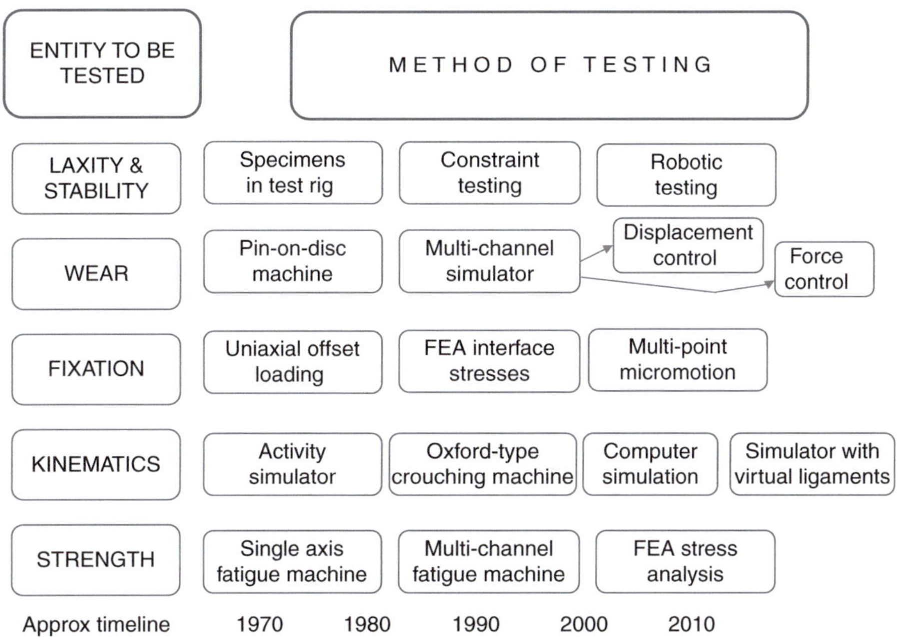

Fig. 13.5 Summary of the most common testing methods of the artificial knee components used from 1970 to the present. The different methods of testing are referred to in the text. FEA finite element analysis

covered the range from high to low conformity, and more experimental data was needed to determine the ideal (Walker et al. 1974). The theory behind the Total Condylar knee was that when it was implanted, the laxity and stability behavior would be the same as when the knee was intact, even though the cruciate ligaments had been resected. To address this, the laxity and stability of anatomic knee specimens were measured by designing test rigs where the knees were mounted into fixtures in an Instron loading machine. Combinations of compressive force, shear force, and torque were applied, and the resulting laxities were measured. All of the ligaments of the specimens were intact so the laxities represented that of the entire knee. Typical laxities for the unloaded knee were a total of 14 mm of anterior-posterior displacement and +/− 15 degrees internal-external rotation. However, when compressive load was applied, the laxity values reduced considerably due to the stability provided by the dishing and compression of the bearing surfaces and the menisci. As a result of this basic research, equations were written from which the radii of the bearing surfaces of the Total Condylar were calculated, in order to produce the same combination of laxity and stability as the anatomic knee.

From the mid-1970s, Keith Markolf PhD developed more elaborate testing methods for measuring the laxity of the knee, both on specimens and on patients, the main application being to sports medicine. The equipment was ingeniously constructed to allow the application of forces and moments but without constraining the resulting motions in other degrees of freedom. He defined laxity, measured in millimeters or degrees, as well as stiffness, being force/displacement. Markolf used his methods to measure the laxity and stability of the Geometric and Anametric artificial knees and the effects of the cruciates (Markolf et al. 1979): "We believe that the characteristics should be correlated with clinical performance and….future designs should be evaluated before they are released for clinical trial." The ASTM have since formulated a standard for characterizing the laxity called "Standard Test Method for Determination of Total Knee Constraint" where the amount of constraint in an artificial knee is measured under different loading conditions. This method was developed in the Orthopaedic Research Laboratories of Seth Greenwald (Postak et al. 1994; Heim et al. 2001). With the femoral component and tibial component set at a prescribed flexion angle, a vertical force was applied to the femoral component. The tibial component was free to move in a horizontal plane. An anterior shear force was applied to the tibia, followed by a medial-lateral force, and finally an axial torque. The maximum forces and torques at the point of dislocation were recorded. Of the six contemporary knee systems tested, there was a wide variation in the forces. These values were compared with those which occurred in functional conditions. The application of the data was to determine whether a particular design could be used without cruciate ligaments or needed preservation of one or both of the cruciates, recognizing that normal function is: "dependent upon load sharing between the implant and the surrounding ligaments…." The authors envisaged that different tibial inserts could be selected depending on the status of each knee: "Implant modularity defines an ability to select different plateau geometries for a specific femoral component and tibial tray design, extending the clinical application of these devices." This is the usual situation with present-day knee systems.

Fixation of Components

Another aspect of total knee design which required a testing methodology was fixation of the tibial component. The experience with the Freeman-Swanson, the Geometric, and the Duo-condylar knees was that interface failure of the tibial component at the cement-bone interface was all too frequent. And yet these designs were all very different, from the solid one-piece construction of the Freeman-Swanson to the crossbridge connection of the Geometric and to the separate plateaus of the Duo-condylar. It could easily have been assumed that the loosening was caused by shear and torque forces, especially due to the conforming geometries of the Freeman-Swanson and Geometric. However, Peter Walker, Chitranjan Ranawat, and John Insall proposed that an important factor was the axial compressive forces acting at a distance from the center of the components, producing a rocking or see-saw effect (Walker et al. 1976). Experiments were conducted in a simple test rig where unicompartmental components were cemented on to resected tibial surfaces, loads applied at different points on the surfaces of the component, and the distractions at the interface measured at the anterior or posterior of the components. It was found that distractions of up to 500 microns (0.5 mm) occurred, especially when there was nonuniform bone density from anterior to posterior. The testing protocol was related to actual surgical cases as follows: "A radiographic study of condylar replacement knees taken at extension and flexion, shows that in many instances the loading point lies outside of the central region of the component." To minimize such interface distractions, the authors determined that anterior and posterior keyholes for cement, or a keel on the base of the tibial component, would be effective.

This work, as well as the clinical experience of designs with one-piece or separate medial and lateral plateaus, led to a complete rethink of tibial component design. A one-piece component would have a more rigid construction, but there would need to be a solid medial-lateral connection, which would eliminate designs which retained both cruciates. Even a one-piece construction would need a rigid connection to the tibia, rather than just drill holes or short keels and pegs. Based on earlier studies of trabecular bone density, the central region of the tibia consisted of relatively soft bone. This led to the idea of a central peg in this region which would be flanked on each of its sides by stronger bone and yet would not require excavating any of the bone on the medial and lateral sides. Such a central peg component was predicted to have more durable fixation than two separate components.

For the fixation of tibial components, another important factor was the effect of repetitive loading, where gradual fatigue failure of the trabecular bone could occur to produce complete loss of fixation, which would not be detected by tests where single loads were applied. This led to the idea of a cyclic load machine which could test multiple samples at the same time (Walker and Hsieh 1977). A nine-channel knee simulating machine was designed, with a flexion-extension arc of 45 degrees and where an axial force of twice body weight was applied for half the cycle. Offsetting the axis of rotation of the femoral component caused the point of force application on the tibia to displace anterior-posterior, reproducing the off-center loading of the earlier static experiments. This multichannel machine allowed for multiple tests to be carried out for millions of cycles in a practical time period. With the one-piece central peg design, there were no interface failures, whereas with the separate plateaus, almost every one failed by fatigue failure of the trabecular bone around the interface.

Following this work, there were few reported studies on tibial fixation in the second half of the 1970s, which is surprising because tibial component loosening was a common problem with the early designs. One study compared the failure modes of two of the earliest designs, the Polycentric and the Geometric knees, when subjected to axial loading (Nogi et al. 1976). The components were cemented into complete knee specimens, the femur and tibia potted in cylinders, and the load applied through a simple press. In both designs, there was fracture of the acrylic cement at the tibial interface. For the Polycentric, in addition, there was sinkage of the tibial components due to compressive failure of the underlying trabecular bone. Examples of both failure modes were seen clinically. Absence of failure of the femoral component was notable, which was later explained qualitatively by the finding that the compressive strength of the trabecular bone in the distal femur was higher than in the proximal tibia (Colley et al. 1978). The interaction of several processes over time was later proposed as failure mechanisms (Ducheyne et al. 1978): varus misalignment leading to medial overload, trabecular failure causing even higher medial loads, and bending of plastic components.

At the Orthopaedic Research Society (ORS) meeting in 1979 (Clement B Sledge MD was President that year), Bill Krause PhD and Joe Miller MD from McGill University in Montreal, Canada, presented their work on the importance of cement penetration into trabecular bone and how to achieve it. The work was published a few years later (Krause et al. 1982). It was proposed that no matter what was the design of the tibial component, unless several millimeters of cement penetration was achieved over the entire interface, bone resorption and fixation failure would occur. Cement penetration was achieved by lavage cleaning and then pressurizing using special nozzles attached to syringes (see Chap. 5). This work led to a major change in the way in which cementing was carried out, but in certain conditions, it was found that there was excessive cement penetration, which was considered undesirable. Several years later, Larry Dorr MD, from the Good Samaritan Hospital in Los Angeles, showed that excessive cement penetration could be avoided, by demonstrating that 2–4 mm was reproducibly achieved using lavage and finger pressing in surgical conditions (Dorr et al. 1984).

Meanwhile there was still no consensus on the optimal design for the tibial component. At the Brigham and Women's Hospital in the early 1980s, an apparatus for fixation testing was constructed where tibial components were fixed to tibial specimens, and a simulated femoral component was loaded from above such that combinations of forces and moments were applied, representing functional loading. Using noncontact transducers, distraction or compression of the tibial component relative to the tibia was measured at points around the periphery (Walker et al. 1981). The criterion was that the least deflections signified the most rigid fixation. Not surprisingly, one-piece components with metal-backing and a central peg were the most successful. Using the same test rig, Peter Brooks MD, a resident at the time, developed wedges to buttress bone deficiencies seen in cases of severe varus or valgus deformity (Brooks et al. 1984).

At the end of the 1980s, after the early experience with uncemented components coated with fiber-metal on sintered beads, there was renewed interest in minimizing the interface micromotion between the porous surface and the trabecular bone. Several laboratories carried out tests where the tibia and its component were mounted in a base, while a vertical rod from a loading machine applied forces to the tibial surface, either centrally or offset to simulate varus loading. Deflections between the component and the bone were measured using transducers. Three examples of such tests are cited here (Volz et al. 1988: Branson et al. 1989; Whiteside and Pafford 1989). Taking a composite of the results, it was found that offset loads usually produced unacceptably high distractions or compressions of the component relative to the bone. Certain combinations of pegs reduced the motions, but screws into the cancellous bone minimized the motions and hence were adopted clinically for most of the uncemented design systems. This is an example where a relatively simple testing method could result in a practical solution which succeeded in practice. However the method did rely on previous basic work which highlighted the importance of interface micromotions as a crucial experimental parameter.

Simulating Machines

We now return to the early 1970s to the development of more elaborate machines which attempted to simulate both the loads and the motions which occurred in walking and other activities. David G Murray MD from Upstate Medical Center in Syracuse, NY, was developing a new type of artificial knee, the Variable Axis. To validate its mechanical efficacy, some type of testing machine was needed to evaluate the wear and fixation strength. Murray collaborated with John Shaw PhD at the Mechanical Engineering Department. They designed and constructed a simulating machine which was based on reproducing normal knee mechanics of the lower extremity (Shaw and Murray 1973). The data of kinematics and forces was already available from James Morrison PhD, which was used in the design of the machine. Instead of loading the femoral or tibial components directly, they applied a vertical body weight to the hip joint and obtained flexion and extension motion across the knee by applying forces to a chain attached to the tibial tubercle, which reproduced the quadriceps mechanism. Since the muscle forces required to perform a specific activity are a function of the joint geometry, physiological joint loading could be achieved for any given external load by ensuring that all forces crossing the joint did so at anatomic locations and directions. The machine was intended to simulate the lower extremity performing a high flexion activity such as walking up and down stairs and crouching. However, due to the limitations of the control system, only approximate wave patterns for motion and forces could be achieved. The concept of the Shaw-Murray dynamic machine was adopted by Ben Hillberry PhD and others at Purdue University, Indiana (Maletsky and Hillberry 2005). The intention was to simulate vigorous activities, which meant high forces and rates of change of joint

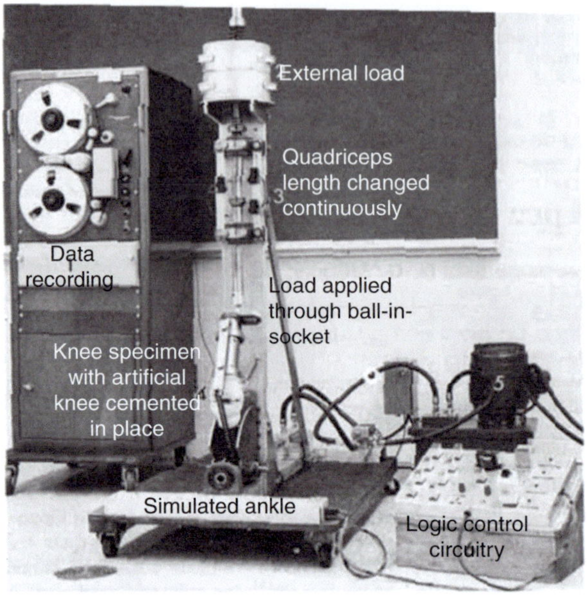

Fig. 13.6 The first knee simulator of its type designed to simulate the loads and motions during walking, such that wear and fixation of an artificial knee could be studied. A vertical external load is applied at the top while the flexion-extension is controlled by changing the quadriceps length during the cycle. A force is generated in the quadriceps cable to equilibrate the external force. The direction of the external force in the frontal plane could be modified to simulate varus or valgus misalignment (Shaw and Murray 1973). (Reprinted with permission from Clinical Orthopaedics & Related Research)

angles, for which data was now available. The machine was also to be used with knee specimens or with artificial joints mounted on fixtures. The authors validated that the tibiofemoral forces were realistic, but even so, the machine simulated quadriceps forces only and did not include the hamstrings, which would have affected the force vectors at the knee. Mechanical complexity limited the application of the machine to short-term tests, such as determining joint forces and contact forces at the knee, rather than long-term fixation or wear studies.

Recognizing the complexity of simulating actual functions, other researchers developed test equipment which was easier to construct and operate yet could still provide meaningful data of some aspect of joint mechanics. Such equipment was first developed at Oxford University, called the Oxford Knee Rig. The Shaw-Murray and the Purdue were machines in that they provided continuous motion and included changing forces and motions. On the other hand, a rig is a construct where a knee is subjected to loading under static conditions, even if the forces are provided by simulated muscle actions. In the Oxford Rig, the tibia was fixed vertically (or at slight flexion), the femur was flexed, a wire was attached to the quadriceps, and the other end of the wire was attached to a weight which was hung over a pulley at the proximal end of the quadriceps. Adjusting the length of the wire produced different

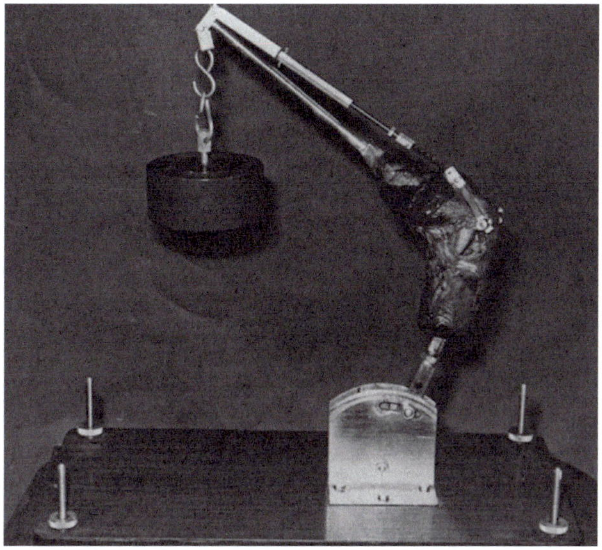

Fig. 13.7 The original Oxford Knee Rig. The forward flexion of the tibia was adjustable from 0 to 30 degrees. The flexion angle was controlled by screw adjustment of the quadriceps length. The rig was used to study the instant centers of rotation of the knee and the contact areas in the patellofemoral joint. A limitation was that the maximum load that could be applied was 75 Newtons (Goodfellow et al. 1976). (Reprinted with permission from Journal of Bone & Joint Surgery B)

flexion angles. The Oxford Rig using this configuration was designed in 1976 to carry out studies of the contact areas in the patellofemoral joint (Goodfellow et al. 1976; Harding et al. 1977). Later, John O'Connor PhD enhanced the functionality by changing the rig to a machine, which simulated the entire lower extremity and where flexion-extension was actively controlled by lengthening and shortening the quadriceps length. This simulated a crouching or squatting activity, useful in that the knee could be studied from full extension to full flexion. The mechanical complexity was greatly reduced from the earlier functional simulating machines. As a result, the Oxford-type machine was widely used in many other laboratories. Using such a machine, Robert Singerman et al. (1995) at Case Western Reserve University, Cleveland, OH, measured the patellofemoral forces and found that the maximum force occurred at 70 degrees flexion and was less than the quadriceps force, peaking at 0.8 times body weight. The center of pressure moved from the lower to the upper patella as flexion increased. They showed the effect of the quadriceps force direction, the Q-angle, giving a tendency for the patella to sublux laterally. This had has application to femoral component design and surgical technique. Some time later, Ezzet et al. (2001) working with Darryl D'Lima MD and others at the Scripps Clinic in San Diego expanded this work to an artificial patella and found improved kinematics with a medialized inset patella. In both of these studies, there was considerable variation in the data between specimens. Other researchers also used the same type of test machine. Miller and Zhang agreed with patella medialization and found no effect on forces when the femoral component was externally rotated, but showed the benefits of a dome patella due to variations in tilting between knees; Rovick and Walker at the Brigham and Women's Hospital determined average knee motion and used the data for the design of an asymmetric total knee.

One of the limitations of the Oxford-type machines was that the hamstring forces were not included, which results in some errors in kinematics. An important aspect of the design of such machines is that the knee joint should be provided with sufficient freedom of motion. This concept was pointed out by Piziali (see Chap. 4). In particular, although flexion-extension is applied by the changing lengths of the quadriceps, the following motions need to be unconstrained so that the femur and tibia continuously find their equilibrium positions: medial-lateral and anterior-posterior displacements and varus-valgus and internal-external rotations. To provide this, Zavatsky (1997) determined that in the design of the test machine, the hip should allow flexion-extension and ab-adduction, while the ankle should allow rotations about three axes. An excellent review of this type of testing machine was written by Kartik Varadarajan (2009). He and Guaon Li compared the data from the machines to data from fluoroscopic studies of normal subjects and artificial knee patients, to determine how relevant was the in vitro data from the Oxford-type machines. Notwithstanding the complexity of making such a comparison due to the numerous studies in the literature and the different designs of the machines and methods of testing, it was concluded: "Results showed that the machines …. can capture certain key features of closed-chain flexion-extension kinematics of both healthy and TKA knees measured in vivo. These systems can replicate the femoral rollback with flexion and screw-home tibial rotation between 0 and 30 degrees flexion seen in healthy subjects, and the reduced femoral rollback and absence of screw home motion in TKA patients."

By the year 2000, a number of researchers had seen the possibilities of using robotic equipment for testing knees. One advantage was that the existing instrumentation and software built into the machines would provide data on 6 degrees of freedom motion and forces. A review of studies carried out using robots was reviewed in the article cited above by Varadarajan and Li. Their robot was used for a number of studies of knee specimens and with specimens where artificial knees were implanted. In one example (Li et al. 2004), the contact pressures between the patella and the femoral trochlea were measured along the neutral path of motion. The method was to position the knee in an unloaded condition at a chosen angle of flexion and to sum the forces along the three axes. At this angle, the robot moved the knee incrementally in all degrees of freedom to find the position where the sum of the forces was a minimum. This defined the neutral position of the femur relative to the tibia at that flexion angle. In this way a neutral path of motion was found for a full flexion range. In subsequent testing where loads were applied, the displacements and rotations were measured relative to the neutral path. In the above example, both quadriceps and hamstrings forces were applied through ropes and pulleys. It was demonstrated that patella pressures changed considerably for both muscles compared with the quadriceps alone, from which the authors proposed that both muscle actions were needed in such testing. One limitation of their robot, and others, was that forces only up to about 200 Newtons could be applied, rather than the much higher forces of activities. This limitation was later overcome by Keith Markolf PhD and colleagues at the UCLA Orthopaedic Biomechanics Laboratory at the UCLA Rehabilitation Center (Lin 2016). Using an industrial robot, their studies

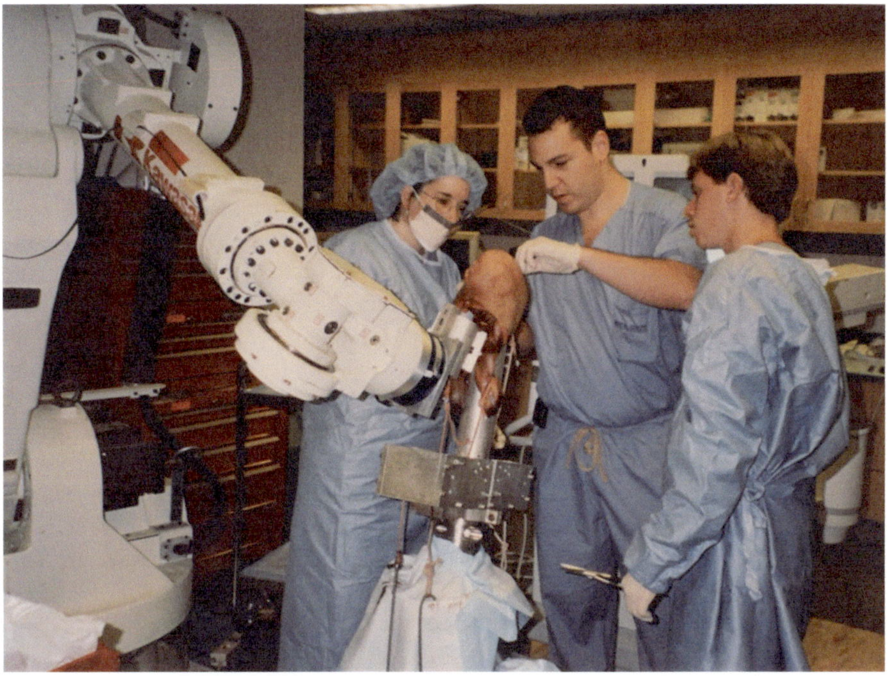

Fig. 13.8 Researchers using a robot arm to carry out biomechanical experiments on knee specimens. The robot applies and measure forces, displacements, and rotations in three dimensions to knee specimens before and after the placement of an artificial knee. This determines how closely the artificial knee replicates the anatomic knee. (Photo taken at the Zimmer Institute, Warsaw, IN c 2006)

are being mainly applied to ligament reconstructions rather than artificial knees: "The 8 foot high 2 ton robot….applies hundreds of pounds of force to a cadaver knee specimen implanted with a custom-designed sensor that measures forces in a knee ligament….Pairing this with a computer program that analyzes every move, the researchers are shedding new light on how the knee works, how it gets injured and how best to repair it. We need a big robot to simulate big forces."

A different mechanical configuration to the above test machines was needed for wear testing, for which physiological loading up to at least five million cycles was required. At one cycle per second, a test would take almost 60 days of continuous running, even more due to the need to make wear measurements at least every million cycles. This demanded a multichannel machine. One of the first such machines was developed in the 1990s at the Royal National Orthopaedic Hospital in Stanmore, England. As a result of the work of John Scales and his staff, there were already a number of test machines in the laboratory being used for fatigue testing. However, in order to provide a more realistic simulation of in vivo conditions, the loading and motion cycles needed to be added to reproduce everyday activities, particularly the most frequent activity of walking. Another factor was that the sliding distances would vary depending on the artificial knee design. For example, a design of low conformity with posterior cruciate preservation would be expected to have greater sliding distances than a more conforming design even if the cruciates were resected. The machines should therefore be designed to account for whatever artificial knee was being tested.

When Peter Walker became Director of Bioengineering in 1987, he decided to design machines which could simulate real-life load and motion conditions. To develop such a wear testing machine, Walker organized a consortium of manufactures to contribute funding, along with the UK's Department of Health. Academic collaborators included Tom Andriacchi (Stanford University), John Paul (Strathclyde University), and David Broome and Mike Dewar (University College London). The result of this endeavor was the four-channel Stanmore Knee Simulator (Walker et al. 1997, 2000). A key feature was that this was a "force-controlled machine," where the prescribed input forces were based on Morrison's data from 25 years ago. This difficult aspect of the machine, accounting for the type of artificial knee design being tested, was solved with the collaboration of Hani Haider PhD, who joined the Department at that stage. In parallel with the mountings for the femoral and tibial components, an arrangement of springs was designed, with strong or weak stiffnesses depending on which of the cruciate ligaments was retained or resected. This concept was in contrast to an alternate scheme called "displacement control" where prescribed anterior-posterior displacements and rotation angles were imposed, along with the flexion-extension angles. With the force-controlled concept, the knee could determine its own displacements and rotations depending on its constraint. The validity of this concept has been borne out by numerous kinematic studies of total knees in patients using fluoroscopy.

John DesJardins PhD, now at Clemson University, SC, who joined the simulator project at the validation stage, carried out studies to demonstrate the efficacy of the method for kinematic comparisons as well as for wear testing (DesJardins et al. 2000). Sixteen of the machines were made by the lab's accomplished technical staff and supplied to companies and laboratories around the world. Hani Haider in his laboratory at the University of Nebraska in Omaha later carried out numerous wear tests of artificial knees for companies, many for FDA requirements, and it was largely due to his efforts that the ASTM testing standard for wear testing was adopted. He has written a comprehensive review of the field of wear testing of artificial knees, explaining the different types of wear machine and the protocols for testing (Haider 2016). Another review article was on the comparison of the wear between fixed bearing knees and mobile bearing knees (Haider and Garvin 2008; Haider and Kaddick 2012). The latter paper, coauthored with Christian Kaddick PhD, includes wear data of many different artificial knee designs, both fixed and mobile bearings. Among the recent studies was a comparison of vitamin E polyethylene compared with previous types of the material (Haider et al. 2012).

Since that time, other knee simulating machines for wear testing have been produced. A notable example is the AMTI (Advanced Mechanical Technologies Inc., Watertown, MA) 6-station Knee Simulating Machine, which can be run in either force control or displacement control modes. While the Stanmore simulator used springs to represent ligaments, the AMTI used virtual soft tissues, a major

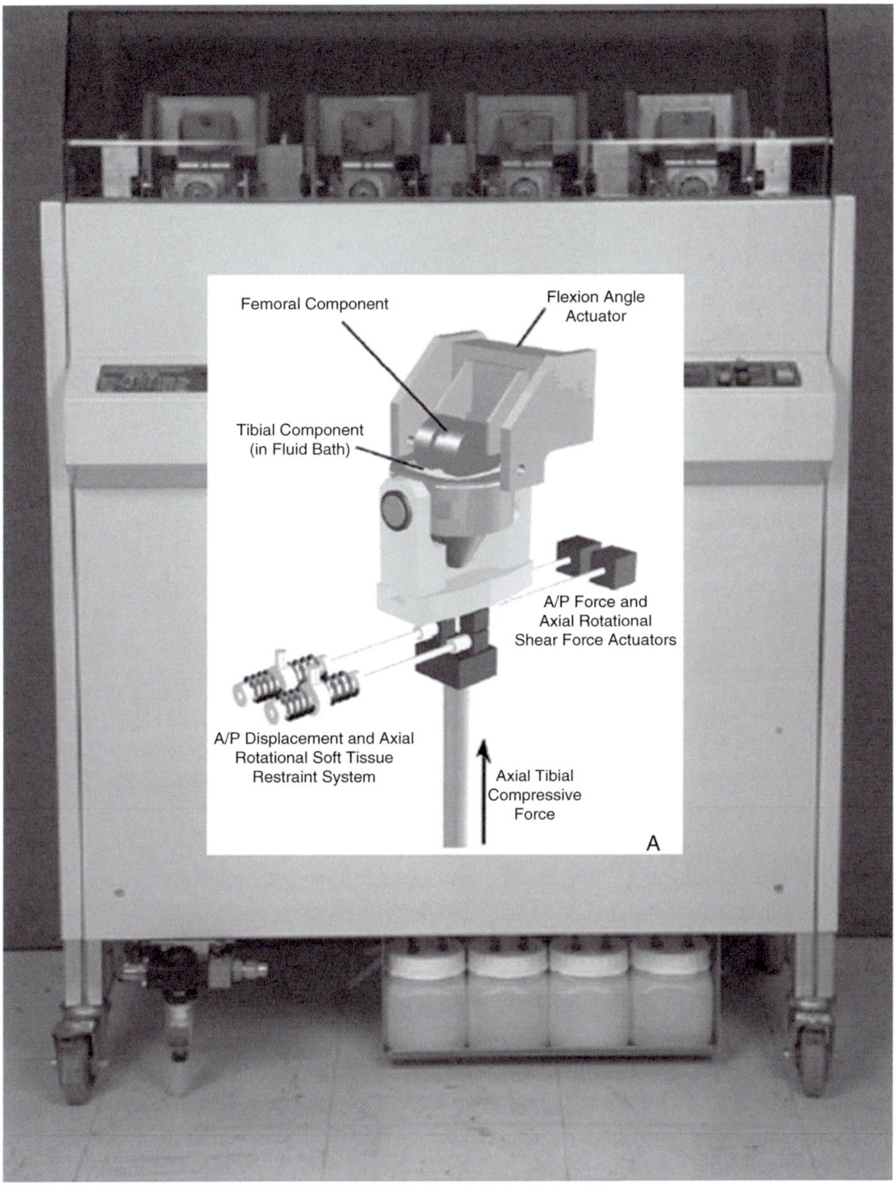

Fig. 13.9 The 4-station force-controlled Stanmore Knee Simulator was designed at the Royal National Orthopaedic Hospital, Stanmore, University College London (Walker et al. 2000). Hani Haider and Peter Walker devised a method for replacing the constraint from soft tissues using a set of springs (inset figure). The principal purpose of the machine was for long-term wear testing over millions of cycles. The machine could also be used for kinematic comparisons between different artificial knee designs (DesJardins et al. 2000). (Reprinted with permission from Elsevier Inc.)

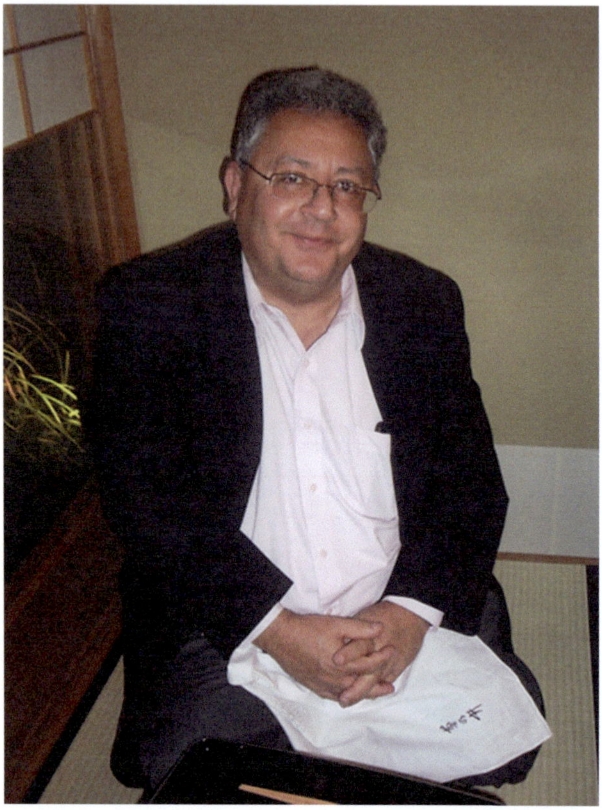

Fig. 13.10 Hani Haider PhD joined Peter Walker's lab at University College London in 1990 where he collaborated on the design of the Stanmore Knee Simulator, used for wear and kinematics testing. In 2000, he became Director of Research at University of Nebraska, Omaha, where he built up a laboratory specializing in wear testing and simulator development. Haider is an active member of the American Society for Testing and Materials (ASTM). (Photo at ISTA conference, Kyoto, Japan, 2014) (© Peter S Walker)

advancement (White et al. 2006). The concept is that each ligament is represented by its attachment points and its stiffness characteristics. As the external forces and motions are applied to the artificial knee being tested, the force vectors from the ligaments are computed in real time and combined vectorially with the applied external forces. To make the wear simulation even more realistic, Bruce White compiled the data of knee forces and kinematics in different activities determined by Georg Bergmann and colleagues (Bergmann et al. 2014). White then proposed a wear test sequence which embodied walking as the main activity, interspersed with stair ascent and descent and other activities. This test scenario was published by ASTM as guidelines but so far has not been incorporated within a standard. There is naturally some reluctance from existing wear test laboratories, to implement major changes to their existing test machines due to technical complexity and cost. Nevertheless, individual experiments have been carried out to investigate the effect of more elaborate and realistic testing conditions.

At the Endolab in Thansau, Germany, Christian Kaddick PhD has for many years carried out standard testing protocols but recently explored machine modifications to simulate highly demanding daily activities (Schwiesau et al. 2013). They

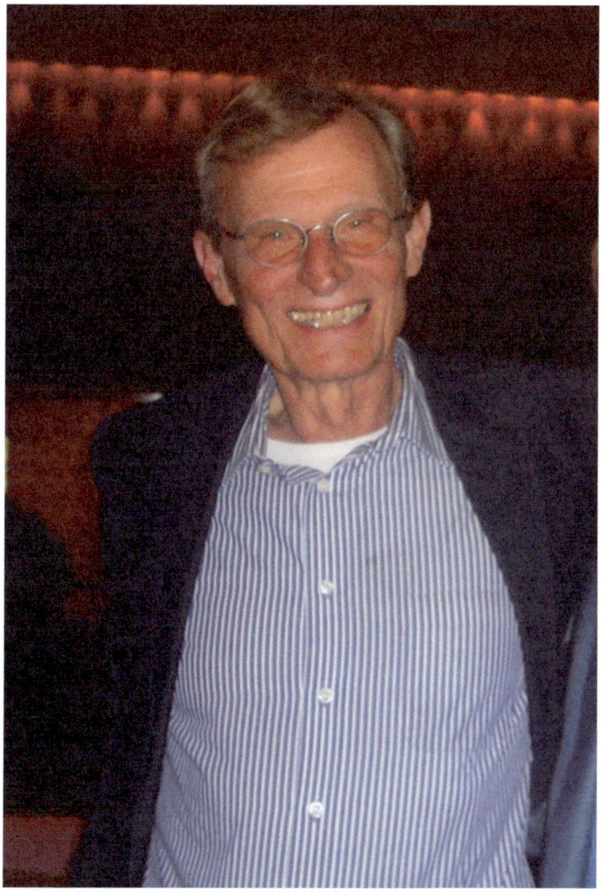

Fig. 13.11 Georg Bergmann PhD, from Charite Hospital, Berlin. He, together with colleagues, developed instrumented artificial knees from which the forces on the knee were determined for a range of activities. His articles summarizing all of the data are an invaluable resource for biomechanical testing and computer modeling. (Photo circa 2005) (© Peter S Walker)

concluded that "further testing is needed to better understand the impact of each activity and the respective influence…." At the Institute of Medical and Biological Engineering, University of Leeds, England, John Fisher and colleagues concluded that sophisticated control systems were needed in their electromechanical machine to carry out such studies (Abdelgaied et al. 2017). Research in the area of wear testing of artificial knee needs to account for technical complexity, high cost of equipment, extended time taken for testing, techniques for accurately measuring exceedingly low wear rates, the lack of complete biomechanical data of a range of activities, variations in function between individual patients, and differences between artificial knee designs and materials. To counteract these problems, studies can be carried out on a comparative basis, for example, comparing the wear between two designs, or a single design with different bearing materials.

A single-channel test machine called the VIVO Joint Simulator for studying the kinematics of the knee was recently designed and introduced by the AMTI company. Forces and flexion-extension are input to the knee based on prescribed cycles,

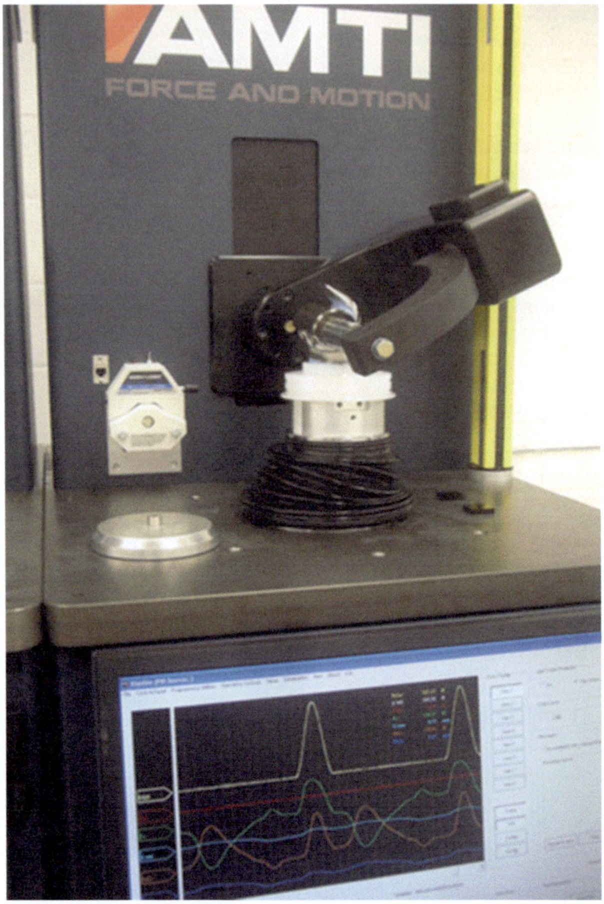

Fig. 13.12 The AMTI VIVO Joint Simulator for testing knee (and other) joints. The machine has a 6-degree-of-freedom system for applying and recording forces and motions, such that different activity cycles can be input and the output displacements and rotations measured. A unique feature is a virtual ligament restraint system where ligaments can be input as defined by their attachment points on the femur and tibia and their elastic properties. Multiple fibers can be defined for a given ligament, such as the medial collateral, to obtain more anatomic realism. (Photo at AMTI Inc., Watertown, MA, with permission c 2015)

but the ligaments are represented virtually, as described above (White et al. 2006). The attachment coordinates and stiffness values of the ligaments are input, while the software computes and applies the force vectors from the ligaments continuously during the motion cycle. Hence the effects of the ligaments on the motion can be readily determined and surgical aspects such as component alignments and soft tissue balancing can be evaluated. This capability of modeling the ligaments virtually is valuable for several reasons. It is not easy to identify a suitable material with a similar load-deflection curve to actual ligaments. Attaching synthetic ligaments at each end is problematic. Conveniently making adjustments in length to simulate varying tightness is difficult. Measuring ligament tensions directly in situ has not been solved in a simple way. Perhaps most importantly, ligaments are multi-bundle with the different parts changing their tensions throughout motion, a property which cannot be simulated practically. These problems can be solved with the virtual ligaments. An example of a study where the VIVO machine has been used for studies on artificial knees has been reported (Willing and Walker 2018).

Long-Term Durability and Wear Particles

A frequently asked question about artificial knees is how long they will last, as if there were a particular time point at which the bearing surfaces wear out or some other definitive failure mode occurs. A better question would be: what is the probability that an artificial knee will still be in place and functioning well after a certain period of time, say 10 years or 20 years? That is the essence of the Kaplan-Meier estimate, a method which has been most frequently used in follow-up studies including large rational databases. The survival probability is (the number of cases at the start – number of failures) ÷ (the number of cases at the start). Another way to express the data is by the revision rate, as shown by the Swedish Knee Registry (see Chap. 1). A 0.95 probability of survival is equivalent to a 5% revision rate. In that graph, for the most recently used artificial knee designs, the probability of survival at 10 years was close to 0.95 and at 20 years, close to 0.92. The next question might well be that because those figures were obtained for artificial knees performed 10 and 20 years ago would not today's artificial knees have an even higher survivorship. The overlap in the curves of the two most recent 10-year groups suggests that the survivorship may be reaching a limit.

In the 1970s and 1980s the most frequent modes of mechanical failure were component loosening, instability, wear-through of the polyethylene, and component fracture. Those problems were significantly reduced by improved cement technique, more accurate alignment, use of designs with inherent stability, more accurate soft tissue balancing, reduced contact stresses and wear-resistant polyethylene, and stronger components which had been thoroughly tested for fatigue strength. In these examples, the association between the causes and the failure modes can easily be seen. In contrast, determining the effect of wear particles has not been so easy. One reason has been that while an accumulation of polyethylene particles could result in bone resorption due to a biological response, resorption could also occur due to stress protection from a component which was too stiff, leading to a reduction in the density of the surrounding bone. Both situations could result in a symptomatically loose component. A further point is that the survivorship values represent the average over a large number of cases, many surgeons and hospitals, and types of artificial knee designs. For a particular case, the probability of survival at 10 years could be higher or lower based on risk factors such as inadequate cementing technique and misalignment, as well as smoking, obesity, and high activity levels.

The design of the artificial knee has until now been in a state of continuous evolution, and there is every sign that this process will continue for some time. In the early stages, many different design configurations were introduced within only a few years. As time went on, early failure of certain designs resulted in withdrawal or redesign. Successful design features were incorporated into new designs. As pointed out earlier in this book, after about only 10 years, the number of design types had been narrowed down to only a few, although the many different manufacturers had their own variations. The same process occurred for the materials, with a convergence to ultrahigh molecular weight polyethylene. Instrumentation too became standardized, with the alignment goals, bony landmarks being more accurately defined, and slotted cutting guides used for the bone cuts. In the ensuing years, the main attention was on the finer points of the design, materials, and techniques. The goal was to achieve the best performance, however, that was specified and measured. The different design concepts were compared in many ways including their stability and functional outcome. Materials were compared for wear and strength. Techniques were compared for consistency of alignment and convenience of use. A crucial measure was the survivorship, how long did artificial knees last before some mode of failure occurred. While some failure modes were evident after only a few years, others took many years to develop.

Complete wear-through of the tibial component, seen in some early designs, was avoided by using bearing thicknesses of at least 6 millimeters, by reducing contact stresses, and by avoiding misalignment. Nevertheless, wear still needed to be minimized because of the vast numbers of particles liberated into the surrounding tissue. In excess, this could cause an inflammatory response, and bone resorption at the interface, leading to loosening. These phenomena were demonstrated in meticulous scientific experiments where titanium fixtures were embedded into rabbit tibiae and responses of bone to both motion and particular debris demonstrated (Goodman 1994). "Both micromotion and particle materials may thus play important roles in prosthetic loosening. If excessive micromotion is present….a fibrous tissue layer will form at the bone-implant interface. This layer may function as a conduit for particles....and elicit an influx of foreign body and chronic inflammatory cells that may initiate bone resorption." Later research showed that particle shape and size also played a role in the magnitude of these processes. The clinical relevance of this work was determined in a 10-year follow-up of almost 400,000 cases in the Australian Registry (Steiger et al. 2015). During that time, there was a steady shift in usage from ultrahigh molecular weight polyethylene (UHMWPE) to crosslinked polyethylene. The crosslinked material was produced by gamma irradiation of the UHMWPE. When the survivorship curves were compared for the two materials at 10 years, there was a much lower failure rate for the crosslinked material. For example, in all of the cases combined, the revision rates were 5.8% for ultrahigh and 3.5% for crosslinked. For patients under 65 years old, the values were a similar proportion but 50% higher. The higher revision rate of ultrahigh molecular weight versus crosslinked polyethylene was attributed to bone lysis and loosening.

For many years it has been a requirement of the FDA that any new design, whether or not it uses a new material, shall have a wear test carried out. The larger companies were equipped to carry out such testing in-house, but independent laboratories developed the special expertise required and offered the service to the field as a whole. The largest such laboratories are at the University of Nebraska (Hani Haider) and the Endolab in Bayern, Germany (Christian Kaddick). They both used similar test methods, force-controlled testing under ISO 14243 specifications. In combination they have measured the wear of 73 different fixed bearing designs and 50 mobile bearing designs (Haider and Kaddick 2012). The expectation was that the mobile bearing would show less wear, because of the higher conformity and hence lower stress of the bearing surfaces. Haider's results were mean wear for fixed 12.7 mg/million cycles, for mobile 7.8. Kaddick's results for mean fixed 5.8, for mobile 5.3. The values had a wide range, however, for example, a range between 1 and 24 for the fixed bearings and from 3 to 13 for the mobile bearings: "....no consistently statistically significant difference was formed that could characterize mobile bearings as having to have lower wear than fixed bearings." Haider did however isolate two designs, one a fixed bearing and the other a mobile bearing, identical in materials and in most design features and showed again no significant difference in wear (Haider and Garvin 2008). One major finding from the combined study however was: "yet such differences were clearly featured....of significantly lower wear in highly crosslinked UHMWPE than in the conventional UHMWPE bearings." This finding was corroborated in an extensive retrieval study.

Implant Retrieval and Wear

Meanwhile, since the 1970s, invaluable data on the wear of polyethylene has been obtained from retrieval studies. Early reports featured wear completely through the plastic insert, usually caused by misalignment and instability. For systematically describing the wear, the early studies defined the types of wear and surface damage, and specified different zones on the tibial component. Burnishing and abrasion occurred due to local fatigue failure of the polyethylene and to entrapped granules of acrylic cement. Later, large surface areas of delamination were shown, as much as several millimeters in depth, due to coalescing of subsurface fatigue cracks beneath the surface, most often seen in designs with low femoral-tibial conformity. Over time, due to improved designs and materials, the wear was seen to reduce. This was recently highlighted in an outstanding scientific exhibit shown at the American Academy of Orthopaedic Surgeons (AAOS) annual meeting in 2018 (Van Citters et al. 2018). The authors were from the longest running retrieval laboratory, at Dartmouth College in Hanover, New Hampshire, founded 30 years ago by John Collier, Professor of Engineering, and Michael Mayor, Professor of Orthopaedic Surgery. So far over 19,000 retrievals have been analyzed, of which over 9000 were artificial knees. They found that the volume of wear increased over time as expected, but that the wear rate reduced when crosslinked polyethylene was introduced. Backside wear, an important contributor to wear, was reduced when the metal tray surface was polished. The overall conclusion was positive: "due to steady improvements in designs and materials, all of the designs included in this study show a large and significant decrease in wear rate compared to the historical reference rate." One caveat was noted, however, the possibility of fatigue damage at longer in vivo times due to oxidation, even of highly crosslinked polyethylene (Currier et al. 2015).

The improvement in wear resistance from crosslinking came with a price, however, loss of ductility and resistance to fatigue crack propagation (Rimnac and Pruitt 2008). In the case of artificial knees, this could lead to fracture of the posts in the PS designs or loosening of the snap-in mechanism of the modular connection in metal-backed tibial components. An extensive body of research to develop a processing method for minimizing wear and oxidation, yet preserving mechanical properties, has been carried out since about the year 2000, at the Harris Orthopaedics

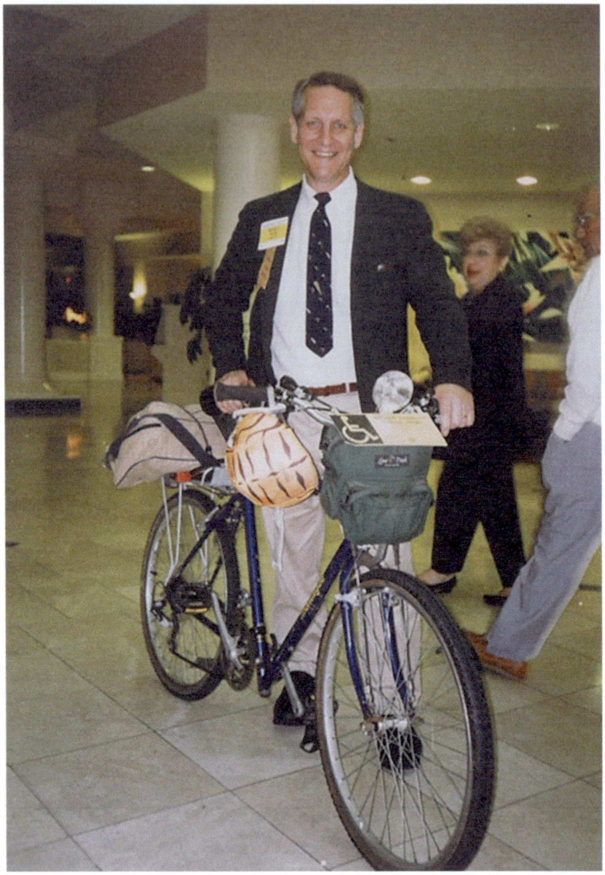

Fig. 13.13 Michael Mayor MD (photo) and John Collier PhD in 1976 founded the implant retrieval program at the Thayer School of Engineering, Dartmouth NH. Since then, over 9000 knees have been studied by the researchers including John Collier, John Currier, and Doug van Citters. A steady reduction in wear has been observed over the years due to improvements in polyethylene processing and implant design. (Photo taken at AAOS Annual conference c 1990) (© Peter S Walker)

Laboratory in Massachusetts General Hospital, by Orhun Muratoglu, Ebru Oral, and their group (Rowell et al. 2015). These authors produced a review article explaining the nuances of their processing methods and verification tests (Oral and Muratoglu 2011). Their conclusion was that while irradiation resulted in a tenfold reduction in wear, there was no method for preventing oxidation over time and maintaining mechanical properties. This dilemma was solved by adding a well-known and biocompatible antioxidant, vitamin E: "The clinical performance will be determined using prospective, randomized clinical studies, which are under way." Such studies may require follow-up times of 5–10 years at least before the effects are seen, considering that long-term prevention of oxidation is one of the proposed benefits of the vitamin E material. Hence while there is strong evidence that crosslinking will reduce the wear compared with UHMWPE, the wear rate of the crosslinked material may start to increase after some years in the body. The time frame is not known, but based on the Australian Registry data above, it seems that there was no acceleration of wear up to 10 years. To verify that the addition of vitamin E will prevent this increase in wear rate in vivo may take 10 years or more

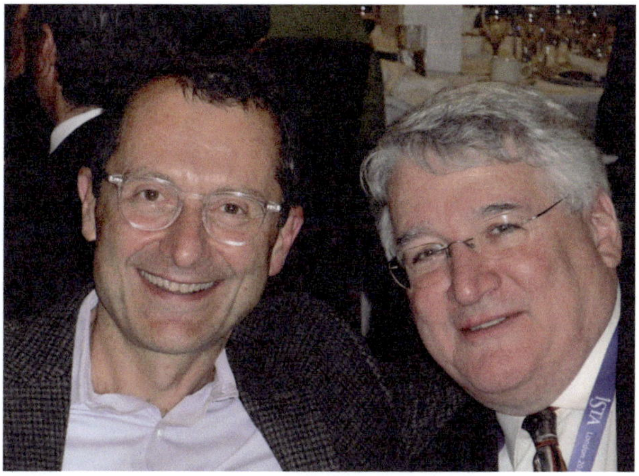

Fig. 13.14 Orhun Muratoglu PhD (left) is Director of the Bill Harris Orthopaedics Laboratory at Mass General Hospital, Boston, and has made major contributions in developing wear-resistant formulations of polyethylene. Joshua Jacobs MD PhD is Chairman of Orthopaedics at Rush University Medical Center in Chicago and is a specialist on the biologic effects of biomaterials used for artificial joints. (Photo taken at the ISTA conference, Boston, 2016) (© Peter S Walker)

of study. Laboratory wear studies have, however, provided indications. In one study (Grupp et al. 2017), a knee simulator was used to test artificial knees, with different materials. The materials were artificially aged at the start of the test, to simulate an extreme oxidative environment. The test were run under loading conditions which included strenuous activities, not limited to the present ASTM test of level walking. Vitamin E addition was found to prevent delamination occurring after several million cycles. Many such tests would have to be carried out to provide a broad spectrum of conditions, but such simulator tests have an advantage of attempting to simulate realistic conditions with a high level of usage, typical of younger more active patients.

Computer Modeling

While the physical testing of artificial knees using equipment such as described above continues to be widely used, much of the kinematic evaluation of artificial knee mechanics has moved to computer simulation in recent years. In one study (Fitzpatrick et al. 2016), the computer model was validated by comparing the output data from a 6-degree-of-freedom test machine, for deep knee bend, gait, and step-down. The model was also shown to be able to differentiate between different designs "performing" these activities. Their computer model was used to carry out constraint testing (Rullkoetter et al. 2017), as described above in relation to an ASTM standard. The computer model was able to extend the testing to the inclusion of soft tissues and then to muscle forces, giving a more realistic evaluation of the

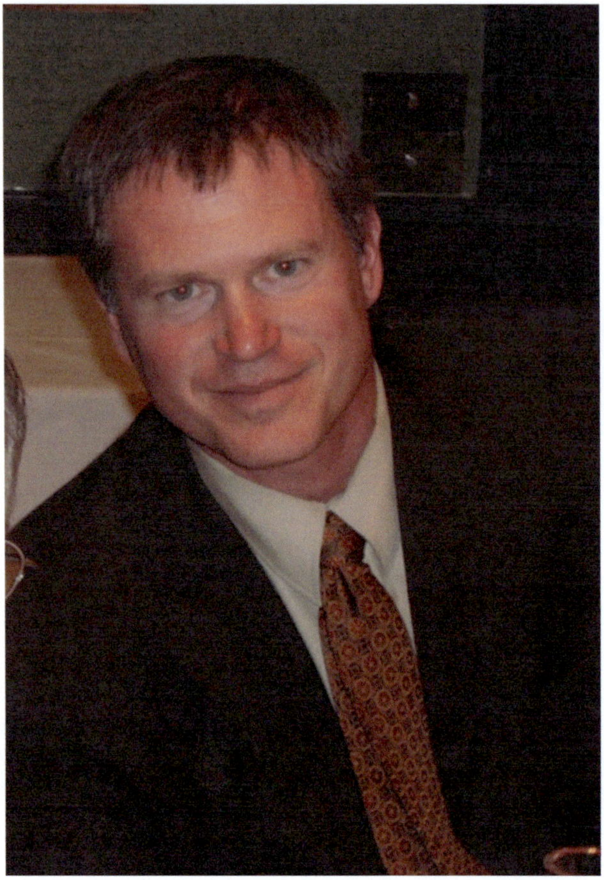

Fig. 13.15 Paul Rullkoetter PhD from the University of Denver, Colorado, along with colleagues including Claire Fitzpatrick, has developed FEA computer models of the knee and lower extremity, for the evaluation of different knee designs in various functions. This is a growing area in joint biomechanics. (Photo taken c 2016) (© Peter S Walker)

in vivo situation in function. A major advantage of computer modeling is that patient variability can be taken into account (Taylor et al. 2013): "Statistical shape models can synthetically generate thousands of representative models from a much smaller training set." If modeling was used to compare different designs, outputs under different service conditions address the goal of robust design (see Chap. 3). In the area of artificial knee design, any design can be optimized. Comparisons can be made between different designs and variations. The effect of patient and surgical variables can be investigated. Different functions can be evaluated. Knees could even be customized given the input data of the patient (Koh et al. 2019). There is a big difference between validating a computer model based on output data from a test machine (which is itself a "model" of sorts) and predicting in vivo behavior. In the first case, the target data is available, and the test machine has well-defined functional behavior. In the second case, the system is far more complex, and the multiple variables are not all known.

This predicament was the main purpose of "The Grand Challenge" organized by Benjamin Fregly et al. (2012). Participants were provided with data sets: "These

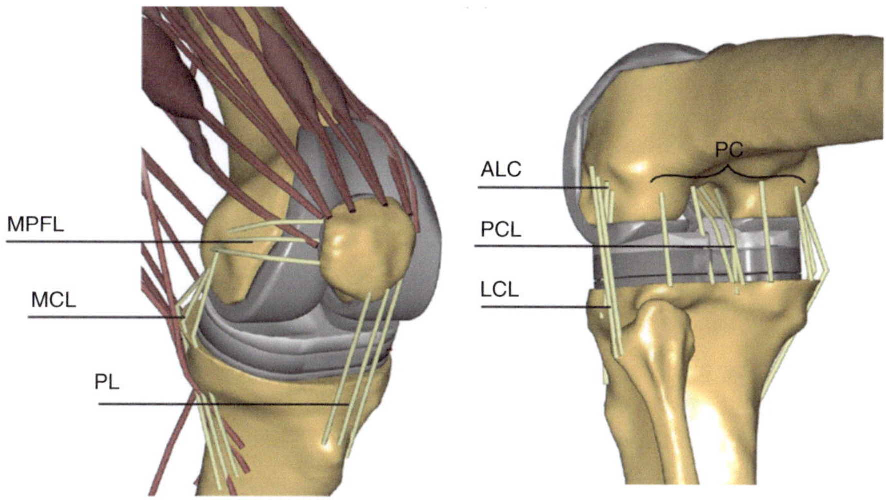

Fig. 13.16 A computer model of the knee with artificial knee implanted, within a full skeletal AnyBody Model of the musculoskeletal system. The model includes multiple bundle models of the ligaments and muscles. Using an inverse kinematic-based analysis, forces and kinematics can be predicted for different activities or artificial knee designs. In this case, the effect of tibial slope was investigated (Marra et al. 2017). (Reprinted with permission from Journal of Biomechanical Engineering)

data sets include tibial contact force, video motion, ground reaction, muscle EMG, muscle strength, static and dynamic imaging, and implant geometry data. Competition participants used their musculoskeletal models to predict tibial contact forces without having access to the corresponding *in vivo* measurements." A crucial point is that the data was obtained from patients who had instrumented tibial components, whether from the Berlin group (Bergmann) or the San Diego group (D'Lima and Colwell). Hence the tibial force data, as well as the data provided to the participants, was available for various functional activities. The results over after several rounds of the Challenge were discussed at a symposium at the Orthopaedic Research Society in 2019. Achieving consistency of results between different computational methodologies was not straightforward due to the complexity of the models, the differences in the models themselves, and the variations of the input data which was needed for the models but not provided. Even today, basic data of soft tissue attachment points and geometries, and their material properties, is conspicuously inadequate, and different studies frequently use different values. In the discussion of the application of the work, there were two extremes. At one extreme, there was the scientific value of a model which was able to accurately predict the tibial forces. At the other extreme, for the purposes of defining a test, for the ASTM, for example, the test itself should be a simple as possible such that it could be easily implemented and be reproducible between different laboratories.

Despite the apparent objectivity of computer modeling, Rullkoetter et al. (2017) pointed out: "Although models typically represent the articular interface well, the interaction with the patient and the surgical process includes significant variability and increase in complexity." It might well be impractical to determine such variables on a given patient, even if it were of benefit to do so. But despite the limitations of computer models, it is clear that there will be increasing application in artificial knee design and evaluation. Rullkoetter stated: "It is evident that future artificial knee designs will be optimized by using preclinical computer models." A limiting factor may be knowing what are the optimal design criteria.

Current Status of Testing and Standards

Today, there are published "standards" for testing all types of materials and products, such that in order to be released to the market, both safety and efficacy must be demonstrated. On a worldwide basis, the International Organization for Standardization (ISO) publishes standards, to ensure that "products are fit for their purpose." In the USA, the American Society for Testing and Materials (ASTM) develops and publishes the standards. The Food and Drug Administration (FDA) determines whether new medical devices can be released to the market based on passing ASTM standards which have been selected by the FDA. The work of developing standards is most often carried out by technical staff from companies and faculty members from universities on a voluntary basis. For artificial knees and the associated materials and instrumentation, the F04 committee on Medical and Surgical Materials and Devices is responsible. Even though most of the applications to the FDA are of devices which are similar to others already on the market, there are often sufficient differences that it is a time-consuming process to complete all of the testing which is necessary and for the FDA to carry out the evaluations. In addition, devices frequently include new design features or improved materials, which adds to the testing which needs to be carried out. Considering the importance of testing devices such as artificial knees, and for advancing the field as expeditiously as possible, it would be an advantage if more resources were available for developing the methodologies for new standards that might be deemed necessary. Advanced simulator studies and computer modeling are among the methods that could be further developed.

In the case of artificial knees, test methods and performance standards are available for material quality, wear of the bearing surfaces, fatigue strength of the components, strength of modular connections, and constraint during shear and torque loading. By the time a new artificial knee has successfully passed the various tests, it is unlikely that the device will fail in vivo for mechanical reasons. Such testing should be regarded as part of the design process in that an unsatisfactory result of any test should require a design modification. Nevertheless, failures still do occur in vivo due to the design itself, to the surgical technique, or related to the patient. For example, excessive instability can occur if the implant has relatively low inherent stability and if the ligaments have not been adequately balanced at surgery and there is weak musculature. Bone collapse or component loosening can occur if the component alignment is incorrect by more than a few degrees and the trabecular bone has been weakened due to the arthritis. In the long term, if the wear is excessive due to a high activity level in a heavy patient, the accumulation of wear particles can cause pain, swelling, and loose components.

How Were Designs Tested for Wear, Strength, and Kinematics?

In the first decade of total knee design, simple test machines were designed primarily for testing laxity and stability, fixation, wear, and strength. Due to the lack of regulations, by no means was every design evaluated. Even so, by 1980, only about 10 years after the first artificial knees were used in patients, there was a high success rate with few designs showing poor results. This can be attributed to the gradual improvement of test methods based on observations of clinical performance, as well as the high incentive to all parties for successful results. Today, for a total knee to be used in patients, extensive testing needs to be carried out as specified by the FDA. The ASTM organization has been the main vehicle for formulating the tests. The tests have largely been the combined work of biomechanics and biomaterials specialists over a period of several decades. While the larger companies have sufficient resources to carry out their own testing, smaller companies contract specialized testing laboratories. These laboratories have developed considerable expertise and experience of a wide range of artificial knee designs. The tests will undoubtedly become more sophisticated and numerous in the future: some may be appropriate as new standards in that they address safety and efficacy, while others will be a means for detailed evaluation of performance. Among the types of testing methods which have a high potential for advancement are wear and strength testing using advanced simulators and functional analyses using fluoroscopy and computer modeling.

References

Abdelgaied A, Fisher J, Jennings LM. A comparison between electromechanical and pneumatic-controlled knee simulators for the investigation of wear of total knee replacements. Proc Inst Mech Eng H J Eng Med. 2017;231(7):643–51.

Bergmann G, Bender A, Graichen F, et al. Standardized loads acting in knee implants. PLoS One. 2014;9(1):e86035.

Branson PJ, Steege JW, Wixson RL, Lewis J, Stulberg SD. Rigidity of initial fixation with uncemented tibial knee implants. J Arthroplast. 1989;4(1):21–6.

Brooks PJ, Walker PS, Scott RD. Tibial component fixation in deficient tibial bone stock. Clin Orthop Relat Res. 1984;184:302–8.

Colley J, Cameron HU, Freeman MA, Swanson SA. Loosening of the femoral component in surface replacement of the knee. Arch Orthop Trauma Surg. 1978;92(1):31–4.

Currier BH, Currier JH, Franklin KJ, Mayor MB, Reinitz SD, Van Citters DW. Comparison of wear and oxidation in retrieved conventional and highly cross-linked UHMWPE tibial inserts. J Arthroplast. 2015;30(12):2349–53.

DesJardins JD, Walker PS, Haider H, Perry J. The use of a force-controlled dynamic knee simulator to quantify the mechanical performance of total knee replacement designs during functional activity. J Biomech. 2000;33(10):1231–42.

Dorr LD, Lindberg JP, Claude-Faugere M, Malluche HH. Factors influencing the intrusion of methylmethacrylate into human tibiae. Clin Orthop Relat Res. 1984;183:147–52.

Ducheyne P, Kagan A 2nd, Lacey JA. Failure of total knee arthroplasty due to loosening and deformation of the tibial component. J Bone Joint Surg Am. 1978;60(3):384–91.

Ezzet KA, Hershey AL, D'Lima DD, Irby SE, Kaufman KR, Colwell CW. Patella tracking in total knee arthroplasty. J Arthroplasty. 2001;16(7):838–43.

Fitzpatrick CK, Maag C, Clary CW, Metcalfe A, Langhorn J, Rullkoetter PJ. Validation of a new computational 6-DOF knee simulator during dynamic activities. J Biomech. 2016;49(14):3177–84.

Freeman MA, Bradley GW, Blaha JD, Insler HP. Cementless fixation of the tibial component for the ICLH knee. J R Soc Med. 1982;75(6):418–24.

Fregly BJ, Besier TF, Lloyd DG, et al. Grand challenge competition to predict in vivo knee loads. J Orthop Res. 2012;30(4):503–13.

Goodfellow J, Hungerford DS, Zindel M. Patello-femoral joint mechanics and pathology. 1. Functional anatomy of the patello-femoral joint. J Bone Joint Surg. 1976;58(3):287–90.

Goodman SB. The effects of micromotion and particulate materials on tissue differentiation: bone chamber studies in rabbits. Acta Orthopaedica Scandinavica. 1994;65(sup258):1–43.

Grupp TM, Fritz B, Kutzner I, Schilling C, Bergmann G, Schwiesau J. Vitamin E stabilised polyethylene for total knee arthroplasty evaluated under highly demanding activities wear simulation. Acta Biomater. 2017;48:415–22.

Gunston FH. Polycentric knee arthroplasty. Prosthetic simulation of normal knee movement. J Bone Joint Surg. 1971;53(2):272–7.

Haider H. Tribological assessment of UHMWPE in the knee, Chapter 32. In: Kurtz SM, editor. UHMWPE biomaterials handbook – ultra-high molecular weight polyethylene in total joint replacement and medical devices. 3rd ed: New York, USA: Elsevier Inc; 2016. p. 559–634.

Haider H, Garvin K. Rotating platform versus fixed-bearing total knees: an in vitro study of wear. Clin Orthop Relat Res. 2008;466(11):2677–85.

Haider H, Kaddick C. Wear of mobile bearing knees: is it necessarily less? J ASTM Int. 2012;9(2):1–10.

Haider H, Weisenburger JN, Kurtz SM, et al. Does vitamin E-stabilized ultrahigh-molecular-weight polyethylene address concerns of cross-linked polyethylene in total knee arthroplasty? J Arthroplast. 2012;27(3):461–9.

Harding ML, Harding L, Goodfellow JW. A preliminary report of a simple rig to aid study of the functional anatomy of the cadaver human knee joint. J Biomech. 1977;10(8):517–23.

Heim CS, Postak PD, Plaxton NA, Greenwald AS. Classification of mobile-bearing knee designs: mobility and constraint. J Bone Joint Surg Am. 2001;83-A Suppl 2(Pt 1):32–7.

Koh YG, Lee JA, Chung PK, Kang KT. Computational analysis of customized cruciate retaining total knee arthroplasty restoration of native knee joint biomechanics. Artif Organs. 2019;43(5):504–14.

Krause WR, Krug W, Miller J. Strength of the cement-bone interface. Clin Orthop Rel Res. 1982;163:290–9.

Li G, DeFrate LE, Zayontz S, Park SE, Gill TJ. The effect of tibiofemoral joint kinematics on patellofemoral contact pressures under simulated muscle loads. J Orthop Res. 2004;22:801–6.

Lin, Judy. 2016. UCLA researchers team up with robot for solutions to debilitating knee injuries http://newsroom.ucla.edu/stories/ucla-researchers-team-up-with-robot-for-solutions-to-debilitating-knee-injuries

Maletsky LP, Hillberry BM. Simulating dynamic activities using a 5-axis simulator. J Biomech Eng. 2005;127:123–33.

Markolf KL, Finerman GM, Amstutz HC. In vitro measurements of knee stability after bicondylar replacement. J Bone Joint Surg Am. 1979;61(4):547–57.

Marra MA, Andersen MS, Damsgaard M, Koopman BFJM, Janssen D, Verdonschot N. Evaluation of a surrogate contact model in force-dependent kinematic simulations of Total knee replacement. J Biomech Eng. 2017;1:139(8).

McCutchen CW. The frictional properties of animal joints. Wear. 1962;5(1):1–17.

Morrison J. The mechanics of the knee joint in relation to normal walking. J Biomech. 1970;3(1):51–61.

Morrison J. Bioengineering analysis of force actions transmitted by the knee joint. Biomed Eng. 1968;3:164–70.

Nogi J, Caldwell JW, Kauzlarich JJ, Thompson RC. Load testing of geometric and polycentric total knee replacements. Clin Orthop Relat Res. 1976;114:235–42.

Oral E, Muratoglu OK. Vitamin E diffused, highly crosslinked UHMWPE: a review. Int Orthop. 2011;35(2):215–23.

Postak PD, Heim CS, Greenwald AS. The role of constraint in contemporary modular knee designs. Surg Technol Int. 1994;3:541–6.

Rimnac C, Pruitt L. How do material properties influence wear and fracture mechanisms? J Am Acad Orthop Surg. 2008;16:S94–S100.

Rowell SL, Reyes CR, Malchau H, Muratoglu OK. In vivo oxidative stability changes of highly cross-linked polyethylene bearings: an ex vivo investigation. J Arthroplast. 2015;30(10):1828–34.

Rullkoetter PJ, Fitzpatrick CK, Clary CW. How can we use computational modeling to improve Total knee arthroplasty? modeling stability and mobility in the implanted knee. J Am Acad Orthop Surg. 2017;25(Suppl 1):S33–s39.

Schwiesau J, Schilling C, Kaddick C, et al. Definition and evaluation of testing scenarios for knee wear simulation under conditions of highly demanding daily activities. Med Eng Phys. 2013;35(5):591–600.

Seedhom B, Dowson D, Wright V. Wear of solid phase formed high density polyethylene in relation to the life of artificial hips and knees. Wear. 1973;24(1):35–51.

Shaw J, Murray D. Knee joint simulator. Clin Orthop Rel Res. 1973;94:15–23.

Singerman R, Berilla J, Davy DT. Direct in vitro determination of the patellofemoral contact force for normal knees. J Biomech Eng. 1995;117:9–14.

Steiger RN, Muratoglu O, Lorimer M, Cuthbert AR, Graves SE. Lower prosthesis-specific 10-year revision rate with crosslinked than with non-crosslinked polyethylene in primary total knee arthroplasty: 386,104 procedures from the Australian Orthopaedic Association National Joint Replacement Registry. Acta Orthop. 2015;86(6):721–7.

Swanson SAV, Freeman MAR, Heath JC. Laboratory tests on total joint replacement prostheses. J Bone J Surg. 1973;55B(4):759–73.

Taylor M, Bryan R, Galloway F. Accounting for patient variability in finite element analysis of the intact and implanted hip and knee: a review. Int J Numer Methods Biomed Eng. 2013;29(2):273–92.

Van Citters DW, Currier JH, Currier BH, Titus AJ, Major MB, Abdul MP, Berry DJ. A retrieval analysis of 1385 tibial inserts for wear, damage and oxidation: What factors are driving performance? Scientific Exhibit SE 10: American Academy of Orthopaedic Surgeons, Annual Meeting March 2018, Las Vegas, NV.

Varadarajan KM, Harry RE, Johnson T, Li G. Can in vitro systems capture the characteristic differences between the flexion-extension kinematics of the healthy and TKA knee? Med Eng Phys. 2009;31(8):899–906.

Volz RG, Nisbet JK, Lee RW, McMurtry MG. The mechanical stability of various noncemented tibial components. Clin Orthop Relat Res. 1988;226:38–42.

Walker PS, Blunn GW, Broome DR, et al. A knee simulating machine for performance evaluation of total knee replacements. J Biomech. 1997;30(1):83–9.

Walker PS, Blunn GW, Perry JP, et al. Methodology for long-term wear testing of total knee replacements. Clin Orthop Relat Res. 2000;372:290–301.

Walker PS, Greene D, Reilly D, Thatcher J, Ben-Dov M, Ewald FC. Fixation of tibial components of knee prostheses. J Bone Joint Surg Am. 1981;63(2):258–67.

Walker PS, Hsieh HH. Conformity in condylar replacement knee prosthesis. J Bone Joint Surg. 1977;59(2):222–8.

Walker PS, Ranawat C, Insall J. Fixation of the tibial components of condylar replacement knee prostheses. J Biomech. 1976;9(4):269–75.

Walker PS, Wang C-J, Masse Y. Joint laxity as a design criterion for the design of condylar knee prostheses. Conference on total knee replacement, Institution of Mechanical Engineers, London UK, 16–18 Sept 1974.

White BF, D'Lima D, Drueding AC, Cox J, Carignan FJ. A simulator study of TKR kinematics using modeled soft-tissue constraint: virtual soft-tissue control for knee simulation. In: Wear of Articulating Surfaces: Understanding Joint Simulation. West Conshohocken: ASTM International; 2006.

Whiteside LA, Pafford J. Load transfer characteristics of a noncemented total knee arthroplasty. Clin orthop rel res. 1989;239:168–77.

Willing R, Walker PS. Measuring the sensitivity of total knee replacement kinematics and laxity to soft tissue imbalances. J Biomech. 2018;77:62–8.

Zavatsky AB. A kinematic-freedom analysis of a flexed knee stance testing rig. J Biomech. 1997;30(3):277–80.

Evaluations of Designs and Techniques

14

Which Evaluation Methods Are Applicable, and Are There Differences Between Designs and Techniques?

Function Measured Using PROMs

According to the Swedish Knee Arthroplasty Register, the survivorship of artificial knees is 92% at 20 years. Because that cannot be improved too much further, there is an increasing focus on the functional performance. From the patient's perspective, apart from a pain-free knee that will last indefinitely, it is not unreasonable to expect a return to the functional level before they developed arthritis. Television advertisements for artificial knees, where the patients are seen running, high-speed cycling, and skiing, do not apply to everybody. However there is the suggestion that when the patient is able to perform those sorts of activities, the artificial knee could safely endure the forces and motions. Concurrent with the introduction of artificial knees, evaluation schemes were devised to assess the function. Such schemes were mostly specific to each investigator or hospital. In evaluating the Polycentric and Geometric knees in the early 1970s, Ilstrup, Coventry, and Skolnick from the Mayo Clinic took a statistical approach to determine the extent to which the patients had improved on their preoperative status in several categories including function. Gshwendt from Zurich devised a chart to show the change from pre-op to post-op, giving a visual impression of how many patients improved and by how much. In the late 1970s, the Hospital for Special Surgery (HSS) Knee Score was introduced, which was based on pain, function, range of motion, muscle strength, flexion deformity, and instability, with subtractions for the use of walking aids. It was not until 1989 that the Knee Society Scoring Systems were formulated for both function and radiographic assessments (Ewald 1989). The scheme recognized that the knee itself should be firstly assessed objectively, by measuring alignments and quality of the interface. Secondly there should be an evaluation of function which depended on many other factors. One of the first studies which attempted to account for the range of activities pertinent to each individual patient was carried out by Philip Noble Ph.D. and associates (Weiss et al. 2002). They first pointed out that "the goals of individual patients will differ with respect to postoperative function and activity."

P. S. Walker, *The Artificial Knee*, https://doi.org/10.1007/978-3-030-38171-4_14

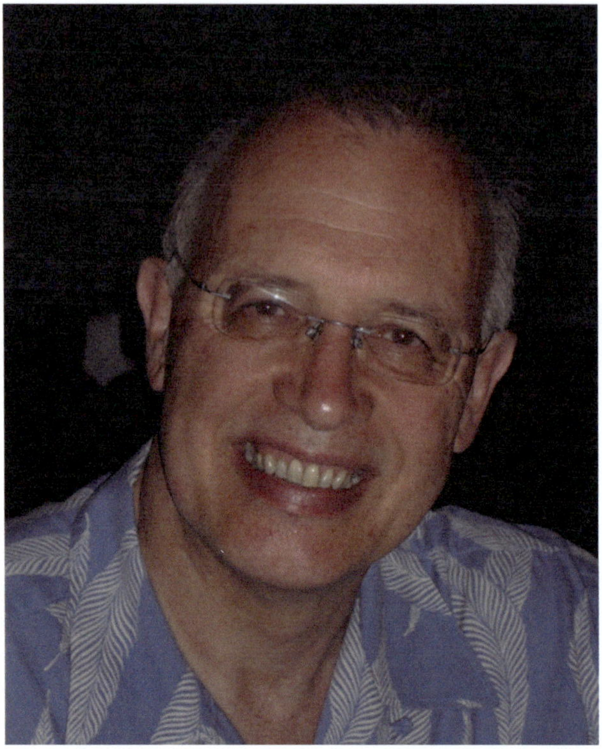

Fig. 14.1 Philip Noble completed his Ph.D. at Strathclyde University, Glasgow, Scotland, and later worked at Baylor College of Medicine and Methodist Hospital, Houston, TX. Working on a Committee of the Knee Society, he advanced the methodology for evaluation of patients with artificial knees by focusing on the preferred activities of each patient and including the ability to perform these activities in the new Knee Society Scoring System. He also devised innovative methodologies for tibial fixation and for evaluating surgical performance. (Photo taken 2015) (© Peter S Walker)

This led them to formulate a questionnaire which divided activities into activities of daily living, movement and lifestyle, and exercise and sports. The patients were asked the importance and frequency of these activities and whether the knee either limited them or bothered them while carrying out the activities. They concluded that "although knee replacement does not prevent patients from doing activities they consider important, the procedure, nonetheless, does not restore the ease associated with normal knee function." The authors also recognized that "Additional work also is needed to compare the responses reported in this study with those of healthy control subjects…" In other words, the patients should be realistic about what is achievable in their particular case. Nevertheless, the study did imply that the artificial knees included in their study were not providing the function and comfort level that the patients would have if they had not developed arthritis. Noble's work then became the starting point for an outcomes subcommittee in The Knee Society, chaired by Giles Scuderi MD, to develop a questionnaire for widespread use in evaluating artificial knees. The result was the Knee Society Scoring System (KSS) (Scuderi et al. 2012). The recorded metrics include both surgeon-reported measures and patient-reported satisfaction and function. After several years of experience with the system, there was a need for a shortened version to improve compliance from patients who otherwise did not have the patience or time to complete the long form (Scuderi et al. 2016).

KNEE SOCIETY SHORT FORM (SECOND HALF)

STANDARD ACTIVITIES

How much does your knee bother you during each of the following activities?	no bother 5	slight 4	moderate 3	severe 2	very severe 1	cannot do (because of knee) 0	I never do this
13- Walking on an uneven surface	o	o	o	o	o	o	o
14- Climbing up or decending a flight of stairs	o	o	o	o	o	o	o
15- Getting up from a low couch or a chair without arms	o	o	o	o	o	o	o
16- Running	o	o	o	o	o	o	o

DISCRETIONARY KNEE ACTIVITIES

Many people consider the following activities important. Of thesse activities, which one is the most important to you?
(please do not write in additional activities)

- ☐ Swimming
- ☐ Golfing (18 holes)
- ☐ Road Cycling (>30mins)
- ☐ Gardening
- ☐ Bowling
- ☐ Racquet Sports (Tennis, Racquetball, etc.)
- ☐ Distance Walking
- ☐ Dancing / Ballet
- ☐ Stretching Exercises (stretching out your muscles)
- ☐ Weight-lifting
- ☐ Leg Extensions
- ☐ Stair-Climber
- ☐ Stationary Biking / Spinning
- ☐ Leg Press
- ☐ Jogging
- ☐ Eliptical Trainer
- ☐ Aerobic Exercises

How much does your knee bother you during the activity checked above?

no bother 5	slight 4	moderate 3	severe 2	very severe 1	cannot do (because of knee) 0
o	o	o	o	o	o

FJS – 12. FORGOTTEN JOINT SCORE

The following 12 questions refer to how aware you are of your artificial knee joint in everyday life.

Please tick one answer from each question.

Are you aware of your artificial joint...

1. ... in bed at night?

o never o almost never o seldom o sometimes o mostly

2 . ... when you are sitting on a chair for more than 1 hour?

3 . ... when you are walking for more than 15 minutes?

4 . ... when you are taking a bath/shower?

5 . ... when you are traveling in a car?

6 . ... when you are climbing stairs?

7 . ... when you are walking on uneven ground?

8 . ... when you are standing up from a low-sitting position?

9 . ... when you are standing for long periods of time?

10 . ... when you are doing housework or gardening?

11 . ... when you are taking a walk/hiking?

12 . ... when you are doing your favorite sport?

A high score 100) indicates a high degree of "forgetting" the artificial joint, that is, a low degree of awareness.

Fig. 14.2 There is a similarity between the Knee Society Short Form (KSS) and the Forgotten Joint Score (FJS). The KSS asks "does your knee bother you in activities?"; the FJS asks if you are aware of your artificial joint in activities. However the KSS allows the patient to choose certain activities, while the FJS provides a list which almost every patient will be able to do. (Left, reprinted with permission The Knee Society; right, reprinted with permission from Journal of Arthroplasty)

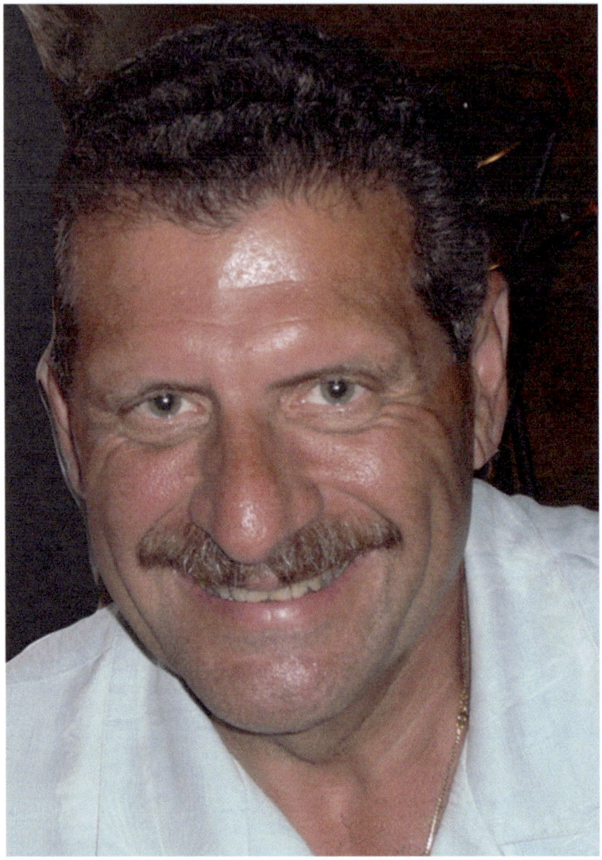

Fig. 14.3 Giles Scuderi MD was a knee fellow with John Insall at the Hospital for Special Surgery, New York, in 1987. Since that time he has been a major educator in multiple forums on the principles of technique of total knee replacement, particular those associated with the PS type of knee. In 2012 Gil Scuderi and other members of The Knee Society formulated the now widely used evaluation method for total knee outcome, the Knee Society Knee Scoring System. (Photo c 2017) (© Peter S Walker)

Today the KSS is but one example of a patient-reported outcome measure (PROM), the most widely used method of evaluating artificial knees. Such measures are simple to carry out, require little time of the physician, include an assessment of function, and produce a numerical score which can be compared with those of other study groups. Typically, a patient checking in to the hospital for an artificial knee will be asked to complete a PROM form on a tablet. Recently a survey was carried out of clinical follow-up studies published in the major orthopedic journals over the past 15 years (Siljander et al. 2018). A previous article was quoted as to what constituted an effective PROM: "…one that adequately measures clinical results, while also being valid, reliable, responsive and easily administered." Siljander et al. found that no less than 42 individual PROMs had been used in previous studies. The Knee Society Score (KSS) was used the most frequently for total knees, but for unicompartmental knees, the Oxford Knee Score (OKS) was mostly used, due to the influence of the originators of the Oxford Knee from the Nuffield Hospital in Oxford, England. Further comments by the authors included the following: "There are many facets to a PROM, and the balance between subjective and objective scores, patient satisfaction, and factors important to the patient vs the surgeons, leave the combination endless… Furthermore an explicit definition of a successful outcome has yet to be determined across all the PROMs."

It is important to define exactly what is being measured in a PROM. As an example of the type of questions, the section of the Knee Society Scoring System (KSS) relating to function, the patient is asked: "how much does your knee bother you during each of the following activities?" covering every day to more strenuous activities (Scuderi et al. 2012). Similarly, in the Knee Injury and Osteoarthritis Outcome Score (KOOS) scoring system for function, another widely used system, the patient is asked for their experience with numerous everyday activities including recreational: "what degree of difficulty have you experienced during the last week due to your knee?" (Roos et al. 1998). The Forgotten Joint Score (FJS) was defined recently to provide a simplified scoring system which focused on what really mattered to the patient (Behrend et al. 2012). "The ability to forget the artificial joint in everyday life can be regarded as the ultimate goal in joint arthroplasty." The patient is asked: "are you aware of your artificial knee when you are walking for more than 15 minutes?" There are 12 such questions covering common activities of everyday living. Such an approach was embodied in Noble's questionnaire cited above (Weiss et al. 2002) in the following question: "does your knee feel normal to you?" PROMs such as the above have been widely used to evaluate the outcomes of groups of patients, with our emphasis being on the functional outcome. The PROMs can readily be used with cohorts of patients to evaluate a new artificial knee design, or to compare one design with another.

In this chapter we will concentrate on the comparisons between designs and also techniques. Given the wide variety of configurations of artificial knees described in previous chapters, it might be expected that some designs would function much better than others and that it would be possible to compile a league table of functional outcomes. Even particular types of design such as a CR or PS made by different manufacturers might be expected to show some differences in function. There are many examples where a manufacturer has a successful knee system, but over the years, a number of improvements are identified. At that point, a new knee system is designed with the improved features. A PROM could be used to determine if the new system produced higher functional scores than the previous system. Such comparisons are now discussed, where PROMs have been the principal method of evaluating the function.

A key question posed in the Introduction was whether any of the newer designs have higher functional scores compared with the cruciate-retaining (CR) and posterior-stabilized (PS) designs. To answer this is not easy for several reasons. There are a large number of studies which have been carried out since 1980. Many of the studies are not comparative, assessing only one particular design. The studies have covered many designs, including different versions of each design, whether CR, PS, or other design types. The evaluation methods have differed, whether the KSS system or one of the other 42 systems (and still more are being added). The conditions of the studies have been different, such as the surgical technique, the rehabilitation regimen, and the length of follow-up. For our purpose, we will preferentially use recent studies, with meta-analyses or reviews being favored, with some attention to the size of the cohorts. Efforts have been made to choose a representative sample of the studies, especially where there is a disparity in the results. Studies which make useful insights or observations are also selected.

Overall Differences Between Designs

In a unique study comparing different knee types, Pritchett (2011) implanted bilateral knees in 492 patients, with different types in opposite knees. At 2-year follow-up, the patients were asked: "which is your better knee overall?" This evaluation method is similar to the Forgotten Joint Score but encapsulates everything into one simple question. The patient had to consider all of their activities combined in giving the answer. Comparing one knee with the other would be easier and more reliable than trying to objectively assess a single knee. The bilateral case study avoided the problem of having two separate groups, each with an artificial knee on one side only.

In Pritchett's study, ACL + PCL preserving (BCS) and medial pivot knees were preferred over standard CR and PS knees. ACL + PCL and medial pivot knees were preferred equally, as were CR and PS. Pritchett offered some explanation of his findings: "…if the implant allows the femur to move forward on the tibia (as occurs with CR and PS) the patient may sense this as an instability…conversely if the prosthesis provides AP stability such as with the ACL + PCL and Medial Pivot prostheses, patients may sense a feeling of stability…in addition patients may prefer ACL + PCL prostheses because of superior proprioception." In this study, Pritchett chose to use a simple test, namely, asking the patients which knee they preferred, to which the patient could provide an assessment covering all conditions.

Unicompartmental vs Total Knee

Unicompartmental knees are expected to show higher functional scores than total knees, based on the preservation of most of the joint except for the medial condyles, and the reduced tissue removed during surgery. In a recent meta-analysis, where most of the publications were since the year 2000, from the 23 selected studies, unicompartmental knees (3254 cases) had a higher range of flexion and higher KSS and WOMAC scores, as well as a quicker return to sports, compared with total knees (10,640 cases) (Migliorini et al. 2019). One of the conclusions was "These results suggest that the UKA implants are more suitable for physically active patients, since they allow better clinical and functional performances." Another recent survey (Pfitzner et al. 2017) showed that while unicompartmental knees did have higher PROM scores in follow-up studies, because their preoperative scores

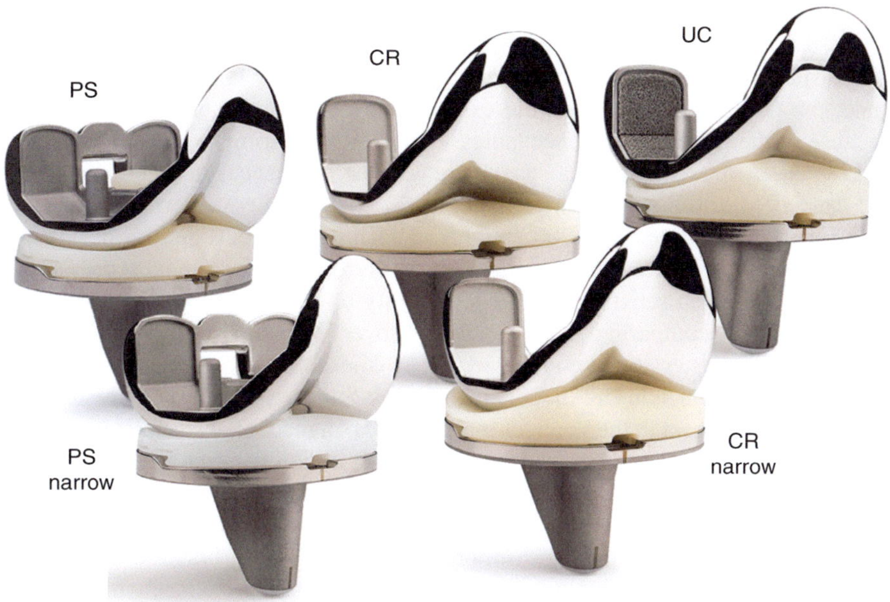

Fig. 14.4 A state-of-the-art knee system consisting of PS (posterior stabilized), CR (posterior cruciate retaining), UC (ultracongruent), and MC (medially congruent). The sizing schemes were based on an analysis of a large CT database, covering gender and race. The PS and CR are in standard and narrow. Comparative outcomes between designs are still being evaluated. (Picture courtesy ZimmerBiomet, Warsaw, IN)

were higher than for total knees, the gains in PROM scores were similar between the two groups. Lyons et al. (2012) reviewed their unicompartmental (219 cases) and total knee (5606 cases) from 1978 to 2009. Their conclusion was "consistent with the literature, we found patients with UKA had higher absolute clinical outcome scores for function preoperatively and at follow-up than patients with TKA. Change in clinical outcome scores were similar in both groups." They emphasized that it was the increase in pre-op to post-op scores that was important; thus, the two groups were similar in outcome. They did surmise however that there was a ceiling effect with some of the evaluation methods. In three other recent studies, the range of flexion was higher after a unicompartmental compared with a total knee, but the functional scores were similar (Hauer et al. 2020; Goh et al. 2018; Kleeblad et al. 2018). Van der List et al. (2017) found that the WOMAC scores were higher for a medial unicompartmental knee with a metal-backed tibial component, compared with a total knee. The point about the metal-backing was that for all-plastic inlay components, deformation and loosening occurred in some cases, causing discomfort and reducing the scores; the rigidity of metal-backing avoided these problems. One unanswered question is that if a particular arthritic knee was treated with a unicompartmental or a total knee, would the outcomes be different?

Cruciate-Retaining (CR) vs Posterior-Stabilized (PS) Knees

It is of particular interest to compare the two most widely used types of artificial knee, the CR and the PS, with the expectation that there would be a difference because of the differences in mechanics. However comparing the WOMAC scores in 1287 cases in a regional data base, there were no differences in functional scores at 5- and 10-year follow-up (Singleton et al. 2019). Also, Serna-Berna et al. (2018) found that in a study of over 200 patients in each group of CR and PS designs, at 10-year follow-up, there were "no significant differences in functional scores, range of motion or patient satisfaction. The superiority of one design over the other was not found." In comparing survivorship of over 133,000 cases in the Dutch Arthroplasty Register, it was concluded that PS knees were 1.5 times more likely to be revised at 8 years than CR knees (Spekenbrink-Spooren et al. 2018). The revision rates were the highest in the younger male group. In a meta-analysis of studies up to 2015, 14 randomized control trials met certain criteria (Jiang et al. 2016). There were 791 CR knees and 622 PS knees, with at least 6-month follow-up. "There were no significant differences in KSS, KSPS, HSS scores… and complications. However the PS provided better total ROM, improvement of ROM and flexion angle." The differences in the flexion angles were 5–10° in the different studies, which can be attributed to the posterior femoral rollback after the cam-post engagement. Beaupre et al. (2017) carried out a randomized study of CR vs PS followed up for 10 years. There were no differences in the pain and function scores, nor the complications, between the two groups. The authors found that there was a gradual reduction in functional scores over time, a function of the aging of the patients rather than related to the artificial knees. This is undoubtedly a factor when analyzing typical artificial age groups where the average age is in the late 60's at the time of the procedure. Finally, in one study it was claimed that a deep-dish tibial insert with a high anterior lip provided a greater pre-op to post-op range of motion than a PS knee, although the mean difference between the designs was only about 3° (Berend et al. 2013). At the same time, if the deep-dish design had advantages over the PS, such as less femoral bone resection and improved patella tracking, the deep-dish insert would not be a disadvantage, at least in flexion range.

In a recent comparative review of CR and PS, Meneghini et al. (2019) combined PROMs and registry data, to conclude the following: "Equivalent functional outcomes in multiple studies comparing CR-type bearings and PS TKA designs, preclude the need for PS TKA designs in the modern health care environment. Based on the available data and modern metrics, traditional PS TKA designs with a cam-and-post articulation are not required for the majority of primary TKA." The authors also pointed out that CR knees with steep anterior tibial surfaces substitute for the posterior cruciate ligament, which brings the CR into the realm of an ultracongruent type where both cruciates are resected. A limitation of this statement is that all CR designs are not likely to be equal, nor all PS designs, nor all ultracongruents.

Rotating Platform Designs

Recently the Forgotten Joint Score was used to compare two rotating platform knee systems, the classic LCS designed by Buechel and Pappas and a recent derivative, the Attune (Behrend et al. 2019). In finding no difference in the Forgotten Joint Scores, as well as WOMAC scores and range of motion, the authors concluded: "The clinical relevance of this study is that it questions the importance of implant design as the single most important factor for patient outcomes." Nobody would question that the type of artificial knee is but one of a number of factors which affect the PROM score, no matter which PROM is being used. But in the example above, the two rotating platform designs were so similar in their configuration and mechanics that it is doubtful if any PROM evaluation method could distinguish between the two designs.

Powell et al. (2018) compared the rotating platform and fixed-bearing designs of the press-fit condylar (PFC) knee using several PROM scores. Their conclusion was "In contrast with the established literature consensus… mobile bearing total knee arthroplasties are superior to identical implants with fixed-bearing inserts…" They attributed their finding to the avoidance of excessive internal rotational position of the fixed-bearing version which evidently caused patella pain and mal-tracking. However the superiority occurred in only some of the PROM evaluations, but not in others. Bailey et al. (2015) reported a randomized study over four centers comparing exactly the same two knee designs. At 1–2 years, there were no differences in any clinical scores including range of flexion, KSS, Oxford, and SF-12. Again using the same designs, although mixing between CR and PS versions, Harrington et al. (2009) found almost identical PROM scores between rotating platform and fixed bearing.

After many years of experience with fixed-bearing and rotating platform designs, a review of their own cases, and of literature reports, White et al. (2015) concluded: "Overall, both kinematic and in-vitro wear studies have highlighted certain benefits of rotating-platforms over fixed-bearing knees in primary TKA. However, the improved axial rotation has failed to show any benefits with respect to clinical outcomes…" This illustrates that there may be advantages of certain designs, in this case patella tracking or rotational placement, that do not alter the PROM score, yet are worthwhile advantages.

Medial Pivot Designs

A medial pivot type of design might be expected to show better function over a symmetric design, considering the asymmetry of anatomic knee motion where the medial side has much less anterior-posterior laxity than the lateral side. An advantage was reported by Pritchett (2011) as described in the above section entitled "Overall Differences Between Designs." Has the advantage been demonstrated in subsequent studies using PROMs as the evaluation tool? In a comparison between 76 medial pivot knees and 88 PS knees at 1 year, the medial pivot showed a significantly higher Forgotten Joint Score (FJS), especially in rising from a seated position (Samy et al. 2018). The authors attributed this to the highly congruent medial side. They found no differences in range of flexion, but no other functional evaluations were carried out. A meta-analysis between medial stabilized (more dished medial side, less dished lateral side) and non-medial stabilized (symmetric) showed the same 90-point Knee Society Score in both groups (Young et al. 2018). The authors stated "…a firm conclusion cannot be reached regarding the comparative clinical performance…" Comparing a medial pivot design (SAIPH) with a fixed-bearing symmetric design (Triathlon), there were no significant differences in KSS or Oxford scores (Benjamin et al. 2018). They raised the question as to why that should be the case, considering the difference in mechanics between the two designs: "The medial pivot design provides anteroposterior stability throughout the entire range of motion. However, it is unclear whether this difference in design translates to clinical and functional improvement." From a large regional database, the 10-year survivorship of the medial pivot knee (Advance) at 96.3% was not statistically different from the other knees in the database, mainly CR and PS, at 95.7% (Bordini et al. 2016). With 150 knees in each group, the Advance medial pivot was compared with a PFC PS knee. There were no differences in the KSS and WOMAC scores or in the range of flexion. The flexion results were impressive at a 9° gain from preoperative. Comparing 261 medial pivot knees with 913 PS knees, there was no difference in range of flexion, or gain in flexion, at 1-year follow-up (Shakespeare et al. 2006). In 98 patients, bilateral cases were analyzed, an Advance medial pivot on one side and a PFC Sigma rotating platform on the other side (Kim et al. 2017). At 2-year follow-up, the rotating platform results were better than for the medial pivot in the KSS scores and the HSS scores. The range of flexion, starting at the same average preoperatively, was higher postoperatively by 12°. There was no explanation given other than the excessive constraint on the medial side. However that does not seem valid because the rotating platform knee has exactly the same anterior-posterior constraint but in a direction along the center of the tibia, rather than along a line on the medial side.

Katchky et al. (2019), a group of surgeons who were part of the initial design team for the Saiph medial pivot knee, together with Michael Tuke, reported on their 5-year follow-up of 81 cases. This was part of the "stepwise introduction" of any new implant, recommended by Henrik Malchau. The average range of flexion was 124°, at the high end of studies of other designs. The conclusion from the study was "Five-year surveillance following limited release demonstrates the safety and efficacy of the SAIPH medial ball and socket total knee arthroplasty. Medial ball and socket kinematics facilitate ligament balancing, while limiting the need for additional soft-tissue release."

Guided Motion Knees

While we have considered the medial pivot and rotating platform designs as 'Guided Motion Knees', those guided motion types which are more biomimetic, have been little used so far. There are two examples which can given at this time. The Aequos G1 design which had a convex lateral tibial surface was tested in 158 patients followed for an average of 1 year (Frosch et al. 2009). Despite the low lateral conformity, the average flexion range was only 107 degrees. The Journey 2 knee with a low conformity lateral side, was followed in a multi-center study in no less than 2000 cases (Harris et al. 2019). The results were similar to those of other more conventional designs as recorded in the Australian National Joint Replacement Registry. However, in neither of these two examples were any biomechanical functional evaluation methods used for analysis.

Surgical Techniques

Using PROMs as the main indicator, there have been inconclusive results concerning the relative merits of different surgical techniques based on a systematic review (Jaffe et al. 2018). With the benchmark of reproducing the mechanical axis in the frontal plane, cases with greater than 2° error had lower KSS functional scores. On this same topic, another author concluded: "...good alignment allows for improved kinematics, stability and range of motion" (Longstaff et al. 2009). However using the mechanical axis as the target has been challenged from two points of view. Firstly, there is a variation in the location of the mechanical axis (line from the center of the femoral head to the center of the ankle) with many male patients having a constitutional varus. Furthermore, there is an inclination of the joint line of 2–3° to the mechanical axis. Following these guidelines in anatomic or kinematic alignment results in variations in the coronal alignment to the mechanical axis, but this made no difference to the Oxford or WOMAC functional scores (Howell et al. 2018). But according to Jaffe et al., "...long-term studies with larger numbers are required before making any conclusions..." On computer navigation, Jaffe et al. concluded that while there was ample evidence for more consistent alignment, there was no evidence of improved KSS scores. Daines and Dennis (2014) reviewed their evidence from two studies for the gap balancing technique versus measured resection. The first study demonstrated that a balanced and rectangular flexion gap during surgery was obtained much more frequently with a gap balanced technique. The second study, using fluoroscopy, demonstrated a much high incidence of femoral condylar lift-off for measured resection. It was concluded that gap balancing provided better frontal plane varus-valgus stability. However in these studies, PROM data was not provided.

Overview of Comparisons Using PROMs

The overall picture is that there are some differences in the PROM outcomes between different designs and surgical techniques, but that in most of the studies, there were no differences. That is surprising considering the mechanical differences between the unicompartmentals, the CR, the PS, the rotating platforms, and the medial pivots. If PROMs do not show functional differences between such extreme designs, it is even more unlikely that differences will be found between different versions of the same design type. In the studies which have not shown significant differences in function between different designs, the reasons could include the following:

- There are indeed no significant differences, so that if a particular patient had received a different artificial knee or technique, the result would have been the same. While it cannot be argued that the PROM result was incorrect, a valid question is was that PROM able to detect differences that would matter clinically?
- The differences are small so that significance cannot be demonstrated with the numbers typically used in studies, the studies being effectively underpowered. A question here is what is the minimal clinically important difference?
- Most of the patients in the study groups are relatively inactive, so that even if a design was capable of better performance, its capabilities would not be realized. One way to counter such a result is to restrict the patient study group to active patients, which is not easy to define, or below a certain age.
- There is a wide range in the condition of the knee preoperatively, and in the general condition of the patient, accounting for the wide range of postoperative scores, so that differences in scores due to the artificial knee design per se cannot be detected. This again relates to the numbers in the study.
- There is a wide range in the condition of the opposite knee, as well as of the hips, such that the PROM outcomes are influenced greatly by the joints other than the artificial knee under study. It is common in follow-up studies that the conditions of the other joint are not documented.
- The PROMs do not ask the questions which really define performance, in that they tend to focus on pain and discomfort in performing activities, rather on the level of performance. This is a plausible explanation and can be countered by focusing on those parts of the scoring system which deal specifically with function.
- The PROMs have a substantial ceiling effect and are not responsive to changes. This is a factor which has been studied by Giesinger et al. (2014).

Such limitations in the use of PROMs have been discussed in an article entitled "The Assessment of Outcome After Total Knee Arthroplasty: Are We There Yet?" (Hossain et al. 2015). The authors focus on the well-recognized requirement of an evaluation system that it accounts for a wide range of more demanding activities: "The lack of depth and breadth in the cover of all aspects of function can lead to imprecision with a skew in the distribution of scores amongst groups of patients. The increasingly younger patients undergoing TKA therefore achieve outcome indices which are near to the ceiling of the measurement scale. At a group level ceiling effects produce Type-2 errors in testing a hypothesis…" In relation to PROMs as they are at present, "there may be limitations to their use at a respondent level which may raise concerns about whether self-reported function adequately reflects actual function. PROM-based methodology is inherently subjective in nature and in the context of function, measures patients' perception of function as opposed to actual ability." As an alternative, "there has hence been an increasing trend by many clinicians to adopt more objective and exclusive methods of measuring function... The advantages offered by such methods compared with PROMs, include greater precision, responsiveness and lack of ceiling effects." This last comment referred to biomechanical methods of evaluation such as video motion analysis, force plates, instrumented treadmills, and accelerometer-based gait analysis. There are signs that such a point of view is gaining more acceptance, where biomechanical measurements are used to distinguish between designs and surgical techniques. The rationale is that the main role of PROMs is to provide an assessment of the patient's function overall, whereas the role of the biomechanical measurements is to focus on quantitative functional aspects which reflect the specific knee being tested. Biomechanical measurements should certainly be considered as an alternate to the use of PROMs alone. If there is evidence of value, biomechanical measurements can be used more extensively in studies where the mechanical aspects of function are the main criteria for comparison. Without this approach, newer designs and techniques which could offer important advantages may be considered ineffective if evaluated on the basis of PROMs alone. That said, some of the limitations of PROMs, listed above, will still apply to biomechanical measurements.

Alternate Evaluation Methods

The following are examples of where alternate methods are applicable. A normal gait pattern is important not only for appearance but for avoiding abnormal forces and motions which could injure other parts of the musculoskeletal system, such as the spine. If a particular artificial knee design was configured to produce normal gait (a unicompartmental, or an ACL + PCL preserving, or a guided motion knee), then gait analysis studies with ground-to-foot force data would be a suitable evaluation method. Another suitable method would be to use mobile fluoroscopy where the x-ray unit remains centered on the patient's knee during the activity. The outcome measure is the movements of the contact points on the lateral and medial condyles, with the pattern in normal knees being the benchmark.

If a particular design or technique was intended to produce accurate soft tissue balancing with infrequent need for recutting the bone or performing soft tissue release, tests at surgery where the soft tissue tensions or the medial and lateral contact forces are measured accurately would be an appropriate experimental method. A new rehabilitation method might be postulated to result in a more rapid return to normal function. Simple evaluations such as the Timed Up and Go (TUG) test or the sit-to-stand (STS) test would be valid methods of measuring the recovery process. Even remote methods such as activity monitoring using inertial measurement units (IMU) electronically recorded could be used. An other example is if a new material to significantly reduce the wear. There is no reason that this would affect the PROM score, but the initial way of testing the wear is by a comparative study using a knee simulating machine.

Hence the proposition is that a PROM should not always be regarded as the only valid measure, rather that other measures can be used which will evaluate some particular parameter which has its own inherent value, even if that parameter might not change the PROM score in a major way.

Function Measured Using Biomechanical Methods

As described above, PROMs provide an overall assessment of which activities the patient can achieve and the extent to which they have difficulties or feel pain during those activities. However they are not designed to distinguish how well or how often or how vigorously the activities take place. Several investigators have suggested that more objective measures should be used in combination with PROMs or even as a substitute in some cases (Mizner et al. 2011; Dobson et al. 2013; Giesinger et al. 2014; Hossain et al. 2015; Parks et al. 2015; Berliner et al. 2017; Graff et al. 2016). The most widely used method has been gait analysis. By using this technique, the joint angles of total knee patients during level walking and going up and down stairs have been measured, as well as the foot-to-ground forces and the moments acting across the knee. In some studies, electromyographic data has been used to identify muscle activity. Such measurements have provided insight into a number of deficiencies in the function of patients with artificial knees. Tom Andriacchi, a

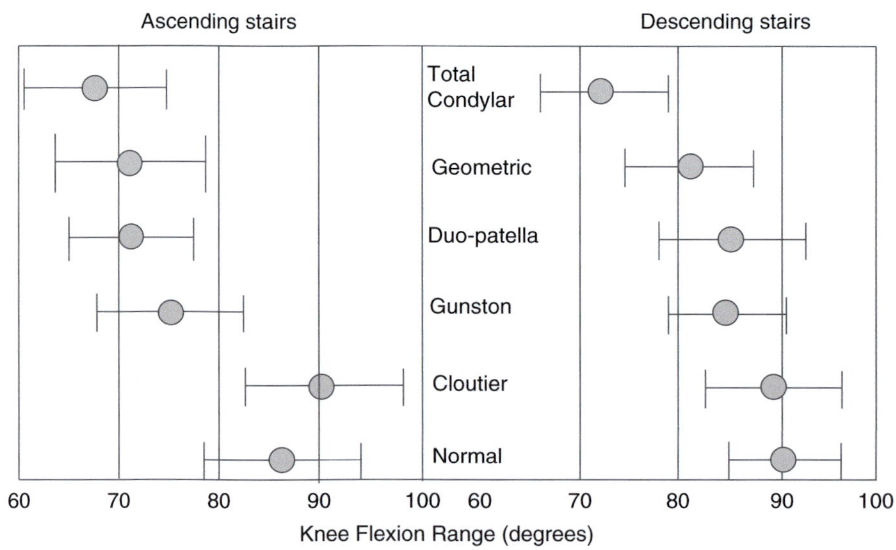

Fig. 14.5 Thomas Andriacchi Ph.D. and colleagues showed that in ascending and descending stairs, some designs of artificial knee had less range of flexion than normal controls. This was attributed to abnormal femoral-tibial contact position in the sagittal plane. The ACL+PCL preserving design with low constraint and soft tissue balancing (Cloutier) had the most normal range. Patients tended to lean forward during ascending to reduce the flexion moment. In level walking, all designs had reduced walking speed and reduced mid-flexion angle (Andriacchi et al. 1982)

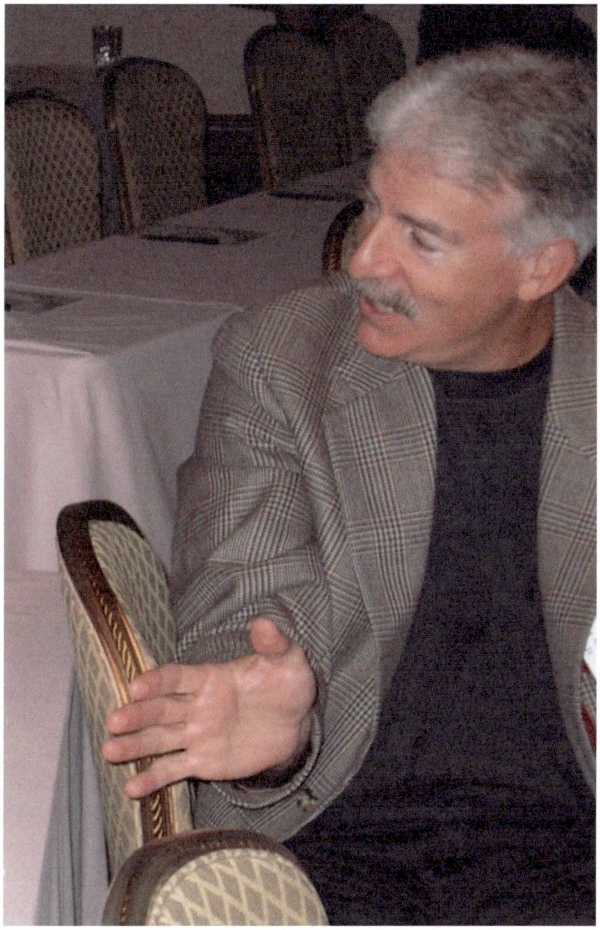

Fig. 14.6 Thomas Andriacchi Ph.D. founded and directed a Kinetics Laboratory at Rush Presbyterian Hospital, Chicago, from 1974 to 1998. He was a major contributor to the Miller-Galante knee and the NexGen CR knee. As a Professor of mechanical engineering and orthopedics at Stanford University since 1998, he has carried out experimental studies which have given new insights into the mechanical factors associated with the development of osteoarthritis. He has developed special footwear for altering the force distribution in the knee for the alleviation of early arthritis. (Photo c 2017) (© Peter S Walker)

biomechanical engineer at Rush Presbyterian in Chicago, and Jorge Galante, chairman of orthopedics, were the first to demonstrate some of the deficiencies of artificial knees in performing activities of daily living (Andriacchi et al. 1980, 1982). While level walking was not impaired in a major way, this was not the case for going up and down stairs. Because the center of gravity of the body was more offset from the center of the knee in the sagittal plane in stair activities, much higher quadriceps muscle forces were needed to balance the external moments which were acting to flex the knee. As a result, the patients had to adapt their posture to reduce the moments. This was especially true if the artificial knee was too constrained such that the contact points did not move posteriorly with flexion. This led Tom Andriacchi and Jorge Galante to favor designs of low constraint with cruciate preservation, and they produced their own design using those principles, the Miller-Galante knee. Andriacchi also pointed out that abnormal muscle function, learned over the time period of the patient's arthritis, as well as weakened muscles, produced abnormal function.

Results of gait analysis studies up to 2007 where artificial knees of various types were compared with normal were reviewed by McClelland et al. (2007). It was found that patients walked at a significantly slower speed than control groups. They also walked with less total range of knee motion and a reduced range of flexion during the loading phase of gait. Patients had less knee flexion during the swing phase of gait compared with healthy controls. Eighty percent of controls showed a biphasic sagittal knee movement pattern where the knee was flexed during the mid-stance phase, compared with less than one third of artificial knee patients.

A recent meta-analysis of gait studies between total knees and unicompartmentals, where differences in kinematics would be expected, showed that most biomechanical factors were similar but that the artificial knee group had significantly shorter stride length than unicompartmental patients (Nha et al. 2018). Not a dramatic finding, although as Andriacchi had already pointed out, level walking is not a major discriminator. In addition, in a review by Komnik et al. (2015), the performance of unicompartmentals is hampered by the patients maintaining their preoperative motion patterns and muscle weakness. In that review, the wide variety of techniques and parameters used in different gait analysis studies was reported. Most studies focused on level walking, whereas more demanding activities were needed to detect kinetic abnormalities. These abnormalities were likely due to impaired muscle activity, based on studies where gait analysis and electromyography were studied simultaneously (Catani et al. 2012). The authors concluded: "The present study supports the evidence that good joint function and nearly physiological muscle activity during gait can be achieved in patients undergoing UKA (unicompartmental knee)." For artificial knees, however, the conclusion was different. Aljehani et al. (2019) demonstrated that in unilateral cases of artificial knee replacement, the status of the opposite knee, often osteoarthritic to a greater or lesser degree, affected the overall gait patterns. In fact, the gait pattern of an artificial knee more closely matched an osteoarthritic opposite knee than a normal opposite knee. This is an unexpected finding which has major implications, that an artificial knee only partially restores the knee to normal from its preoperative arthritic condition.

Measurements of muscle strength on kinetic test machines have provided information about the preoperative and postoperative condition of the total knee patient (Skoffer et al. 2015). Reduced muscle strength and abnormal neuromuscular patterns were considered the reasons why patient function after a total knee was deficient (Yoshida et al. 2013). In studies over many years in the Physical Therapy Department in Newark, Delaware, Lynn Snyder-Mackler Ph.D. and associates have focused on the major effect that muscle strength and coordination have on the functional outcomes after total knee replacement. They concluded that appropriate rehabilitation programs pre- and postoperatively are effective in improving functional outcomes (Pozzi et al. 2020). At 1-year follow-up, their conclusion was "on average, TKA does not restore functional ability to the levels of age-matched subjects without joint pathology…but…a greater proportion of patients who participated in the progressive strengthening protocol achieved what could be considered normal clinical and

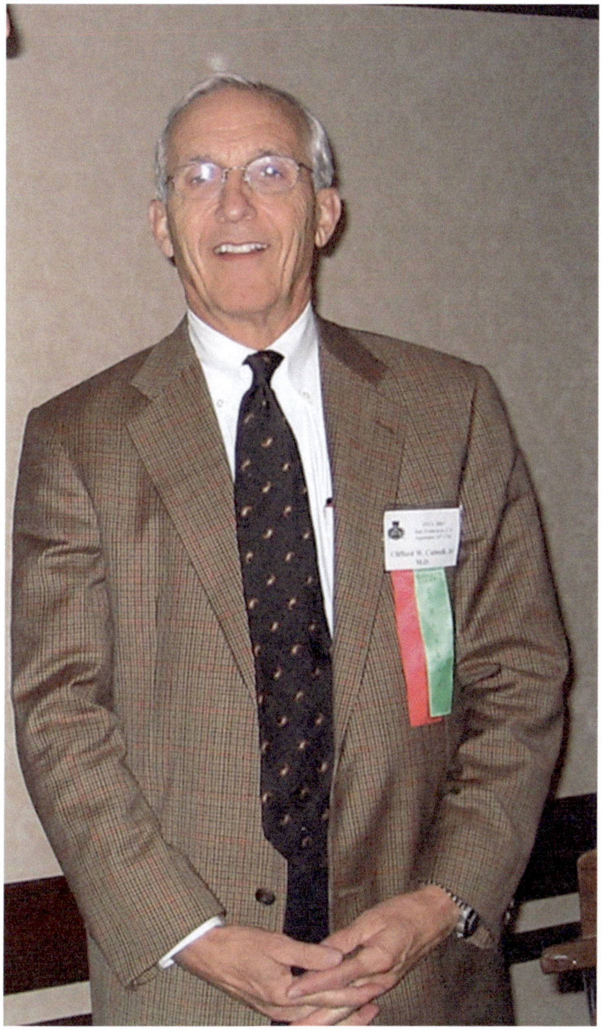

Fig. 14.7 Clifford Colwell MD (left), from the Scripps Clinic, Ja Jolla, CA, has made major contributions in research into the biomechanics of the knee. He collaborated with Darryl D'Lima in the design of implanted instrumented artificial knees, carried out surgical implantations, and measured forces in multiple activities, including sports. This focused attention on the possibilities of the artificial knee to allow an active and healthy lifestyle as well as relieve pain and restore basic functions. (Photo taken at the ISTA meeting, San Francisco, 2003) (© Peter S Walker)

functional scores." As well as muscle strength per se, one role of an artificial knee is to provide the optimal lever arm for the joint to effectively balance external moments and produce desired motions. Equally important were the rehabilitation protocols.

The most striking example of research of technical and organizational excellence in recent years was the measurement of forces in the knee by instrumented tibial components. This was implemented in two centers, the Charite Hospital in Berlin, Germany, and Scripps Clinic, San Diego. The work in Berlin has been described previously in relation to the testing of implants for wear (see Chap. 13). The work at the Scripps Clinic, led by Darryl D'Lima MD and Cliff Colwell MD focused on the forces during everyday and sporting activities (D'Lima et al. 2011). Peak forces in walking averaged 2.6 body weight (BW), increasing to 4 BW in jogging. Surprisingly, similar high forces as well as high shear and torque forces occurred

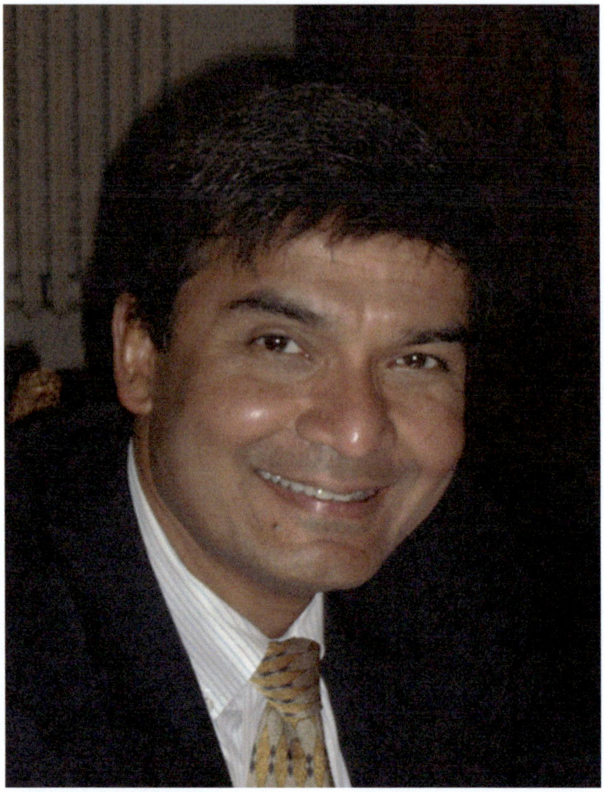

Fig. 14.8 Darryl D'Lima MD Ph.D. is director of orthopedic research at the Shiley Center for Orthopaedics, Scripps Clinic, San Diego. He was the main designer of the "Lab-in-a-knee" which was an instrumented tibial component for measuring knee forces in vivo. That work has resulted in several awards from major research organizations. Other research areas include soft tissue balancing and cartilage injury and regeneration. (Photo taken c 2018) (© Peter S Walker)

while performing golf strokes. Stationary cycling produced only 1 BW, indicating its suitability for those with an arthritic knee. Wearing special variable insole shoes offloaded the medial side of the knee by up to 19%, potentially valuable in relieving pain in osteoarthritis. New sensor technology could make it possible to monitor joint forces on a more routine basis.

Fluoroscopic Evaluation of Kinematics

One evaluation method for revealing the kinematics within the joint itself has been fluoroscopy, which was first developed at the Massachusetts Institute of Technology by Scott Banks Ph.D. and Andy Hodge MD (1996). Their purpose in developing the method was as follows: "Accurate measurements of knee replacement kinematics during functional activities would provide the basis for assessing the performance of current designs and for objectively designing devices with improved kinematics." The method consisted of taking successive fluoroscopic images of the knee in motion. Knowing the three-dimensional geometry of the implant components and the relative motion between the femur and tibia could be calculated and expressed as three rotations and three

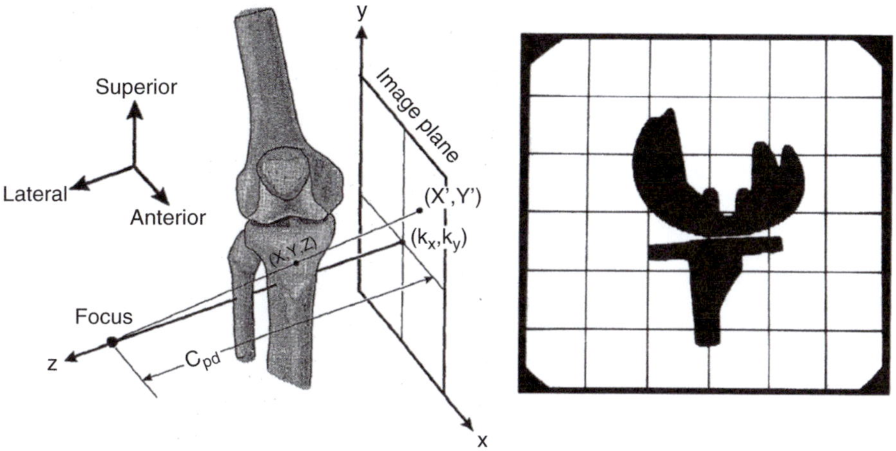

Fig. 14.9 Fluoroscopic imaging to determine the kinematics of the knee, often described by the path of the contact points on the tibial surface or by movement of the transverse femoral axis relative to the tibia. A radiographic image is produced in the plane of the x-ray plate, from the point source (focus). After correction for distortions, the orientation of each component in the global axis frame and the orientation of the femur relative to the tibia are computed (Banks and Hodge 1996). (Reprinted with permission IEEE Transactions in Biomedical Engineering)

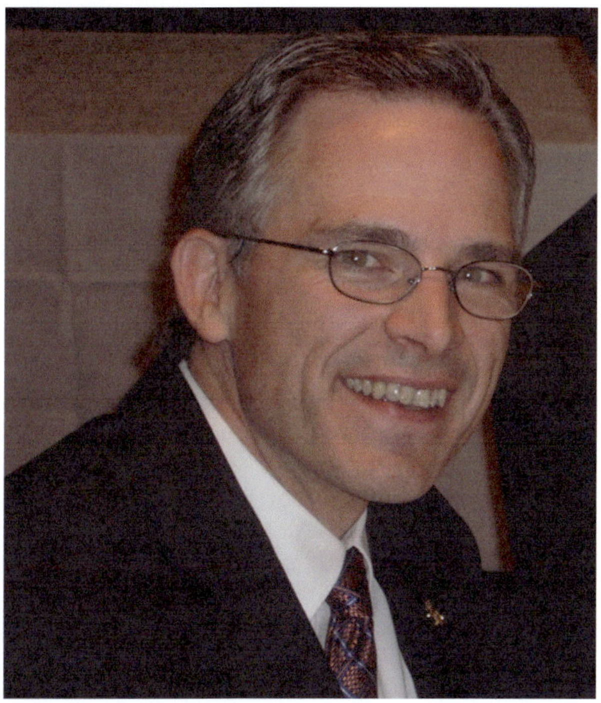

Fig. 14.10 Scott Banks Ph.D. from University of Florida in Gainesville, working with Andy Hodge MD from Massachusetts General Hospital, developed the first fluoroscopic system for determining the relative three-dimensional positions of the femoral and tibial components, enabling the tracking of motion during activity. The work was first published in Banks' Ph.D. thesis at Massachusetts Institute of Technology in 1992. (Photo taken c 2015) (© Peter S Walker)

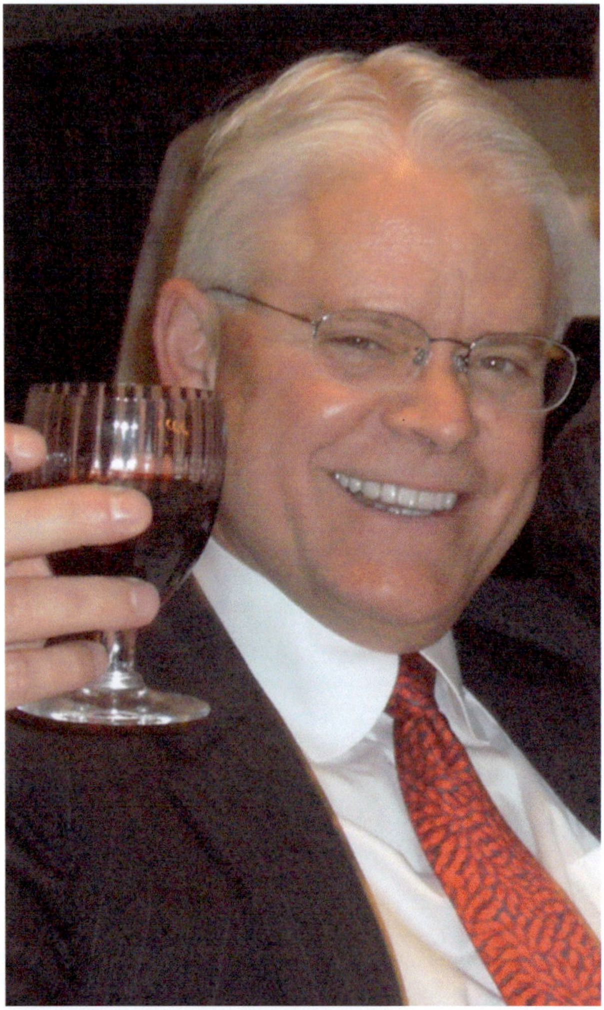

Fig. 14.11 Douglas Dennis MD works at the Colorado Joint Replacement Center in Denver, Colorado, a specialist high-volume center in knee and hip replacement. He holds academic affiliations with the universities of Colorado and Tennessee, in order to conduct research on the kinematics of joints. His fluoroscopic research with Rick Komistek has produced invaluable data, which have been widely propagated at conferences around the world. (Photo taken c 2017) (© Peter S Walker)

displacements. A requirement was that the knee had to stay in the frame of the x-ray cameras, so the motions studied were mainly a lunge through a full flexion angle, rising from a seated position and walking on a treadmill which is not the same as normal walking. Important insights were discovered about total knee function by Banks and Hodge. Many surgeons collaborated in using their methodology for the evaluation of a new design or surgical technique; as examples, "how is high flexion achieved in the anatomic and artificial knee?", "what is the role of femoral rollback and tibial slope?", "do bicruciate (ACL+PCL) and medial pivot artificial knees move similarly to the anatomic knee?", and "why do CR and PS knees have such variable centers of internal-external rotation?". Richard Komistek Ph.D. adopted the method a few years later while working in Denver, Colorado, and carried out numerous collaborative studies with Doug

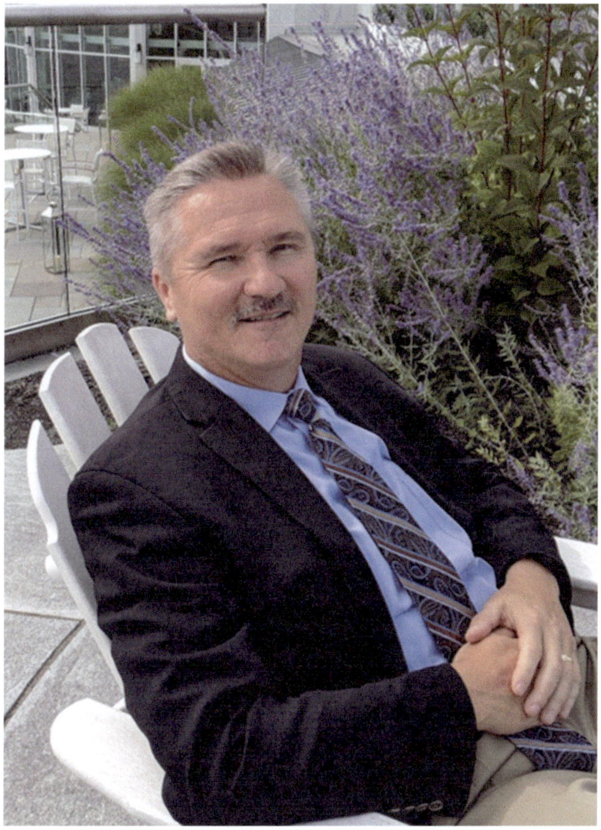

Fig. 14.12 After starting off as a designer in industry, Rik Komistek Ph.D. moved to the University of Colorado in Denver in 1994 where he established a fluoroscopic evaluation laboratory in collaboration with Doug Dennis MD and Jim Stiehl MD. They carried out groundbreaking influential studies on the motion of different types of total knee in various activities. In 2002 Rik moved to Knoxville where he continued this work, expanding it in engineering sophistication with the application of Kane's Dynamics to analyze the forces in the musculoskeletal system. Recently his lab developed the first mobile fluoroscopic unit for studying the kinetics of functional activities. (Photo taken 2019) (© Peter S Walker)

Dennis MD and Jim Stiehl MD. Subsequently many other surgeons sent their fluoroscopic data for analysis using their software system. After moving his laboratory to Knoxville, Tennessee, Rick Komistek extended his work in several directions such as analysis using Kane's dynamics, but still including fluoroscopy as the core technology.

Depicting three-dimensional motion data in a way that can be readily interpreted is not easy. However for artificial knees, this was solved by plotting the succession of femoral-tibial contact points on to the lateral and medial tibial surface, connected with straight lines. This provided visualization of position, whether anterior or posterior; rollback, whether uniform or different laterally and medially; and internal-external rotation, together with the center of rotation. Possibly the most influential fluoroscopic study was a comparison of over 800 CR and PS knees in the stance phase of walking and deep knee bend (Dennis et al. 2003). The motion patterns of artificial knee motions were compared with those of normal intact knees. In gait, from heel strike to toe-off, normal knees showed posterior displacement laterally but small medial displacements. The artificial knees showed highly variable patterns of motion, but generally with less lateral displacement than normal. In some knees there was anterior displacement of contacts, opposite to normal behavior. In deep

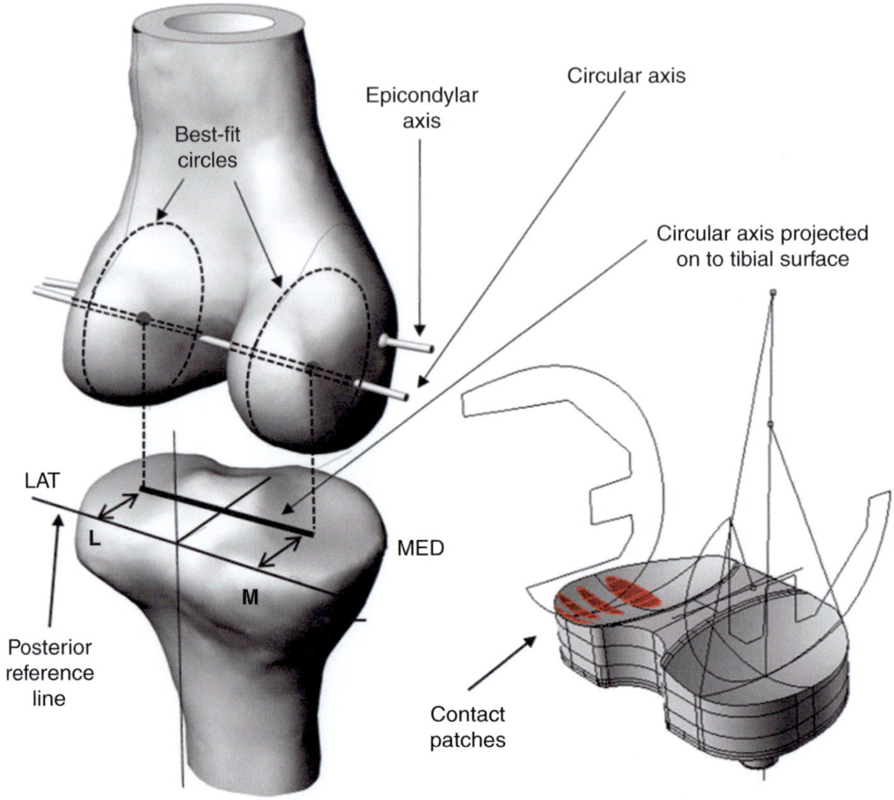

Fig. 14.13 Method for describing the motion of the femur on the tibia during flexion. The circular axis is projected on to the tibial surface plane. At a particular flexion angle, distances L and M describe the femoral position on the tibia. The succession of the circular axis projections at a succession of discrete flexion angles describes the motion path. For a total knee, this method is similar to describing the centers of the lateral and medial contact patches, if the circular axis of the condyles of the femoral component is used. The epicondylar axis in general will not be coincident with the circular axis

knee bend, normal knees showed 19 mm posterior lateral displacement and 3 mm posterior medial displacement, resembling a medial pivot action. Artificial knees with ACL + PCL showed similar patterns to normal knees. In contrast, CR knees showed a highly variable pattern, but on average there were equal lateral and medial displacements of the contact points. Up to 90° flexion, in 70% of cases, there was more than 3 mm anterior femoral displacement during flexion, with an average of 8 mm, so-called paradoxical sliding. In PS knees there were again almost equal lateral and medial displacements on average, with paradoxical sliding in only 43% of cases, average 6 mm. The authors considered that this sliding reduced the maximum flexion achieved and reduced the quadriceps moment arm, reducing efficiency. The authors concluded that "The sagittal plane translation patterns after an artificial knee usually do not duplicate those of the normal knee." The relative magnitude of the displacements between the different designs tested could be explained largely by the relative amount of dishing of the tibial bearing surface, the most displacement for the ACL + PCL preserving, intermediate for the CR, and least for the PS. These relative sliding distances can be explained by the different dishing between the three types of designs. The lack of a medial pivot action as in normal anatomic knees could be explained by the symmetric condyle shapes of the artificial knees, compared with the asymmetric geometry in the normal knee. Recently, Rick Komistek in Knoxville, Marcus Pandy Ph.D. in Melbourne, and William Taylor Ph.D. in Zurich developed a mobile fluoroscopy system where the x-ray cameras followed the center the knee. These extraordinary machines allow many types of everyday activities to be studied, and data is just now beginning to emerge. A recent article has reviewed numerous fluoroscopic studies which have showed characteristic, and variable, patterns of motion for different implant designs and examined whether the motion was associated with outcomes (Angerame et al. 2019). The general findings were that there were few relations even when some functional effect of motion might be expected.

Biomechanical Evaluation Methods for the Clinic

Due to the expense, time taken, specialized equipment, and expertise required for the above gait analysis and fluoroscopic methodologies, they have been used mainly in a research setting rather than in general clinical practice. Nevertheless for evaluating a new artificial knee design or technique, such studies provide in-depth data about the function of the knee. For general clinical evaluations however, as an alternative, a number of simpler tests have been developed and used extensively, so far used mainly in physical therapy and rehabilitation rather than in the orthopedics clinic. In the Timed Up and Go (TUG) test, the test subject starts from a seated position, they then rise, walk 3 m, turn around, walk back to the chair, and sit down again. The test is described by Dobson (2015): "The TUG is a transition test that assesses strength, agility and dynamic balance during multiple activities including Sit-to-Stand, walking short distances and changing direction whilst walking." The measure is the time taken to complete the test. The test is simple to carry out and has a single number to quantify the result. The sit-to-stand (STS) test has three versions, testing knee strength or endurance, important indicators of function. In the 30-second test, the subject stands up and sits down as many times as possible. The normal value for somebody of average total knee age is 12–18 times. In the five-times sit-to-stand test, the time is measured for the subject to stand-sit five times. In the right-left comparison test, the right/left force ratio is calculated. In recent years, with the increasing availability of wearable sensors, biomechanical methods such as a "portable gait lab" using accelerometers have been conveniently implemented in a clinical setting (Parks et al. 2015). Ground-to-foot forces and pressures, as well as cadence and stance times, have been measured using instrumented insoles (Stöggl and Martiner 2017). The thin insoles only 3 mm in thickness are placed into the normal footwear used by the test subject, with the data being transmitted wirelessly

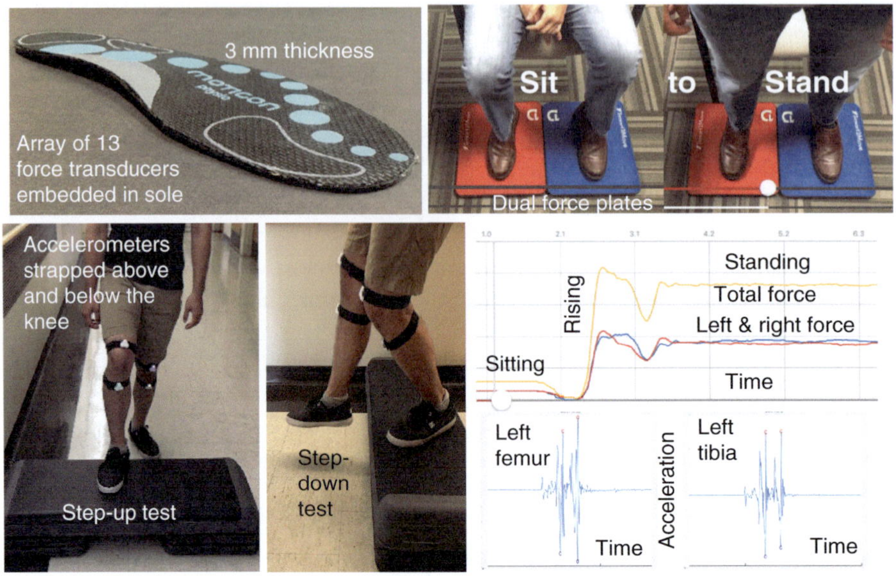

Fig. 14.14 Equipment is now available for carrying out simple biomechanical tests in the clinic. The Instrumented Insoles are used for measuring right and left forces and force ratios, in a Timed Up and Go test, in walking, and in step-up/step-down tests. The dual force plates are used in a sit-to-stand test, to measure right-left force ratios in rising and standing. The IMUs (inertial measuring units) are used for measuring joint angles during activities and the accelerations below and above the knee

to a computer. Several activity monitors have been introduced in recent years, with the idea of accumulating the types and frequency of activities that the subject carries out over a prescribed time period. These devices, which attach to a location on the body, have the advantage of quantifying activity and alerting the physician or therapist if progress is deficient by linking the data through a cell phone (Lipperts et al. 2017). In the following section, examples will be given of the application of the evaluation methods described above, to compare different artificial knee designs.

In the above study to compare rehabilitation methods, Pozzi et al. (2020) used the Timed Up and Go test, the stair climb test, and the 6-minute walk test. Parks et al. (2015) used similar tests as well as a portable gait lab to track the progress of recovery after a total knee, finding that most of the measures had peaked at the 4-month follow-up time, although in general, 1 year is generally used as the minimum time where close to full recovery has been reached. Such tests, particularly the TUG test, have been used primarily to monitor or compare the progress of a particular therapy or to compare one therapy to another. Examples are as follows: surgical balancing of the medial side of the knee to avoid looseness was found to produce shorter TUG times than when the MCL was loose; TUG times up to 3 months after surgery were used to compare whether using a tourniquet or not at surgery made any difference to functional recovery; recovery trajectories after different therapies, high intensity or low intensity, were measured using TUG times; and whether there was a greater variation in function within a patient group, before and after artificial knee surgery. The advantage of this type of measure over a PROM is that it provides an objective measurable quantity which signifies functional ability and is not subject to interpretation by the patient. However, at this time there are relatively few available studies where these measures have been used as the principal method to compare different artificial knee designs or surgical procedures. Based on those studies which have used the methods however, they do appear to be a useful adjunct to the use of PROMs. In certain evaluations, they have been used as the primary indicator.

Function Measured in the Laboratory

To evaluate the function of an artificial knee design, the most objective method may be a mechanical test or a computer model. This might seem to be unreasonable in that how can an artificial knee be evaluated without being in the patient? There is however some rationale. An automobile has performance measures of the engine and suspension, which can be tested objectively in the factory or on a test track. Put the car in the hands of 20 drivers, and the way the car performs will be completely different in every case. A Maserati in the hands of a cautious driver would be driven similarly to a family sedan. Yet each type of car will have its own objective performance measures, no matter who drives the car or how. One obvious way in which an artificial knee can be tested is in a knee simulating machine, which can be used for both wear and kinematics. The Stanmore knee simulator was used by John DesJardins, now at Clemson University, South Carolina, to test the kinematics of different designs of artificial knee and also to study the effects of different stiffnesses of ligament constraints as well as ligament resections (Desjardins et al. 2000). The results revealed that certain designs might be over-constrained, while at the other extreme, loose ligaments could result in instability in a low-conformity design. In a recent paper, Hani Haider (2017) stated: "The future will carry exciting developments into more sophisticated soft tissue simulation for the force-control methodology. More daily activities beyond walking will be simulated…" Crouching machines, a derivative of the original Oxford test rig, as well as modern robotic arms, have been used in comparisons between knee designs and found to give realistic data (Varadarajan et al. 2009). An authoritative summary paper has been written of the knee forces during different activities measured by instrumented tibial components in vivo (Bergmann et al. 2014). This data has been submitted to the American Society for Testing and Materials (ASTM) as the basis for a new standard by ASTM. Although not yet implemented, the data acts as a guideline for advanced simulation experiments. In terms of motion inputs, it seems logical to input only the flexion-extension cycle for the different activities. The other displacements and rotations will be determined mainly by the restraints from the bearing surfaces of the artificial knee and the soft tissues, which is the principle of a force-controlled machine. Advanced Mechanical Technology (AMTI) in Watertown, MA, recently introduced the VIVO machine for studying the kinematics of the knee. Forces and flexion-extension are input to the knee, while the ligaments are represented virtually. With such a machine, using the Bergmann data, the kinematics of any artificial knee can be determined under a sequence of ligament properties, alignments, and activity scenarios. This will evaluate laxity, stability (and instability), and robustness of designs to extreme loading and alignment conditions. An example of how the machine can be used to study the effects of soft tissue variations was recently published (Willing and Walker 2018).

Which Evaluation Methods Are Applicable, and Are There Differences Between Designs and Techniques?

Patient-reported outcome measures (PROMs) have been by far the most frequently used method for evaluating artificial knees or surgical techniques. PROMs provide an overall assessment of the function of the patient and are suitable for databases of large numbers of patients. However for evaluating specific aspects of function in a more quantitative way, a broad range of biomechanical evaluation methods is available. The methods include radiographic techniques, particularly fluoroscopy but also MRI and RSA; gait and force analysis and muscle force measurements; simple clinical tests such as TUG, STS, and activity monitoring; and finally, computer simulations. Based on PROM data, it has been difficult to detect systematic differences between different designs in function. However the biomechanical evaluation methods have detected differences between designs and techniques, in gait, kinematics, forces, and other factors. Their results have provided pointers to improvements in design, technique, and rehabilitation methods. Biomechanical evaluation methods, whether complex and used in specialist laboratories, or simple and used in a clinical setting, can provide yet further insights.

References

Aljehani M, Madara K, Snyder-Mackler L, Christiansen C, Zeni JA Jr. The contralateral knee may not be a valid control for biomechanical outcomes after unilateral total knee arthroplasty. Gait Posture. 2019;70:179–84.

Andriacchi TP, Andersson GB, Fermier RW, Stern D, Galante JO. A study of lower-limb mechanics during stair-climbing. J Bone Joint Surg Am. 1980;62(5):749–57.

Andriacchi TP, Galante JO, Fermier RW. The influence of total knee-replacement design on walking and stair-climbing. J Bone Joint Surg Am. 1982;64(9):1328–35.

Angerame MR, Holst DC, Jennings JM, Komistek RD, Dennis DA. Total knee arthroplasty kinematics. J Arthroplast. 2019;34(10):2502–10.

Bailey O, Ferguson K, Crawfurd E, James P, May PA, Brown S, Blyth M, Leach WJ. No clinical difference between fixed- and mobile-bearing cruciate-retaining total knee arthroplasty: a prospective randomized study. Knee Surg Sports Traumatol Arthrosc. 2015;23(6):1653–9.

Banks SA, Hodge WA. Accurate measurement of 3-dimensional knee replacement kinematics using single-plane fluoroscopy. IEEE Trans Biomed Eng. 1996;43(6):638–49.

Beaupre LA, Sharifi B, Johnston DWC. A randomized clinical trial comparing Posterior-Cruciate Stabilizing vs Posterior Cruciate-Retaining Prostheses in primary total knee. J Arthroplasty. 2017;32(3):819–23.

Behrend H, Giesinger K, Giesinger JM, Kuster MS. The "forgotten joint" as the ultimate goal in joint arthroplasty: validation of a new patient-reported outcome measure. J Arthroplasty. 2012;27(3):430–436.e431.

Behrend H, Zdravkovic V, Bosch M, Hochreiter B. No difference in joint awareness after TKA: a matched-pair analysis of a classic implant and its evolutional design. Knee Surg Sports Traumatol Arthrosc. 2019;27(7):2124–9.

Benjamin B, Pietrzak JRT, Tahmassebi J, Haddad FS. A functional comparison of medial pivot and condylar knee designs based on patient outcomes and parameters of gait. Bone Joint J. 2018;100-b(1 Supple A):76–82.

Berend KR, Lombardi AV, Adams JB. Which total knee replacement implant should I pick? Correcting the pathology: the role of knee bearing designs. Bone Joint J. 2013;95-B(11 Suppl A):129–32.

Bergmann G, Bender A, Graichen F, et al. Standardized loads acting in knee implants. PLoS One. 2014;9(1):e86035.

Berliner JL, Brodke DJ, Chan V, SooHoo NF, Bozic KJ. Can preoperative patient-reported outcome measures be used to predict meaningful improvement in function after TKA? Clin Orthop Relat Res. 2017;475(1):149–57.

Bordini B, Ancarani C, Fitch DA. Long-term survivorship of a medial-pivot total knee system compared with other cemented designs in an arthroplasty registry. J Orthop Surg Res. 2016;11:44.

Catani F, Benedetti MG, Bianchi L, Marchionni V, Giannini S, Leardini A. Muscle activity around the knee and gait performance in unicompartmental knee arthroplasty patients: a comparative study on fixed- and mobile-bearing designs. Knee Surg Sports Traumatol Arthrosc. 2012;20(6):1042–8.

D'Lima DD, Patil S, Steklov N, Colwell CW Jr. The 2011 ABJS Nicolas Andry award: 'Lab'-in-a-knee: in vivo knee forces, kinematics, and contact analysis. Clin Orthop Relat Res. 2011;469(10):2953–70.

Daines BK, Dennis DA. Gap balancing vs. measured resection technique in total knee arthroplasty. Clin Orthop Surg. 2014;6(1):1–8.

Dennis DA, Komistek RD, Mahfouz MR, Haas BD, Stiehl JB. Multicenter determination of in vivo kinematics after total knee arthroplasty. Clin Orthop Relat Res. 2003;416:37–57.

DesJardins JD, Walker PS, Haider H, Perry J. The use of a force-controlled dynamic knee simulator to quantify the mechanical performance of total knee replacement designs during functional activity. J Biomech. 2000;33(10):1231–42.

Dobson F. Timed up and go test in musculoskeletal conditions. J Physiother. 2015;61(1):47.

Dobson F, Hinman RS, Roos EM, Abbott JH, Stratford P, Davis AM, Buchbinder R, Snyder-Mackler L, Henrotin Y, Thumboo J, Hansen P, Benell K. OARSI recommended performance-based tests to assess physical function in people diagnosed with hip or knee osteoarthritis. Osteoarthr Cartil. 2013;21(8):1042–52.

Ewald FC. The knee society total knee arthroplasty roentgenographic evaluation and scoring system. Clin Orthop Relat Res. 1989;248:9–12.

Frosch KH, Nägerl H, Kubein-Meesenburg D, Buchholz J, Dörner J, Dathe H, Hellerer O, Dumont C, Stürmer KM. A new total knee arthroplasty with physiologically shaped surfaces. Part 2: first clinical results. Unfallchirurg. 2009;112(2):176–84.

Giesinger K, Hamilton DF, Jost B, Holzner B, Giesinger JM. Comparative responsiveness of outcome measures for total knee arthroplasty. Osteoarthr Cartil. 2014;22(2):184–9.

Goh GS, Bin Abd Razak HR, Tay DK, Chia SL, Lo NN, Yeo SJ. Unicompartmental knee arthroplasty achieves greater flexion with no difference in functional outcome, quality of life, and satisfaction vs total knee arthroplasty in patients younger than 55 years. A propensity score-matched cohort analysis. J Arthroplast. 2018;33(2):355–61.

Graff C, Hohmann E, Bryant AL, Tetsworth K. Subjective and objective outcome measures after total knee replacement: is there a correlation? ANZ J Surg. 2016;86(11):921–5.

Haider H. Chapter 7.10: Wear: knee joint arthroplasty. In: Ducheyne P, Grainger DW, Healy KE, Hutmacher DW, Kirkpatrick CJ, editors. Comprehensive biomaterials II, vol. 7. Oxford: Elsevier; 2017. p. 152–74.

Harrington MA, Hopkinson WJ, Hsu P, Manion L. Fixed- vs mobile-bearing total knee arthroplasty: does it make a difference?--a prospective randomized study. J Arthroplast. 2009;24(6 Suppl):24–7.

Harris AI, Christen B, Malcorps JJ, O'Grady CP, Kopjar B, Sensiba PR, Vandenneucker H, Huang BK, Cates HE, Hur J, Marra DA. Midterm performance of a Guided-Motion bicruciate-stabilized total knee system: rseults from the International study of over 2000 consevutive primary total knee arthroplasties. J Arthroplasty. 2019;34(7S):S201–S208.

Hauer G, Sadoghi P, Bernhardt GA, Wolf M, Ruckenstuhl P, Fink A, Leithner A, Gruber G. Greater activity, better range of motion and higher quality of life following unicompartmental knee arthroplasty: a comparative case-control study. Arch Orthop Trauma Surg. 2020;140(2):231–7.

Hossain FS, Konan S, Patel S, Rodriguez-Merchan EC, Haddad FS. The assessment of outcome after total knee arthroplasty: are we there yet? Bone Joint J. 2015;97-b(1):3–9.

Howell SM, Shelton TJ, Hull ML. Implant survival and function ten years after kinematically aligned total knee arthroplasty. J Arthroplast. 2018;33(12):3678–84.

Jaffe WL, Dundon JM, Camus T. Alignment and balance methods in total knee arthroplasty. J Am Acad Orthop Surg. 2018;26(20):709–16.

Jiang C, Liu Z, Wang Y, Bian Y, Feng B, Weng X. Posterior cruciate ligament retention versus posterior stabilization for total knee arthroplasty: a meta-analysis. PLoS One. 2016;11(1):e0147865.

Katchky AM, Jones CW, Walter WL, Shimmin AJ. Medial ball and socket total knee arthroplasty five-year clinical results. Bone Joint J. 2019;101B(1_Supple_A):59–65.

Kim YH, Park JW, Kim JS. Clinical outcome of medial pivot compared with press-fit condylar sigma cruciate-retaining mobile-bearing total knee arthroplasty. J Arthroplast. 2017;32(10):3016–23.

Kleeblad LJ, van der List JP, Zuiderbaan HA, Pearle AD. Larger range of motion and increased return to activity, but higher revision rates following unicompartmental versus total knee arthroplasty in patients under 65: a systematic review. Knee Surg Sports Traumatol Arthrosc. 2018;26(6):1811–22.

Komnik I, Weiss S, Pagani CF, Potthast W. Motion analysis of patients after knee arthroplasty during activities of daily living–a systematic review. Gait Posture. 2015;41(2):370–7.

Lipperts M, Laarhoven SV, Senden R, Heyligers I, Grimm B. Clinical validation of a body-fixed 3D accelerometer and algorithm for activity monitoring in orthopaedic patients. J Orthop Transl. 2017;11:19–29.

Longstaff LM, Sloan K, Stamp N, Scaddan M, Beaver R. Good alignment after total knee arthroplasty leads to faster rehabilitation and better function. J Arthroplast. 2009;24(4):570–8.

Lyons MC, MacDonald SJ, Somerville LE, Naudie DD, McCalden RW. Unicompartmental versus total knee arthroplasty database analysis: is there a winner? Clin Orthop Relat Res. 2012;470(1):84–90.

McClelland JA, Webster KE, Feller JA. Gait analysis of patients following total knee replacement: a systematic review. Knee. 2007;14(4):253–63.

Meneghini RM, Stefl MD, Hodge WA, Banks SA. A cam–post mechanism is no longer necessary in modern primary total knee arthroplasty. J Knee Surg. 2019;32:710–3.

Migliorini F, Tingart M, Niewiera M, Rath B, Eschweiler J. Unicompartmental versus total knee arthroplasty for knee osteoarthritis. Eur J Orthop Surg Traumatol. 2019;29(4):947–55.

Mizner RL, Petterson SC, Clements KE, Zeni JA Jr, Irrgang JJ, Snyder-Mackler L. Measuring functional improvement after total knee arthroplasty requires both performance-based and patient-report assessments: a longitudinal analysis of outcomes. J Arthroplast. 2011;26(5):728–37.

Nha K-W, Shon O-J, Kong B-S, Shin Y-S. Gait comparison of unicompartmental knee arthroplasty and total knee arthroplasty during level walking. PLoS One. 2018;13(8):e0203310.

Parks NL, Whitney CE, Engh GA. Can we quantify functional improvement following total knee arthroplasty in the clinical setting? J Knee Surg. 2015;28(6):475–82.

Pfitzner T, Perka C, von Roth P. Unicompartmental vs. total knee arthroplasty for medial osteoarthritis. Zeitschrift fur Orthopadie und Unfallchirurgie. 2017;155(5):527–33.

Powell AJ, Crua E, Chong BC, et al. A randomized prospective study comparing mobile-bearing against fixed-bearing PFC Sigma cruciate-retaining total knee arthroplasties with ten-year minimum follow-up. Bone Joint J. 2018;100-b(10):1336–44.

Pozzi F, White DK, Snyder-Mackler L, Zeni JA. Restoring physical function after knee replacement: a cross sectional comparison of progressive strengthening vs standard physical therapy. Physiother Theory Pract. 2020;36(1):122–33.
Pritchett JW. Patients prefer a bicruciate-retaining or the medial pivot total knee prosthesis. J Arthroplast. 2011;26(2):224–8.
Roos EM, Roos HP, Lohmander LS, Ekdahl C, Beynnon BD. Knee Injury and Osteoarthritis Outcome Score (KOOS)–development of a self-administered outcome measure. J Orthop Sports Phys Ther. 1998;28(2):88–96.
Samy DA, Wolfstadt JI, Vaidee I, Backstein DJ. A retrospective comparison of a medial pivot and posterior-stabilized total knee arthroplasty with respect to patient-reported and radiographic outcomes. J Arthroplast. 2018;33(5):1379–83.
Scuderi GR, Bourne RB, Noble PC, Benjamin JB, Lonner JH, Scott WN. The new knee society knee scoring system. Clin Orthop Relat Res. 2012;470(1):3–19.
Scuderi GR, Sikorskii A, Bourne RB, Lonner JH, Benjamin JB, Noble PC. The knee society short form reduces respondent burden in the assessment of patient-reported outcomes. Clin Orthop Relat Res. 2016;474(1):134–42.
Serna-Berna R, Lizaur-Utrilla A, Vizcaya-Moreno MF, Miralles Muñoz FA, Gonzalez-Navarro B, Lopez-Prats FA. Cruciate-retaining vs posterior-stabilized primary total arthroplasty. Clinical outcome comparison with a minimum follow-up of 10 years. J Arthroplast. 2018;33(8):2491–5.
Shakespeare D, Ledger M, Kinzel V. Flexion after total knee replacement. A comparison between the Medial Pivot knee and a posterior stabilised implant. Knee. 2006;13(5):371–3.
Siljander MP, McQuivey KS, Fahs AM, Galasso LA, Serdahely KJ, Karadsheh MS. Current trends in patient-reported outcome measures in total joint arthroplasty: a study of 4 major orthopaedic journals. J Arthroplast. 2018;33(11):3416–21.
Singleton N, Nicholas B, Gormack N, Stokes A. Differences in outcome after cruciate retaining and posterior stabilized total knee arthroplasty. J Orthop Surg (Hong Kong). 2019;27(2):2309499019848154.
Skoffer B, Dalgas U, Mechlenburg I, Soballe K, Maribo T. Functional performance is associated with both knee extensor and flexor muscle strength in patients scheduled for total knee arthroplasty: a cross-sectional study. J Rehabil Med. 2015;47(5):454–9.
Spekenbrink-Spooren A, Van Steenbergen LN, Denissen GAW, Swierstra BA, Poolman RW, Nelissen RGHH. Higher mid-term revision rates of posterior stabilized compared with cruciate retaining total knee arthroplasties: 133,841 cemented arthroplasties for osteoarthritis in the Netherlands in 2007-2016. Acta Orthop. 2018;89(6):640–5.
Stöggl T, Martiner A. Validation of Moticon's OpenGo sensor insoles during gait, jumps, balance and cross-country skiing specific imitation movements. J Sports Sci. 2017;35(2):196–206.
Van der List JP, Kleeblad LJ, Zuiderbaan HA, Pearle AD. Mid-term outcomes of metal-backed unicompartmental knee arthroplasty show superiority to all-polyethylene unicompartmental and total knee arthroplasty. HSS J. 2017;13(3):232–40.
Varadarajan KM, Harry RE, Johnson T, Li G. Can in vitro systems capture the characteristic differences between the flexion–extension kinematics of the healthy and TKA knee? Med Eng Phys. 2009;31(8):899–906.
Weiss JM, Noble PC, Conditt MA, et al. What functional activities are important to patients with knee replacements? Clin Orthop Relat Res. 2002;404:172–88.
White PB, Ranawat AS, Ranawat CS. Fixed bearings versus rotating platforms in total knee arthroplasty. J Knee Surg. 2015;28(5):358–62.
Willing R, Walker PS. Measuring the sensitivity of total knee replacement kinematics and laxity to soft tissue imbalances. J Biomech. 2018;77:62–8.
Yoshida Y, Mizner RL, Snyder-Mackler L. Association between long-term quadriceps weakness and early walking muscle co-contraction after total knee arthroplasty. Knee. 2013;20(6):426–31.
Young T, Dowsey MM, Pandy M, Choong PF. A systematic review of clinical functional outcomes after medial stabilized versus non-medial stabilized total knee joint replacement. Front Surg. 2018;5:25.

Discussion and Future Possibilities

15

How Has the Present Status Been Reached, and What Further Advances Can Be Made?

It is now more than 50 years since the first cemented cobalt-chrome on polyethylene total knees were invented. Some of the earliest designs functioned well and achieved a high level of survivorship. For the original Total Condylar knee, of 220 knees performed in the mid-1970s, only 14 revisions were required at an average of 11.4-year follow-up (Rodriguez et al. 2001). For the Townley knee, survivorship was 89% at 23 years with an average flexion of 117°, the main reason for failure being polyethylene wear (Pritchett 2015). For the AGC knee, there was 96% survivorship at 15 years in a large cohort of over 1500 knees (Atrey et al. 2014). Over 3000 early knee designs, including Total Condylar, Press-fit Condylar, Kinematic, Kinemax, and AMK, performed at the Wrightington Hospital in England, showed a survivorship of 89% at 10 years (Pradhan et al. 2006). For 99 cases of the Insall-Burstein knee, the survivorship was 92% at 10 years with an average flexion of 106° (Aglietti et al. 1999). From multiple registries, with many different designs over different time periods, pooled data showed that 82% of knees lasted for 25 years (Evans et al. 2019). Overall, this was a remarkable achievement after little more than 10 years of development.

By 1980, two particular design types, the posterior cruciate retaining (CR) and the posterior stabilized (PS), were widely used and were considered successful in terms of function and durability. Several companies manufactured their versions of the CR and PS. These two designs dominated the market, although other design types had not been abandoned. Designs which preserved both the ACL and PCL were being used. Unicompartmental knees maintained their place, mainly for medial osteoarthritis. The rotating platform mobile bearing knee had recently been introduced and had gained a following. Stabilized designs with intercondylar varus-valgus stability were used for severe instability or for revisions.

Since 1980, due to the continuous stream of research, clinical follow-up studies, advances in technology, surgical specialization, and education, the quality of the designs and techniques has steadily advanced. This has produced not only further improvements in functional results but more consistency with fewer outliers. Various problems and deficiencies have been identified and largely resolved. For

P. S. Walker, *The Artificial Knee*, https://doi.org/10.1007/978-3-030-38171-4_15

example, some of the early tibial components fractured due to stress concentrations or misalignment. Serious polyethylene wear was caused by excessive contact stresses, often in conjunction with uncontrolled sliding. In the longer term, wear was exacerbated by gradual oxidation of the polyethylene. Instability resulted from bearing surfaces which were inadequately constrained in combination with soft tissues which were too loose. Misalignments, most commonly excessive varus, led to elevated medial loading, causing bone collapse, component loosening, and polyethylene wear. Loosening at the cement-bone interface, one of the most common problems, was due to inadequate cementing technique, misalignment, or inadequate bone coverage. Patella pain and even dislocation were due to a shallow trochlea groove on the femoral component or erroneous rotational positioning of the femoral or tibial components. Inadequate range of flexion was caused by a femoral component which was incorrectly sized, by a tibial component with too much posterior constraint, or where the posterior tibial tilt angle was insufficient. "Clicking and clunking" noises occurred, especially on PS designs, due to cam-post engagements and to soft tissue entrapment in the intercondylar region, as well as by impacting of the metal on the plastic, although this problem has not been associated with diminished function. Most knee designs which were prone to such problems as the above were either removed from the market, modified, or replaced by newer designs, with the result that the problems have been reduced to a much lower level. For example, the NexGen CR and PS knees had a survivorship of 100% and 98% at 15-year follow-up (Sartawi et al. 2018). The Triathlon knee had 98% survivorship at 10 years (Scott et al. 2019).

The situation today (2020) is that most artificial knees are part of a system consisting of several different design types, often ranging from primaries to revisions. The American Joint Replacement Registry (AJRR), founded in 2010 and affiliated with the American Academy of Orthopaedic Surgeons (AAOS), is accumulating invaluable data on artificial knee usage in the USA. The data is based on about one third of the knees used today, and the proportion continues to grow as more institutions participate. Up to this time, the mean age of the patients is 66.8 years with a standard deviation of 9.6 years. This indicates that about 16% of patients are below 57 years old, a challenging group due to their higher activity and expectation levels. As expected, there are more female than male patients, at 59% and 41%. The distributions of design types for primary knee cases confirm the persistence of types invented in the 1970s: 50% are posterior stabilized (PS), and 40% are posterior cruciate retaining (CR). The remaining 10% is divided between rotating platforms (7%) and ultracongruent (3%). Unicompartmental knees are only at about 3% of total knees despite the more conservative procedure, quicker recovery, and better functional outcomes, although the durability has been less than that for total knees in some series (Pfitzner et al. 2017).

The commercial exhibits at the major orthopedic conferences, notably the American Academy of Orthopaedic Surgeons (AAOS), the European Federation of National Associations of Orthopaedics and Traumatology (EFORT), and major Asian meetings, show that a majority of the market is serviced by a few large companies. However there are still numerous smaller companies. Many of their designs

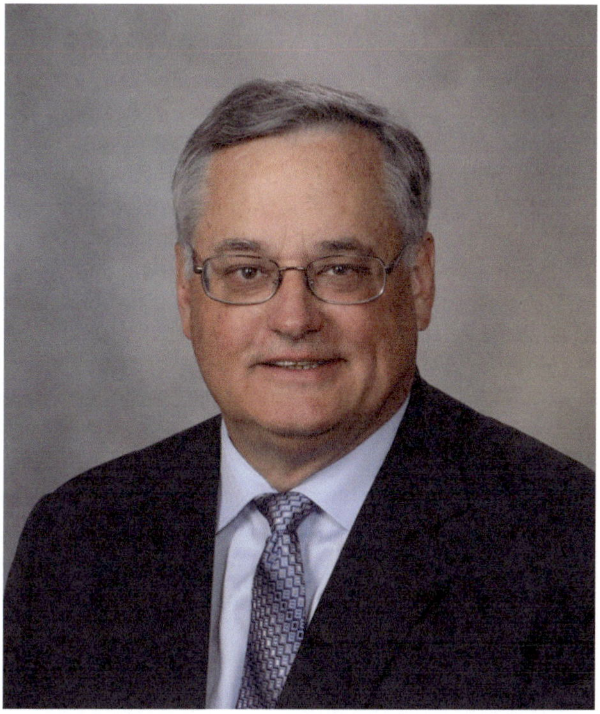

Fig. 15.1 David G. Lewallen MD from the Mayo Clinic, Rochester, MN, is the Medical Director of the American Joint Replacement Registry (AJRR). This organization collects performance data of artificial joints from numerous hospitals in the USA. The purpose is to improve the long-term outcomes and the quality of care. (Photo courtesy David Lewallen)

are standard CR or PS, where the designs are obtained from previous versions which have a successful clinical history. In some cases, minor improvements or advancements in instrumentation have been made. Other smaller companies offer specialized designs such as medial pivots, mobile bearings, and guided motion types, while one company specializes in custom-made knees.

Today's CR and PS designs, descendants of designs from the 1970s, do have certain differences. Some are close to being anatomic in their general shape, including the radii of the sagittal profiles of the femoral component and the peripheral shape of the tibial component. Other designs are more geometric, such as having a constant sagittal radius of the femoral bearing surfaces. Several systems offer a large number of sizes and shapes to closely match any particular knee, where gender and ethnic shape differences have been taken into account (Mahfouz et al. 2012). Some cam-post geometries engage in early flexion in an effort to maintain stability and provide a high flexion angle due to femoral rollback. Though many of these differences are important, there is a general similarity in the CR and PS designs produced by the different companies, such that there is a perception that the designs have become generic. Typically, clinical follow-up studies of a particular CR or PS design are often taken to represent the class as a whole. The justification is that for the most part, the results between different CR designs or PS designs have been similar, while even between CR and PS themselves, major differences have not been demonstrated. This is remarkable considering the fundamental differences in design and mechanics between a CR and a PS.

Obviously today's designs are not exactly the same models as in the 1970s, as there have been numerous modifications since then, but the basic design configurations are clearly recognizable. How has this situation been reached? After all, there are few products in today's world which have remained the same over such a long period of time. One only has to look at automobiles, bicycles, cameras, and cell phones to realize that. Part of the answer can be found in the way in which specific knee designs became widely used and maintained their standing.

It is instructive to identify the reasons for the success of certain designs in the initial time period from the late 1960s up to 1980:

- A prestigious institution. In such institutions, there was invariably a well-organized total knee service with a high volume of cases, a trainee and fellowship program for carrying out follow-up studies, research facilities, and affiliation with a university. There were resources available for new developments as well as ongoing evaluation. Even if the institution did not originate the design themselves, if their surgeons used a high volume of a particular design and reported on results at conferences, that represented strong support for the design. In this case, the support would be strengthened because of the objectivity and lack of any direct gain for that institution.
- A well-known and authoritative surgeon-designer. This was essential in presenting the design to surgeon groups at conferences and in producing publications. An enthusiastic and confident presentation manner was also a positive factor. It certainly helped that artificial knees were just beginning and were seen as an important new breakthrough in the treatment of osteoarthritis of the knee, as had already been demonstrated for the hip.
- Collaboration between surgeon and bioengineer. This combined both surgical and technical expertise, together with the characteristic thinking patterns of the different professions. Technical aspects of design and materials were unfamiliar to most surgeons, while experimental and analytical support would add to the credibility and understanding of the design. The manufacturers themselves, while having expertise in production and materials, were generally unfamiliar with testing methods and did not possess suitable equipment.
- A team of reputable surgeons. This signified a broad consensus of the positive design features of the particular design. In parallel there would be less likelihood of design flaws. Another advantage was a wider representation of the design at conferences.
- A well-established company. This was a major factor simply because of the manufacturing facilities and expertise and the sales exposure across the country. Also the company could more easily develop relations with prominent surgeons. Such relations were not subject to the regulatory restrictions as they are today.
- Strong company support for the design. This was a major factor, especially from a well-established company. If the design was promoted as the flagship knee of the company, it received high prominence on the company's exhibit at conferences, which elevated the confidence of potential surgeon users. David Fitzgerald,

President of Howmedica in the 1970s and 1980s, considered that this factor signified the company's confidence that the product would be a clinical and commercial success.

- A convincing design rationale. In the early days of artificial knee design, sound concepts backed up by logical thinking and experimental data, as well as ideas which related to anatomic mechanics, carried a great deal of weight. In this arena, technical experts such as materials scientists and biomechanical engineers played an important role. In contrast, a "new" or "different" idea without a great deal of background evidence might attract attention, but surgeons were reluctant to use on patients.
- A well-thought-out technique with accurate and easy-to-use instruments. While skilled surgeons were capable of inserting components requiring "hand-fitting," it was obvious that components with straight edges using instruments to guide the saw cuts would result in more consistent accuracy and a shorter operating time. Techniques that were targeted to correct alignment as well as to soft tissue balancing were favored.
- Few problems such as loosening or instability during early clinical application by the developers. It was in everybody's interests to use a design that would work well with few problems. There were many instances of designs being withdrawn due to short-term problems, unless a convincing change in design or technique had been introduced to solve the problem. But even this was not always easy due to lack of confidence in the design and the availability of more successful designs on the market.

With all of the above factors at play, it is understandable that there was a high turnover of designs and a large disparity in the sales between one design and another in the same company as well as between one company and another. In the early days, some companies would even produce a design for a particular surgeon mainly because they had a high volume of cases and the company wished to maintain good relations with that surgeon. However some of these designs were not well thought out and had to be withdrawn. Even the most popular designs were only made in two or three sizes for economic reasons and because the advantages of closely matching the anatomy were not appreciated. At conferences, there was intense rivalry between the proponents of different concepts, such as cruciate retaining versus cruciate sacrificing, high or low conformity between the bearing surfaces, the best fixation peg design for the tibial component, cement versus porous coated fixation, and whether or not the patella should be replaced.

During the 1970s the designs gradually improved, more sizes were made, and different design concepts were put together in "systems." The idea of a design team came into play as a result, combining the expertise of several surgeons and designers with different areas of specialization. Knee systems typically consisted of designs from unicompartmental to revision hinges, presented as being progressive depending on the severity of the arthritis, especially the level of deformity and instability. Because of the large investment required to produce a system, the number of separate design types tended to remain static.

In general, the clinical results improved, and there were no major differences apparent in the performance between design types, although each type did have its own nuances. By and large, there were two main "camps," one for posterior cruciate retention and one for posterior cruciate substitution with smaller support groups for bi-cruciate retention, mobile bearing, and unicompartmental. In a similar way, there were supporters of different surgical techniques, the main two approaches being gap balancing where preference was given to equality of soft tissue tensions, and measured resection where placement of components based on anatomic landmarks was the main goal followed by soft tissue adjustments.

By 1980, the CR and PS had become well established. The CR represented surgeons who preferred an anatomic approach, with the posterior cruciate seen as an important stabilizer which would provide femoral rollback and produce a higher range of flexion, and freedom of motion between the bearing surfaces to account for a range of activities and differences between patients. The PS represented surgeons who preferred a more mechanistic approach, where the surgical technique was easier and more reproducible, where stability was taken care of by the bearing surfaces themselves, and where the cam-post would produce the rollback to increase flexion. In parallel a great deal of attention had been given to tibial fixation, wear of the polyethylene, stability, soft tissue balancing, and alignment, essentially refining the designs and techniques.

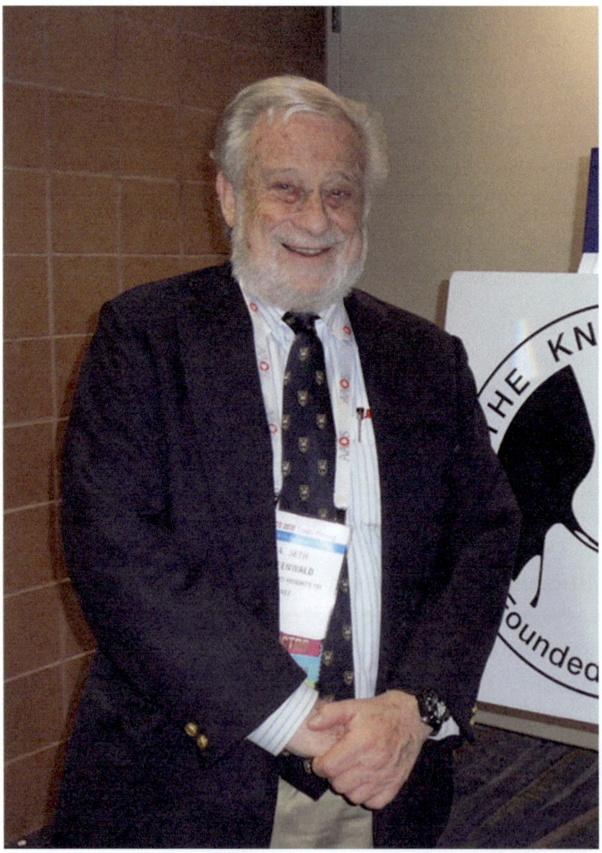

Fig. 15.2 Seth Greenwald Ph.D. founded Current Concepts in Joint Replacement (CCJR) in 1983, with the goal of providing continuing education for reconstructive joint surgeons, taught by the experts in the field. Over 36 years, CCJR has been a leading educator to tens of thousands of surgeons from the USA and around the world. Seth also founded a laboratory at Cleveland, OH, dedicated to the development of ASTM standard tests for evaluating contemporary artificial knees. (Photo taken at Specialty Day, AAOS, 2018) (© Peter S Walker)

By now, an additional criterion for the success of a new knee design had become apparent:

- The design team. This expanded beyond a surgeon working with an engineer, or a small group of surgeons. Now, the emphasis was on a larger group of experts, from a number of institutions and countries. Many surgeons had gained considerable experience and were well known, while the same applied to biomechanical engineers and materials scientists. The team would consist of such members. The company would hold regular design meetings, where the team would be divided into groups to deal with each type of design, and testing requirements would be assigned to laboratories in the company or at universities. Some companies had set up surgical skills facilities where instruments could be developed and knee designs tested on specimens.

Barriers and Possibilities for Alternate Designs and Techniques

The pervasiveness of the posterior cruciate retaining (CR) design and the posterior stabilized (PS) design with cruciate resection continued through the 1980s and 1990s. During that time, there were steady improvements in the designs and techniques but not in terms of changing the designs in any major way or introducing other design types. Comprehensive knee systems from the larger companies dominated the market, which included revision components, in some cases using porous materials as space fillers. The systems often included rotating platform versions of both CR and PS designs because of the expectation that the wear would be reduced and the function improved. While rotating platforms did gain some popularity, by no means did it approach the volume of the standard fixed bearing CR and PS designs. The main reasons for this were that the rotating platform versions were more expensive and there was no clear indication from follow-ups and experiments that function was improved or that wear was reduced. However function started to gain more attention as a priority because 10-year follow-up studies were available on some designs, showing failure rates of only a few percent. Durability had therefore become a prerequisite in any design, which it was thought could be attained by not deviating too far from the previous successful design types. In reality, it was probably the quality of the polyethylene and the improved cementing techniques that led to the durability, as much as the designs themselves.

In the late 1990s, the ultracongruent design concept was introduced by Aaron Hofmann and Roy Bloebaum from Salt Lake City (see Chap. 10 entitled "Posterior Stabilized"). This design, with its "deep-dish" tibial surface, not requiring cruciate preservation, was a direct challenge to the PS knee with its cam-post. The ultracongruent gained some support but still did not alter the predominance of the standard PS. It was generally considered to be too constrained with a higher risk of tibial loosening and with a likely reduction in flexion range due to the height of the plastic posteriorly and the lack of a mechanism for femoral "rollback" in flexion.

Nevertheless it did maintain a following and was increasingly regarded as a viable design concept. The concept was embodied first in the Natural knee.

In the late 1990s, another new artificial knee design type, the medial pivot, was introduced by Mike Freeman and Mike Tuke in the UK and by David Blaha in the USA (see Chap. 11 entitled "Guided Motion Knees"). In this design, rather than both the lateral and medial sides having the same amount of laxity, the medial side was a ball-in-socket eliminating the anterior-posterior laxity altogether, while the lateral side allowed almost unrestricted anterior-posterior laxity. There was biomechanical support for the concept in that it reproduced to a large extent the mechanics of the normal knee as demonstrated by MRI studies on specimens and on the living knee. At the same time, those studies did not show an absolutely fixed medial pivot, but some deviation of the contact point on the medial side due to the deformability of the medial meniscus and the lack of complete femoral-tibial conformity. In contrast, the medial pivot knee had a fully constrained ball-in-socket medially. Nevertheless the resemblance to anatomic mechanics was an attractive feature, together with the anterior-posterior stability it provided. Because of this, the medial pivot was a viable option to the standard CR and PS designs. There were several reasons why the knee did not achieve widespread adoption. In surgery, there was some difficulty with soft tissue balancing, especially when the posterior cruciate ligament was retained. The company which manufactured the design in the USA was relatively small, without a prior background in artificial knees. But the major factor was that the existing designs had a great deal of inertia, consisting of impressive medium-term results from prominent institutions and individual surgeons. As a result there was limited market penetration of the medial pivot, and this has persisted up to this time.

Another factor which acted as a deterrent to the introduction of new design types was the procedure specified by the Food and Drug Administration (FDA) to introduce a new design to the market. Since 1976, a new device could be introduced to the market if it could be shown to be substantially equivalent to a previously marketed device. The FDA's definition was: "A 510(k) requires demonstration of substantial equivalence to another legally U.S. marketed device. Substantial equivalence means that the new device is at least as safe and effective as the predicate." (This regulation has recently been changed to a device which was introduced in the past 10 years.) This regulation made it relatively easy to introduce a new PS or CR knee, even though mechanical testing was still necessary. If the new device was not substantially equivalent to a prior device, this meant complying with a complex pre-market approval (PMA) process which included limited clinical trials, which was expensive and which could take around 3 years or more to implement. This requirement undoubtedly limited the introduction of more innovative designs of artificial knees. However a well-established company with a successful total knee system already could decide to invest in a new design if it was considered to have a strong market potential. The rotating platform design was an example of this, and indeed the 7–9% of the US market, higher in certain other countries, is a sizeable market share which justified the process.

Another factor which inhibited the emergence of a design other than the CR and PS was the high development cost. It was necessary to have multiple sizes, right and left, and many tibial thicknesses. Revision components also had to be provided, which were expensive to produce and yet with a much smaller demand than the primary knee. Hence if a company was designing and introducing a new system, the designs that took precedence were the CR and PS. Nevertheless, the company and the design group would often have the intention of including a "high-performance" knee in the system, but this would be put "on the back burner" due to the sheer volume of work, time, and expense in dealing with the standard designs. In some cases, the new standard designs were but modifications of the previous system, but with enhancements based on the accumulated clinical experience and recent research. A major advantage was that the new system could build on the long and successful clinical record of the previous system. It would then be an easy transition for a surgeon to move to the new system. To maintain continuity, there could be similar bearing surfaces between the new and previous designs, to the point where there could be intermixing. On the other hand, a totally new design concept would be unfamiliar, and many surgeons would be reluctant to use it immediately. This would make the introduction slow, without any guarantee of it reaching economic levels.

Also linked to the high cost of developing a new design was the need for "legacy," being able to show that the design had a successful history in patients. This would require a number of studies from different institutions, of a sizeable number of patients, for a sufficient length of time. This led to the preference for improving an existing design, rather than developing a new design which was substantially different. There can be a fine line between an improvement and something novel.

Despite the above obstacles to the introduction of a new design or technique, if the advantages were sufficiently convincing, there is the likelihood of gradual acceptance even if the process might be slow. There are several designs already available which are potential candidates. Unicompartmental knees have been available almost for as long as total knees, but some convincing reason would have to emerge for an increase in usage to occur. The indications may have reached their limit, although there is one study which suggested that 21% of arthritic knees which were treated with a total knee could have been treated with a uni (Arno et al. 2011). Robotic surgery for unis, with intraoperative planning to assure ideal placement and soft tissue balancing, may increase usage to some extent. The impressive long-term results of the Oxford group with their mobile bearing uni design have demonstrated viability, but the results were achieved with an expert group, specializing in unis. Few centers or individuals have so far taken that route. Using bi-unicompartmental knees, in some cases with a separate patella flange, has the attraction of accurately reproducing the original bearing surfaces (Romagnoli et al. 2015), but again there are limited indications and the procedure is surgically challenging. A robotic technique could make the surgery easier.

The ACL + PCL type, sometimes called bi-cruciate retaining (BCR), has been available since the early 1970s with the Townley and later the Cloutier. However a ccurate component positioning is required so that all four ligaments function optimally, requiring an anatomic design in sufficient sizes. Preserving the anterior

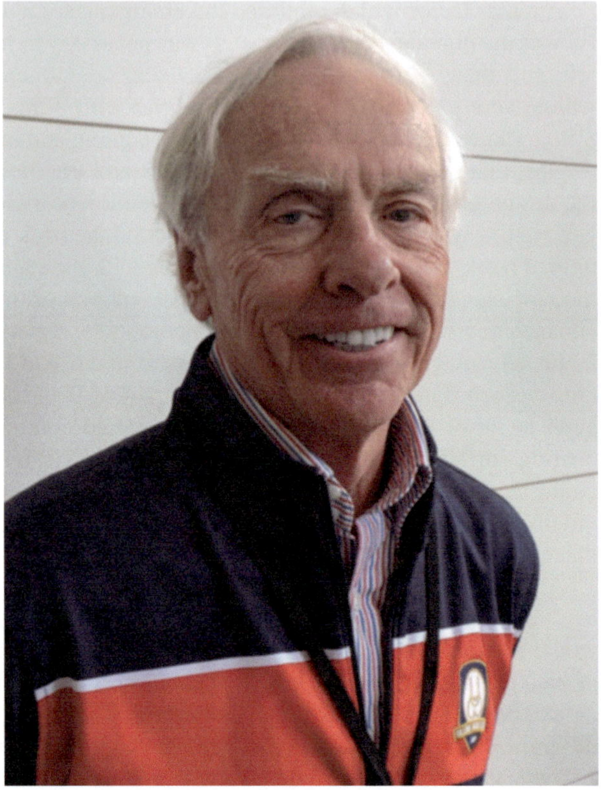

Fig. 15.3 W Norman Scott MD was a Fellow of John Insall in the early 1970s and contributed to early knee designs as well as editing several editions of John Insall's book *Surgery of the Knee*. Norman Scott was a founding member of the International Congress for Joint Reconstruction (ICJR) with worldwide instructional courses organized by local experts. Norman focuses on resident and fellow training, not only through ICJR but by his organization of the Insall Traveling Fellowship and the Insall Scott Kelly Fellowship. He is currently a Professor at NYU Langone Orthopedic Hospital. (Photo taken at the Knee Society Annual meeting 2019) (© Peter S Walker)

cruciate without problems has not been easy. Although there is evidence that excellent results can be achieved, this has not been a consistent finding.

Rotating platform designs may have reached a stable level now that wear is no longer regarded a major problem in CR and PS designs, but the freedom of rotational position and better patella tracking are still regarded as advantages. It is possible that the early Eftekhar and UCI tibial designs with their rotatable tibial tracks would function the same as a rotating platform, but with a lower cost of manufacture.

Medial pivot designs still have potential based on positive results from many users, but the smaller companies that produce these at present have much less marketing force compared with the major established companies. Ultracongruent designs are an attractive concept due to their mechanical simplicity and inherent stability. Furthermore, the tibial inserts can conveniently fit into existing knee systems using the same tibial tray as a CR or PS. One company has produced a hybrid design where a tibial insert has a more congruent medial side and a less congruent lateral side, equivalent to a "loose medial pivot." This may gain some traction because of the convenience of being able to use it in an existing well-established system.

There is a high potential for Guided Motion knees, where the goal is to restore the anatomic characteristics of the normal knee joint, both in the geometry and in the kinematics. This can be called a biomimetic approach. The guided motion knee can achieve this due to the interaction of the femoral-tibial bearing surfaces without requiring the cruciate ligaments. The collaterals are still required to ensure varus-valgus stability. The guided motion knee can provide the stability normally provided by the cruciates, but with the same laxity as in the normal knee. While there is only a small degree of laxity medially, on the lateral side, there is high laxity but with a mechanism for inducing lateral roll forwards in extension and rollback in flexion. Other advantages of a guided motion knee as described above are normality of the "flow" of soft tissues around the anatomically shaped boundaries and the anatomical "feel" to the kinematics.

This brings up the approach of custom implants, which does have a strong rationale. One question is the extent of customization which is needed. Is it sufficient to match the patient's main bone dimensions only, or do the components need to be anatomically shaped also? Should the inherent stability of the bearing surfaces match the ideal for that patient, and how is that to be measured? Wide adoption of custom knees over time will likely depend upon showing improved functional results of some type.

In the area of technique, standard mechanical instruments provide satisfactory results and are generally reliable and easy to use, but there is still room for improvement. They could be made much simpler and less expensive to make. The intramedullary rod system for defining the frontal plane angle could be made more accurate for all canal diameters. Centering the tibial cutting guide on the ankle could be made more accurate. The use of smart tools is a low cost and convenient way of improving performance of mechanical instruments.

Computer-assisted soft tissue balancing devices address a need in achieving the goals of medial-lateral tightness in extension and flexion and have by no means reached their full potential. It has been emphasized from the early days of knee replacement that "it is a soft tissue operation" which means that no matter how the components are positioned on the bones, unless the soft tissue tensions around the knee are uniform during the full flexion range, the knee will not function optimally. Inadequate soft tissue balancing can result in pain, tightness, a low flexion range, and instability. Assessment of soft tissue tensions by the "feel" of the surgeon, no matter how experienced the surgeon, has been shown to be inaccurate. Use of an instrumented device shows that even small gap differences between the medial and lateral sides result in sizeable differences in soft tissue tensions. This points to the need for a quantitative means of assessment, which is likely to be more and more recognized over time.

Computer-assisted navigation has been available for about 10 years and seems to have reached a limit, unless it can be modified to make it easier and quicker to use. However, experienced advocates of the system are likely to continue to use navigation as an accurate way of carrying out the surgery. There is currently a movement towards robotics because of its many capabilities. For example, in New York State, in 2008, only 4.3% of artificial knee surgeries used navigation or robotics, which increased to 11.6% by 2015 (Boylan et al. 2018). Most of the use was in high-volume hospitals, because most "early adopters" of new technology work there. Robotic systems can offer surgical planning before or at the time of surgery, analysis of the effect of varying bone cut levels and angles, soft tissue balancing assessment, and validation of the surgical plan. It is not easy to predict the growth and level of acceptance of robotic knee surgery because of the interplay between the advantages and disadvantages. Other computer-assisted technologies such as virtual reality await evaluation.

There are many factors involved with the successful introduction of a new artificial knee design or surgical technique, but certain criteria must be met. Anything new has to compete with whatever is already available and therefore has to offer demonstrable advantages. These advantages can apply to the patient (the most important criterion), the surgeon, the hospital, and the health-care system as a whole. Combining these, it is suggested that a new or improved artificial knee design or technique needs to offer one or more of the following, if it is to be successful:

- Improved durability
- Improved functional performance
- Quicker recovery time
- Increased flexion angle
- Reduced time, complexity, and cost of surgical procedure
- Research and educational support

Improved Durability

The survivorship of today's designs is likely to be in the mid-90 percentile at 20 years, based on follow-up studies and joint registries. The first step in determining which factors will reduce failure is to examine the main causes. A recent paper from the Hospital for Special Surgery (Pitta et al. 2018) reported that the main causes of revision from 18,000 artificial knees performed between 2007 and 2012 were; in order of percentage; infection, instability, loosening, and stiffness. Revisions for other reasons were at a much lower level. Infection is being addressed by a universal decolonization protocol, control of operating room traffic, air disinfection, air recirculation, lavages, and antibacterial coatings on the implants. In terms of the other factors, the authors pointed out that: "The reasons for failure for primary TKA have evolved as implant designs, materials, and surgical techniques have improved... New forms of polyethylene... have improved the material's wear behavior and thus decreased the rate of polyethylene-related failures." In particular, the reduction in wear rates of newer polyethylenes reduced the outright failures due to wear-through as well as component loosening caused by polyethylene debris. Those findings were in general agreement with other studies.

It is notable that the polyethylene improvements were widely accepted in a matter of a few years, rather than waiting for evaluations after many years of follow-up. The initial demonstration of reduced wear was based on testing on simple reciprocating test machines, while specific knee designs were tested on knee simulating machines, taking only a few months for 5 or 10 million cycles of testing. In reality the wear test protocols do not fully simulate the variable activities typical of patients, but since the tests compared the new material versus the previously used material, that provided a high level of credibility. The main material improvement was polyethylene with increased cross-linking, with processing methods to maintain the mechanical properties. Later, the addition of vitamin E was shown to maintain a low wear rate and, in addition, to reduce oxidation over time and therefore not be subject to increased wear in the long term. While the results of such testing have been considered sufficient to justify clinical application, in vivo wear has been monitored at progressive time intervals by retrieval studies (Rowell et al. 2015). Gradually, the evidence is building to confirm the efficacy of these materials. An alternative way to reduce polyethylene wear is by using oxidized zirconium-coated femoral components, which showed reduced wear in knee simulator tests. In retrieval studies, there was less damage on both the femoral and tibial components, validating the concept, at least in the time frame of the study (Heyse et al. 2011). Another example of reducing wear was a tri-condylar design where the femoral component and the tibial baseplate were made from alumina ceramic, with a compression-molded polyethylene bearing, showing that ceramic was a promising alternate material for the femoral component (Nakamura et al. 2017).

Tibial component loosening is now relatively infrequent with presently used tibial components and techniques. However in order to sustain this, new fixation post designs must follow known principles for success; otherwise early failure can occur as has been found in recent years. Minimizing long-term bone loss due to stress shielding can be avoided by avoiding excessive stiffness of the tibial baseplate (Srinivasan et al. 2017). Adequate bonding or mechanical keying of pegs and fins to the cement mantle can prevent interface motion and premature failure. There are many cases where radiolucent lines develop over time, and while most do not develop sufficient symptoms to require revision, some go on to failure. At the same time, many of these cases may experience some pain on activity and limitation of function. These problems can be addressed by meticulous cement technique at surgery, where cancellous bone is exposed, fluid material is cleaned from the surface, and sufficient pressurization is applied to obtain cement penetration to a depth of 2–3 mm across the entire interface, including the peripheries.

Uncemented fixation can potentially reduce long-term loosening should cemented fixation be shown to be at risk in active patients. Assuring initial rigidity of fixation is essential for the bone ingrowth to occur. Newer porous materials, including those fabricated using 3D printing technologies, may further enhance ingrowth capabilities. Some long-term loosening failures are due to misalignment, most commonly where the knee has been in too much varus or where the joint line has deviated too far from the horizontal. The misalignment has caused progressive collapse of the bone with further misalignment and fixation failure. Such outliers of

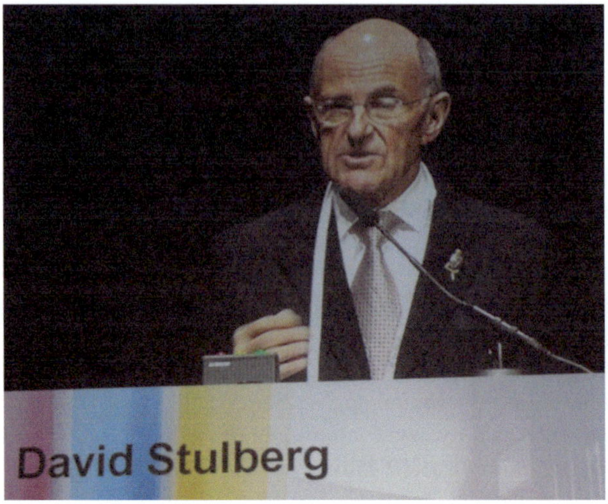

Fig. 15.4 David Stulberg MD from Northwestern University, Chicago, has been a strong proponent of the potential value of technology in arthroplasty from the 1990s when custom implants were prominent, to today's expansion of computer-assisted surgery. For many years David Stulberg has been the Secretary General of the International Society for Technology in Arthroplasty (ISTA) which has organized conferences around the world and is the largest society focusing on the technology area. (Photo taken at an ISTA meeting) (© Peter S Walker)

alignment could be reduced in number by improved surgical planning procedures and by improved surgical techniques including computer-assisted surgery.

Instability can be due to the use of a relatively unconstrained knee in combination with inadequate soft tissue balancing (Wilson et al. 2017). Meticulous surgery, using computer-assisted methods for bone cutting and balancing, can reduce the instability. However, especially when mechanical instrumentation is used, artificial knees which have built-in constraint, such as PS or guided motion types, will provide stability more consistently. At the same time, accurate soft tissue balancing is still needed for varus-valgus stability. Stiffness, the opposite of instability, can again be due to inadequate balancing or to incorrect placement of the components. In addition, there are indications that biological factors play a role.

In summary, durability can potentially be improved by the use of low wear polyethylenes, by tibial component designs which do not cause excessive stress protection of the underlying trabecular bone, by selection of implants with adequate femoral-tibial stability, by a systematic technique when cement is used, by uncemented designs with rigid initial fixation, by accurate balancing techniques at surgery, and by instrumentation which routinely provides accurate alignments.

Even then, it is hard to imagine more than a small gain in survivorship percentages, due to unpredictable and outlier situations. Much of the potential gain in durability may already be embodied in today's designs and techniques. A further point is that there is now more evidence of risk factors for implant failure (Bosco et al. 2018) such as weak bone, smoking, overweight, and impact sports, allowing behavior modification or pre-habilitation to be implemented prior to surgery and hence reducing failures, especially those which might have occurred in the short term.

Improved Functional Performance

In the previous chapter (Chap. 14 entitled "Comparisons and Evaluations"), methods for measuring function were discussed. At this time, PROMs are regarded as the gold standard and are included in most joint registries. For a more objective evaluation, biomechanical measures can be used. Thirdly, the function can be modeled objectively as a property of the artificial knee in isolation or in combination with the knee into which it is implanted. Many studies have shown that the factor which has the greatest influence on the functional outcome is the overall physical condition of the patient, in particular the muscular status of the lower extremities. For example, in a study of 200 patients, half subjected to standard of care therapy and half to progressive quadriceps-strengthening interventions, it was found that the latter showed "enhanced clinical improvement in short and long-term, approaching the functional level of healthy older adults. Conventional rehab did not yield similar outcomes" (Petterson et al. 2009). In a later review of this type of therapy, it was concluded: "Progressive exercise is critical to recovery after TKA. There is a large decrease in quadriceps strength immediately after TKA, which is attributed to activation deficits and atrophy. This loss of strength is related to functional impairments and biomechanical asymmetries. Progressive exercise protocols and early application of neuromuscular electrical stimulation (NMES) should be used to attenuate early quadriceps weakness and the associated impairments" (Pozzi et al. 2013). The evaluation methods in the above studies, as well as PROMs, were the TUG test, stair-climbing test, 6-minute walk test, and sit-to-stand balance test. Despite the improved function that has been achieved with such high-intensity rehabilitation methods, implementation involves increased physiotherapy resources, increased cost, and compliance from the patient. The latter is impacted by the extra time commitment as well as the discomfort of the therapy. Some of these disadvantages can be overcome by the use of wearable activity monitors together with mobile applications (Chughtai et al. 2019). Such systems provide more motivation to the patient, while monitoring the data to the physician can alert to any deficiencies. In the system reported by Chughtai et al., KSS pain and function scores and WOMAC scores improved substantially more than for conventional therapy.

An important question is to what extent the function can be improved by the design of the artificial knee. In the previous chapter, several studies were cited showing that there were no significant differences in PROMs, but yet there were differences in biomechanical parameters. Designs which more closely simulated normal anatomy, or which avoided excess anterior-posterior sliding, showed superior performance. To achieve a high level of function, Romagnoli et al. (2015) have advocated the use of modular components including unicompartmental and patella resurfacing. They point out that an accurate fit can be more readily achieved with small components, compared with using conventional artificial knees: "…the versatility of these implants is such that they can be adapted to almost all knees, allowing the creation of custom-made prostheses that preserve, as much as possible, the intact parts of the native knee… including the cruciate ligaments…" They propose using modular components for broader indications than medial osteoarthritis. Curved runners for the femoral condyles can be fitted so that the original surface shapes of the femoral condyles are closely reproduced, given appropriate instrumentation and cutting tools. Special attention is needed to ensure reliable fixation of the tibial components, but this is within the scope of today's technologies. Despite the resistance to expanding the use of even unicompartmental knees, the use of small modular components should be considered further given the likely benefits to function.

For artificial knees covering all of the bearing surfaces, custom knees designed to match the bony geometry of the individual knee offer the possibility of improved function due to maintaining the anatomic soft tissue envelope and muscle lever arms. A convincing case has been made based on a dimensional analysis of 24,000 CT scans which showed that even for the multi-sized systems available today, around 25% of cases would have errors of fit of the femoral component more than 3 mm (Meier et al. 2019). However, the custom knee design itself needs to be of a type that would optimize function, but there have been some positive results from recent studies.

Are there types of artificial knee designs available which will provide superior function to the CR and PS? The alternate designs readily available today are mobile bearing versions of the CR and PS, ACL + PCL preserving knees, ultra-congruent knees, and medial pivot knees. So far ACL + PCL knees have not fulfilled their promise according to a recent review paper (Barrett et al. 2017). While acknowledging patient preference determined in the studies by James Pritchett, this advantage has been offset by the surgical difficulties and other complications. Medial pivot knees, also preferred by patients in the Pritchett studies, have shown improved functional scores attributed to the AP stability. Ultracongruent knees, including a medially congruent version, have shown at least equal functional results compared with CR and PS, without loss of range of flexion. It has also been shown in laboratory studies that a type of guided motion knee can provide an even closer representation of anatomic laxity and stability, implying that the functional performance should be further enhanced. Guided motion knees are at the opposite extreme to the modular components in that the ideal blend of laxity and stability is provided by mechanical interactions in the artificial knee. An advantage of this mechanistic approach is that it requires less accuracy of surgery and the artificial knee is therefore a more robust design. On the other hand, there could be an issue with joint proprioception, although after reviewing the literature, Takasaki et al. (2019) concluded that: "More high-quality studies are required to achieve a comprehensive understanding of the effect of Proprioceptive Neuromuscular Facilitation on the Joint Position Sense" while Wautier and Thienpont (2017) found that proprioceptive testing with different types of total knees was inconclusive. Implementation of both approaches, small modular components and a guided motion knee, would require investment from companies and objective monitoring of the functional results using both PROMs and biomechanical methods.

Quicker Recovery Time

In the early days of knee replacement, continuous passive motion (CPM) was seen as a potential method of restoring the motion of the knee and assisting with the healing of surrounding soft tissues at their optimal physiological lengths (Salter et al. 1980). Originally intended for healing cartilage defects, CPM was soon applied to other applications including total knees. The patient's leg was fitted in a fixture which slowly flexed and extended the joint over a time period, repeated several times each day. It seemed a logical way to speed up recovery, reduce pain and discomfort, and achieve a higher flexion angle. Initial results showed less thrombophlebitis and more rapid attainment of flexion after surgery, but with the ultimate flexion angle being unchanged from conventional methods (Vince et al. 1987). After many years of trials, a review of 24 articles comprising 1445 cases concluded: "CPM does not have clinically important effects on active knee flexion ROM, pain, function or quality of life to justify its routine use" (Harvey et al. 2014).

Addressing the earlier time period after surgery, a major advance in the control of pain and swelling was introduced for application to both artificial hips and knees (Parvataneni et al. 2007). The idea behind the treatment was that local periarticular

SESSION TOPICS IN THE 36TH ANNUAL CCJR. WINTER 2019.
(IN PARTNERSHIP WITH THE HIP AND KNEE SOCIETIES)
Ethics, Economics & OR Efficiency
Why Knees Fail: Recognizing Causality Leads to Avoidance
The PCL in Contemporary TKA
Examining Knee Arthroplasty Technologies
The Medial Uni-Compartment Alternative: Fixed or Mobile
Mechanical Alignment Optimizes Patient Outcome
The Cemented All Poly Tibia: Regardless of Age & BMI
The Medial Stabilized Knee: The Emerging Choice for TKA
Periprosthetic Joint Infection
Big Data: The Where, the What & the How
The Unstable Knee: Manifestations, Reasons & Corrective Actions
Smart Trials: Taking Soft Tissue Balancing from an Art to a Science
Maximizing Cement Interdigitation During TKA
Patient Dissatisfaction Following TKA

INTERNATIONAL SOCIETY FOR TECHNOLOGY
IN ARTHROPLASTY - ANNUAL MEETING 2019
Innovations in TKA Kinematics
TKA Limb Alignment
Modeling and Preoperative Planning
Novel Technology for Treating Infections
TKA Wear and Retrievals
TKA Robotics & Navigation Outcomes
Ensuring Fixation of Arthroplasty Implants
Clinical Pathways to Enhance Patient Outcomes
Biomechanics and Preclinical Testing
TKA Tissue Balancing Techniques
Rapid Recovery and Pain Management
Role of Implant Design on TKA Biomechanics
Computational Models for Innovations in Arthroplasty
Design & Evaluation of 3D Printed Devices

Fig. 15.5 Typical program topics of a CCJR meeting organized by Seth Greenwald. The program focuses on practical issues relevant to orthopedic surgeons specializing in artificial joints. This is contrasted with a recent program of ISTA, where many of the topics relate to new developments which are currently in the early stages of clinical evaluation; the attendance at the ISTA meeting is typically divided between surgeons, researchers, and company staff

injections at various sites in and around the knee at the time of surgery would be effective as a substitute for the then current perioperative pain control modalities. "Analgesics and anti-inflammatories acting via different pathways is emphasized for a multi-modal approach." This new method was shown to have advantages including lower pain scores from the first day onwards, quicker to straight leg raise, going home earlier, and reduction of side effects. Adjunct measures are multimodal pain management including regional blocks, periarticular injections, and opioid-sparing medication protocols.

Also related to the postoperative period are programs such as the Perioperative Orthopaedic Surgical Home (POSH) initiative. In a retrospective study of over 4000 total joint patients, patients who were assessed for modifiable risk factors and then were treated accordingly were compared with patients who were not examined. There was a significantly lower number of readmissions in the assessed group (Kim et al. 2019).

In a review paper, Rutherford et al. (2017) discussed the multiple factors which could improve the rehabilitation process. The first step was patient optimization: "Recognising which patients are at risk for adverse outcomes after total knee is the first step in preventing them." This was accompanied by behavior modification and support. Preoperative education was useful in preparing patients for the entire process and what was expected of them. Intraoperative measures were important with incisions which preserved quadriceps function being important. Rehabilitation was recognized as being important, but "There is no consensus regarding the appropriate frequency, duration or intensity of physical therapy protocols after TKA." There is clearly a need for additional research on methods for muscle strengthening and coordination, which will overcome problems of patient compliance. Yet the prolonged time and discomfort of recovery period after an artificial knee remain as an area for potential improvement. The tennis player referred to at the beginning of this book, while able to walk after about 2 weeks and return to work shortly thereafter, found it was more than 6 months before he was able to return to active sports. In the early recovery period, he imagined 100 elastic bands around his knee giving the sensation of tightness. Even now, several years later, he feels that the shock absorbers are gone. A woman patient, whose functional requirements were less ambitious than those of the tennis player, was nonetheless surprised and disappointed at the level of discomfort after the procedure and the protracted recovery time. Even now at 2 years after surgery, the range of flexion is only 100°, and she feels that the knee is still not as good as her near-normal opposite side, especially in flexion range. This is a perceptive observation because restoration to an almost normal condition is not an unreasonable expectation. Retrospectively neither of these patients would have changed their decision to undergo artificial knee surgery due to their severe pain and disability. Their rehabilitation experiences were mirrored to a large extent by those of Kevin Bozic MD, recounted in the monthly *AAOS Now* newsletter (2019). The days after the procedure were "a lot more painful than I expected… I couldn't even travel in a car across town 2 weeks after surgery… I had pain past 6 weeks and wasn't fully recovered or functional by that time." In his case, there was a positive end result: "Less than a year after surgery, a hiking trip for 8–10 hours a day in rugged terrain."

Increased Flexion Angle

The normal knee achieves a high degree of flexion by the interaction of the bearing surfaces and the menisci (Pinskerova et al. 2009). Firstly, there is a small posterior displacement of the medial femoral condyle followed by lateral femoral displacement down the slope of the lateral tibial plateau, the lateral menisci being pushed posteriorly and downwards. Flexion from 120 to 160° was considered as a separate arc, which the authors considered would be difficult to reproduce with an artificial knee. The benefits of high flexion were clearly demonstrated in a study of more than 5000 cases (Ritter et al. 2008). Pain, walking ability, and stair climbing ability were enhanced for a flexion greater than 128° with a distinct falloff below 118°.

The design of the tibial insert is expected to affect the maximum flexion angle achieved. An insert with a high posterior lip could block the femur from flexing by impingement against the posterior cortex. However in a clinical trial with the same femoral component, using a high-lip ultracongruent insert, and a lower lip PS insert, gave the same mean flexion angle of 116° at follow-up (Laskin et al. 2000). It has been shown that artificial knee designs that allow for high flexion by modifications to the posterior bearing surfaces of the femoral condyles and tibial insert do not necessarily produce higher flexion. However if this type of implant is combined with quadriceps releases from the anterior femur when necessary, high flexion values can be achieved (Tarabichi et al. 2010). In a series of 218 NexGen LPS-Flex mobile bearing designs in 125 Asian and Middle East patients (most bilateral), 54 males and 71 females, average age 64 years, the initial average flexion angle was 125°; the range of flexion at 3–5 years follow-up was 140°. This does however need be seen in the context of gain in flexion from pre-op, 15°. However it is still higher than typical series of Western patients where the preoperative and postoperative values are close to equal.

A study using fluoroscopy showed there were multiple factors affecting range of flexion (Dennis et al. 2007): "over-stuffing of the patellofemoral joint during TKA may have adverse effects on postoperative knee flexion… a pattern of progressive posterior femoral translation with increasing knee flexion has been observed… in our analysis amounting to about 1.4° flexion for every millimeter posterior femoral translation." Posterior tibial slope produced a similar increase in flexion. It is evident that these different factors are either design related, technique related, or a combination. However there has not been a specific design change which has been able to reproducibly increase flexion by a substantial amount, say at least 10°. Nevertheless, high flexion remains an important goal for an artificial knee in that it makes many activities of daily living much easier to perform. Identifying the factors which affect the range of flexion and evaluating therapies which can increase flexion is a worthwhile area of continuing research.

Reduced Time, Complexity, and Cost of Surgical Procedure

Considering the importance of this area, there is relatively little literature. A positive start was made 25 years ago in a study which identified 42 steps which were carried out during a typical procedure, from positioning the patient to closing the wound (Dunbar and Gross 1995). Eight of the steps took significantly larger than the other steps, but there was considerable variation in the times and between surgeons. The need to repeat certain steps was an important factor. Robert Booth, from Jefferson Health in Philadelphia, combined all facets of the procedure into a systematic work flow (unpublished data). At the start of the day, the plan for each patient was discussed with the entire team. For the procedure itself, the assistants were thoroughly familiar with the instruments and the order of the steps, so that going from one step to the next was a seamless process. With this system the time per case was minimized and the quality optimized. It would be an advantage if such a system could be implemented in major centers, but the extensive range of procedures and the varying staff assignments are barriers. There is benefit in the organization of the instruments in the operating room (von Eiff et al. 2019). If the sizing of implants for each case can be determined, the instrument trays can be supplied with far fewer instruments, resulting in time savings in preparation, cleaning, and repackaging, as well as during the procedure itself. This was termed size-specific trays as opposed to standardized trays. The main conclusion was: "Performing 4 TKA's in sequence generates time saving of approximately 54 minutes which can be used for an additional procedure."

Can there be a reduction of time based on the type of artificial knee? Designs that do not require meticulous accuracy and balancing will keep the time at the lower end of the scale. Simpler instruments without unnecessary sub-components and adjustments will reduce time and improve ease of surgery. The use of uncemented components could reduce the time, provided the bone preparation time was the same as that for cemented components. The use of 3D printed instruments has been considered and is available in a limited way with some designs (Hooper et al. 2019). There are now polymeric materials available which are biocompatible and sufficiently strong and wear resistant to be used as cutting guides. The ideal is to develop a set of single-use 3D printed instruments which could be used for any design of artificial knee. The instruments would be provided in a pre-sterilized pack or even sterilized by autoclave. This is feasible for the primary bone cuts of the distal femur and proximal tibia, but is problematic for the femoral AP and chamfer cuts which are in multiple sizes and different between manufacturers. Furthermore the trial components need to be replicas of the actual final components. The concept would however be feasible for a particular design of artificial knee.

Can computer-assisted instrumentation reduce time, complexity, and cost? The challenge ahead was expressed succinctly in an article entitled "The impact of smart tools on total knee arthroplasty" (Scuderi 2007): "…there has been an exponential rise in the number of TKA's performed annually. The resulting demand… will necessitate improving technology so that it can be used to treat more patients while

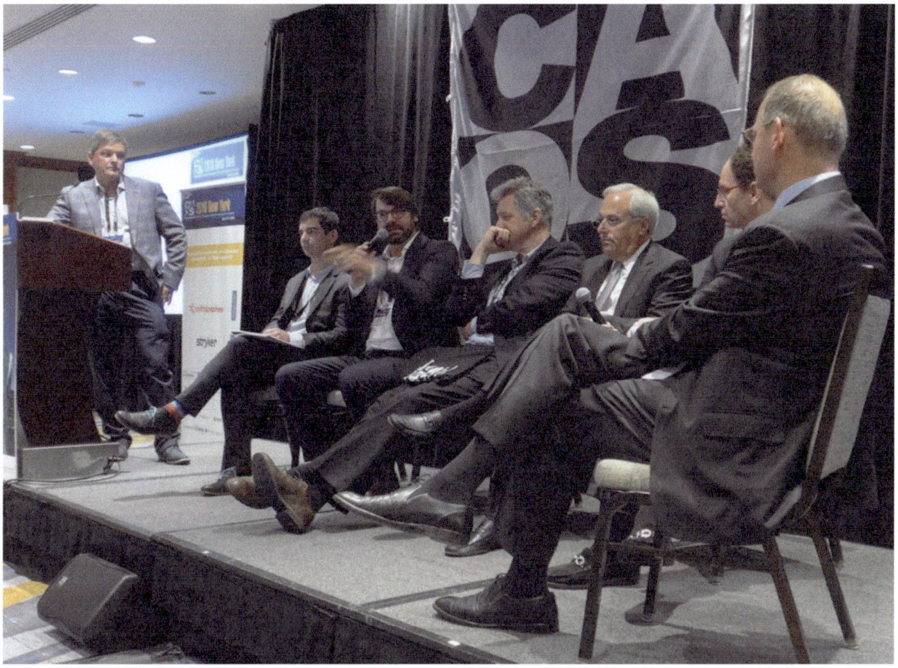

Fig. 15.6 A panel discussion held at the Computer-Assisted Orthopaedic Surgery (CAOS) annual conference in New York in 2019. Such panels, with different specialists including those from industry, are typical of today's conferences. From left to right: Martin Roche, Chris Plaskos, Branislav Jaramaz, Pierre Couture, Robert Cohen, Stefan Kreuzer, and Patrick Meere. (President of CAOS 2019)

maintaining quality of care. Smart tools and robotics surgery may represent one answer to this demand." In other words the challenge of computer-assisted surgery is to enable a faster procedure with greater accuracy. At this date (2019), there is evidence that the computer-assisted smart tools have slightly reduced the surgical time and improved the accuracy. However the robotic systems, while improving the accuracy, have increased both the time and the cost of each procedure. It can also be argued that complexity has been increased due to the higher technical skill and training required both of the surgeon and the supporting staff. Imaging does allow the surgeon greater flexibility of positioning and balancing of the implant components, early evidence showing that this will result in better outcomes.

Another way in which computer-assisted surgery could make a difference is in the concept of minimally invasive surgery. At present robots are being used to perform the same tasks as mechanical instruments. Could they be used in a new way with newly designed components that could be inserted through very small incisions?

Is there a possibility for a custom-made implant for every patient, made by 3D printing either in the hospital itself or in a local facility? With newer bearing materials, this might be possible in the not too distant future.

Research and Educational Support

The process by which new artificial knee designs and techniques become accepted and used clinically is multifactorial, but the associated research studies and the extent of publications and presentations at conferences are an essential ingredient. This is typically a process which can take many years. Embedded within this are the separate factors which determine the end result. These factors were listed at the beginning of this chapter for the success of designs up to 1980: prestigious institution, authoritative designer(s), collaboration between surgeon and bioengineer, reputable design group, well-established company, strong company support, convincing design rationale, well-thought-out technique, and minimum problems in early trials. These are all relevant today, with a greater emphasis on design teams rather than on individuals and on a greater role for companies, particularly where large investments are needed such as in robotic surgery. Basic research plays a role, especially in new materials development or in biomechanical evaluations, while large databases such as the national registries rely on new statistical methods, including machine learning. There is a high output of research studies from universities and hospitals, funded from a wide variety of sources. Such output provides most of the content for the lectures at conferences and publications. Based on the increasing numbers of papers being written, it might be thought that the funding for such work is adequate. However there is justification for a higher level of funding from the NIH, where most of the funding for orthopedics in general is derived. Studies of the biomechanics of the knee can be considered fundamental, which provides a basis for the design of treatments for the arthritic knees. Devising experimental methods or computer models for the evaluation of artificial knees is an area which can minimize problems and enhance clinical results. New materials for the bearing surfaces, for the structure of the components, and for uncemented fixation all require basic research studies. The possibility of economically fabricating custom joints for every patient requires research in computer technology and manufacturing methods. The crucially important area of recovery and rehabilitation needs further basic research.

Today, there are several educational vehicles for the presentation and evaluation of research on artificial knees. The American Academy of Orthopaedic Surgeons (AAOS), the largest orthopedic conference in the world, provides a holistic forum of lectures, instructional media, scientific exhibits, and posters which include basic and applied research studies and displays of products by companies. The annual meeting of the American Association of Hip and Knee Surgeons (AAHKS) is a scientific forum for implant design, outcomes, surgical technique, complications, and socioeconomic issues. The courses held during the year by the International Congress for Joint Reconstruction (ICJR) and the Current Concepts in Joint Replacement (CCJR) present the state of the art of the field, intended for the specialist surgeon in artificial knees, as well as other joints. The CCJR includes debate scenarios on such topics as CR vs PS, cemented fixation vs porous and coated, whether or not to resurface the patella, and mechanical vs kinematic alignment. The presentations usually recognize that each alternative is valid, but it provides the surgeon with a deeper understanding of the nuances to enable a rational choice to be made. The ICJR often includes live interactive surgeries which can reveal fine points and ways of overcoming problems and choices which might arise. Most companies run instructional laboratories where expert surgeons demonstrate new designs and techniques.

For the most part, in the above organizations, the large majority of the attendees are orthopedic surgeons. In contrast, in the field of artificial joints, there are two societies which represent more technical aspects and the boundary between today and tomorrow, ISTA and CAOS. The general purpose of these societies is to showcase and evaluate new possibilities, whether it be in methods of outcome measurement, new materials and designs, or alternate surgical techniques, particularly computer-assisted. The attendance at these conferences is divided roughly into thirds: orthopedic surgeons, researchers and academics, and company representatives. These meetings are invaluable in that they provide a multidisciplinary perspective of what might eventually enter the mainstream of joint replacement practice or find a useful niche in a special application. One of the features of the meetings is that the technical aspects can be covered in considerable depth. An important issue is the interface between such meetings and those which deal mainly with surgical practice. To some extent there is a dividing line where practicing surgeons do not encounter the scientific or developmental activity. This is to a large degree inevitable due to time constraints alone, although some understanding of basic biomechanical principles should be regarded as essential, in order to appreciate the functional aspects of artificial knees. The main interface needs to be with those orthopedic surgeons who are considered the opinion leaders and who make presentations at clinical conferences. Such individuals provide an objective interface in transferring appropriate new technology to a broader front.

The ORS is also involved in the area of new technology, attracting scientific researchers mainly from academia. Computer modeling is currently a major area of interest for determining the relative influence of variables such as geometry and soft tissue balancing and on its potential for personalizing artificial knee design. Recently an Implants Section was formed which has separate sessions, as well as the sessions on implants in the general program. However, there is a greater focus on biology at the ORS rather than on the physical sciences. A debate was recently held at the ORS on the alternate solutions of biology versus mechanical for osteoarthritis of the knee and hip. This is detailed below.

Biological Treatments

The possibility is often brought up that biological treatments will solve arthritis and that artificial knees will be unnecessary. In 2017, the Orthopedic Research Society held a debate entitled "Will Regenerative Medicine Make Orthopaedic Implants Obsolete in Our Time?" (Johnstone et al. 2018). The title could apply to all types of implants although the main focus was on artificial hips and knees.

For the proposition, Brian Johnstone stated as an overview: "The reality is that orthopedic surgeons, and the orthopaedic industry, had better become smarter biologists soon, because we are underestimating the myriad of things that regenerative medicine will do in the long run." He defined the purpose of regenerative medicine as "the repair, regrowth, or replacement of damaged or diseased cells, tissues, or organs." With gene therapies, cell therapies, tissue engineering, and production of artificial organs, "it is hard for me to believe that regenerative medicine will not make plastic and metal implants obsolete in our time." "We have to transition from traditional engineering and metallurgy-based therapies to biology and biomedical engineering-based ones." Johnstone summarized as follows: "... metal and plastic orthopedic implants are without question, a success story... they have plateaued in terms of significant improvement, providing a stimulus for developing new technologies."

Against the proposition, Joshua Jacobs stated: "Fabricating complex biological structures to replace or restore diseased organs has been the holy grail for decades... for orthopedic applications such as total joint replacement, there are no viable regenerative medicine alternatives at the present time." Jacobs then emphasized the high performance of artificial joints: "... total joint arthroplasty with engineering materials has set a very high bar for performance that will be difficult for regenerative medicine to exceed." Why should it not be the case that a structure made from durable synthetic materials will surpass biological materials in a system such as a knee joint? Jacobs also pointed out that the arthritis was, in most cases, caused by a deficient biomechanical system: "If the aberrant biomechanics, whether static or dynamic, are not corrected, tissue engineered constructs will likely be overloaded and degraded as was the native tissue." This crucial last point was made by Brandt et al. (2008), after decades of research into osteoarthritis: "The importance of abnormal joint mechanics in the etiopathogenesis of OA cannot be overemphasized. The authors view OA as a process that is attempting to contain a mechanical problem in the joint; OA is best defined as failed repair of joint damage that has been caused by excessive mechanical stress. Because the body's innate mechanisms for repairing damaged cartilage cannot deal with the underlying mechanical abnormality, they cannot solve the problem of OA... The common mechanical factor underlying OA is a pathologic increase in intra-articular stress."

Concluding Points

Today, there are well-established designs and techniques, a steadily increasing demand worldwide, and good functional results with few complications. In this chapter, possibilities of further advances have been discussed based on evidence from recent published studies. These advances would improve the durability and functional performance, provide a quicker recovery time with an increased flexion angle, and require less time for a more accurate procedure. The most likely possibilities, based on the advantages that will be obtained, are a gradual shift in the design types used most frequently, from the CR and PS to designs such as ultracongruent, medially congruent, medial pivot, and guided motion; more use of uncemented implants with porous coatings; and a change from manual instrumentation to manual plus smart tools and to robotic surgery, although the latter may be focused on major centers and for young active patients. If such changes do occur, they are

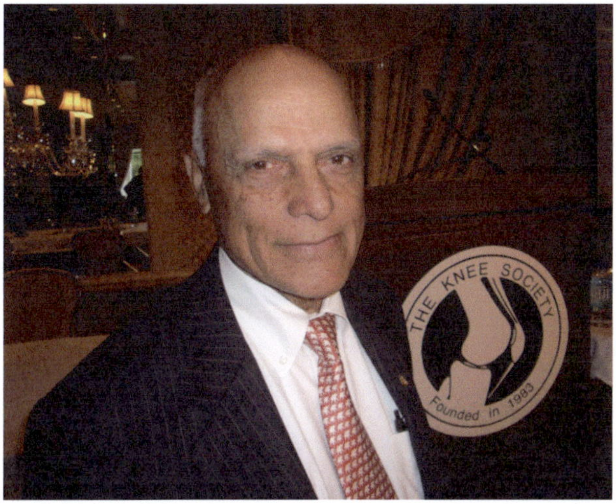

Fig. 15.7 Chitranjan S Ranawat MD has been a highly recognized surgeon at the Hospital for Special Surgery in New York since the late 1960s. Since being one of the designers of the first condylar knees in the early 1970s, he has continued to be a major force in the areas of design, surgical technique, clinical follow-up, and pain management to this day. He was the main founder of the Knee Society in 1983. His educational excellence to residents and fellows and at numerous conferences, has been unparalleled. (Photo taken 2018) (© Peter S Walker)

likely to take a number of years to take effect due to the time taken to reach a consensus that there are worthwhile benefits without any downsides. The way in which such changes will take effect is through the well-organized and extensive research and educational infrastructure. The increasing use of biomechanical evaluation methods will play an important role in accelerating the decision-making, in providing more convincing functional data. Companies too will play a role in funding and promoting the designs and techniques which are the most successful. Finance will however play a pervasive role through the system, with some conflict between obtaining high quality but without an increase in cost.

Are there likely to be any revolutionary changes in treating the artificial knee? Custom knees and disposable instrumentation could be designed and made on-site using a CNC machine for polyethylene tibial components and 3D printing for PEEK femoral components. Implant manufacturing units would be a product sold to hospitals. The regulatory and liability questions are however formidable, while on-site technical expertise would be essential. Furthermore, the functional benefits would have to be well demonstrated. Components made from deformable polymeric materials such as polyurethane or hydrogels are another possibility for making joints which are deformable, allow fluid film lubrication, and giving a more natural feel to the patient, but the wear and strength properties required may be beyond what is possible at this time. Minimally invasive surgical techniques, widely used for internal medicine, could result in a procedure with a much more rapid recovery and higher flexion, but this would require a major change in the design of the components and the way they are fitted to the femur and tibia. Could arthritis be prevented in many cases by detection at an early stage and carrying out a procedure to treat a biomechanical abnormality such as misalignment? Or if the knee had a ligament or meniscal injury, could the treatment be restricted to those tissues rather than the entire joint? There is evidence from the sports medicine area that this approach has some possibilities. Whatever changes are made in the next few years or even the next decade, based on the changes over the past three decades since 1980, further changes may take considerable time, but one can but expect that the best solutions will come to the forefront and that new possibilities will be explored.

References

Aglietti P, Buzzi R, De Felice R, Giron F. The Insall-Burstein total knee replacement in osteoarthritis: a 10-year minimum follow-up. J Arthroplast. 1999;14(5):560–5.

Arno S, Maffei D, Walker PS, Schwarzkopf R, Desai P, Steiner GC. Retrospective analysis of total knee arthroplasty cases for visual, histological, and clinical eligibility of unicompartmental knee arthroplasties. J Arthroplast. 2011;26(8):1396–403.

Atrey A, Edmondson MC, East D, Miles K, Butler-Manuel A, Ellens N. A retrospective medium-to long-term results of 1500 AGC total knee replacements - an independent Centre functional follow up and survivorship. J Orthop. 2014;11(1):37–42.

Barrett TJ, Shi L, Parsley BS. Bicruciate-retaining total knee arthroplasty, a promising technology, that's not quite there. Ann Transl Med. 2017;5(Suppl 1):S17.

Bosco JA, Harty JH, Iorio R. Bundled payment arrangements: keys to success. J Am Acad Orthop Surg. 2018;26(23):817–22.

Boylan M, Suchman K, Vigdorchik J, Slover J, Bosco J. Technology-assisted hip and knee arthroplasties: an analysis of utilization trends. J Arthroplast. 2018;33(4):1019–23.

Bozic KJ. My own joint replacement was a reality check. AAOS Now, Aug 2019.

Brandt KD, Dieppe P, Radin EL. Etiopathogenesis of osteoarthritis. Rheum Dis Clin N Am. 2008;34:531–59.

Chughtai M, Kelly JJ, Newman JM, et al. The role of virtual rehabilitation in total and unicompartmental knee arthroplasty. J Knee Surg. 2019;32(01):105–10.

Dennis DA, Komistek RD, Scuderi GR, Zingde S. Factors affecting flexion after total knee arthroplasty. Clin Orthop Relat Res. 2007;464:53–60.

Dunbar M, Gross M. Critical steps in total knee arthroplasty. Int Orthop. 1995;19(5):265–8.

Evans JT, Walker RW, Evans JP, Blom AW, Sayers A, Whitehouse MR. How long does a knee replacement last? A systematic review and meta-analysis of case series and national registry reports with more than 15 years of follow-up. Lancet (London, England). 2019;393(10172):655–63.

Harvey LA, Brosseau L, Herbert RD. Continuous passive motion following total knee arthroplasty in people with arthritis. Cochrane Database Syst Rev. 2014;(2):Cd004260.

Heyse TJ, Chen DX, Kelly N, Boettner F, Wright TM, Haas SB. Matched-pair total knee arthroplasty retrieval analysis: oxidized zirconium vs. CoCrMo. Knee. 2011;18(6):448–52.

Hooper J, Schwarzkopf R, Fernandez E, Buckland A, Werner J, Einhorn T, Walker PS. Feasibility of single-use 3D-printed instruments for total knee arthroplasty. Bone Joint J. 2019;101-B(7_Supple_C):115–20.

Johnstone B, Jacobs JJ, Sandell LJ, Wilkinson LM. Regenerative medicine will make orthopaedic implants obsolete in our time. J Orthop Res. 2018;36:2579–85.

Kim KY, Anoushiravani AA, Chen KK, Li R, Bosco JA, Slover JD, Iorio R. Perioperative orthopedic surgical home: optimizing total joint arthroplasty candidates and preventing readmission. J Arthroplast. 2019;34(7S):S91–6.

Laskin RS, Maruyama Y, Villaneuva M, Bourne R. Deep-dish congruent tibial component use in total knee arthroplasty: a randomized prospective study. Clin Orthop Relat Res. 2000;380:36–44.

Mahfouz M, Fatah EEA, Bowers LS, Scuderi G. Three-dimensional morphology of the knee reveals ethnic differences. Clin Orthop Relat Res. 2012;470:172–85.

Meier M, Zingde S, Steinert A, Kurtz W, Koeck F, Beckmann J. What is the possible impact of high variability of distal femoral geometry on TKA? A CT data analysis of 24,042 knees. Clin Orthop Relat Res. 2019;477(3):561–70.

Nakamura S, Ito H, Nakamura K, Kuriyama S, Furu M, Matsuda S. Long-term durability of ceramic tri-condylar knee implants: a minimum 15-year follow-up. J Arthroplast. 2017;32(6):1874–9.

Parvataneni HK, Shah VP, Howard H, Cole N, Ranawat AS, Ranawat CS. Controlling pain after total hip and knee arthroplasty using a multimodal protocol with local periarticular injections: a prospective randomized study. J Arthroplast. 2007;22(6 Suppl 2):33–8.

Petterson SC, Mizner RL, Stevens JE, et al. Improved function from progressive strengthening interventions after total knee arthroplasty: a randomized clinical trial with an imbedded prospective cohort. Arthritis Care Res. 2009;61(2):174–83.

Pfitzner T, Perca C, Roth P. Unicompartmental vs total knee arthroplasty for medial osteoarthritis. Z Orthop Unfall. 2017;155(5):527–33.

Pinskerova V, Samuelson KM, Stammers J, Maruthainar K, Sosna A, Freeman MA. The knee in full flexion: an anatomical study. J Bone Joint Surg. 2009;91(6):830–4.

Pitta M, Esposito DCI, Li DZ, Lee MDY, Wright TM, Padgett DE. Failure after modern total knee arthroplasty: a prospective study of 18,065 knees. J Arthroplast. 2018;33(2):407–14.

Pozzi F, Snyder-Mackler L, Zeni J. Physical exercise after knee arthroplasty: a systematic review of controlled trials. Eur J Phys Rehabil Med. 2013;49(6):877.

Pradhan NR, Gambhir A, Porter ML. Survivorship analysis of 3234 primary knee arthroplasties implanted over a 26 year period. Knee. 2006;13:7–11.

Pritchett JW. Bicruciate-retaining total knee replacement provides a satisfactory function and implant survivorship at 23 years. Clin Orthop Relat Res. 2015;473(7):2327–33.

Ritter MA, Lutgring JD, Davis KE, Berend ME. The effect of postoperative range of motion on functional activities after posterior cruciate-retaining total knee arthroplasty. JBJS. 2008;90(4):777–84.

Rodriguez JA, Bhende H, Ranawat CS. Total condylar knee replacement: a 20-year followup study. Clin Orthop Relat Res. 2001;388:10–7.

Romagnoli S, Marullo M, Massaro M, Rustemi E, D'Amario F, Corbella M. Bi-unicompartmental and combined uni plus patellofemoral replacement: indications and surgical technique. Joints. 2015;3(1):42–8.

Rowell SL, Reyes CR, Malchau H, Muratoglu OK. In vivo oxidative stability changes of highly cross-linked polyethylene bearings: an ex vivo investigation. J Arthroplast. 2015;30(10):1828–34.

Rutherford RW, Jennings JM, Dennis DA. Enhancing recovery after Total knee arthroplasty. Orthop Clin North Am. 2017;48(4):391–400.

Salter RB, Simmonds DF, Malcolm BW, Rumble EJ, MacMichael D, Clements ND. The biological effect of continuous passive motion on the healing of full-thickness defects in articular cartilage. An experimental investigation in the rabbit. J Bone Joint Surg Am. 1980;62(8):1232–51.

Sartawi M, Zurakowski D, Rosenberg A. Implant survivorship and complication rates after total knee arthroplasty with a third-generation cemented system: 15-year follow-up. Am J Orthop (Belle Mead, NJ). 2018;47(3). https://doi.org/10.12788/ajo.2018.0018

Scott CEH, Bell KR, Ng RT, MacDonald DJ, Patton JT, Burnett R. Excellent 10-year patient-reported outcomes and survival in a single-radius, cruciate-retaining total knee arthroplasty. Knee Surg Sports Traumatol Arthrosc. 2019;27(4):1106–15.

Scuderi G. The impact of smart tools on total knee arthroplasty. Am J Orthop (Belle Mead NJ). 2007;36(9 Suppl):8–10.

Srinivasan P, Miller MA, Verdonschot N, Mann KA, Janssen D. Strain shielding in trabecular bone at the tibial cement-bone interface. J Mech Behav Biomed Mater. 2017;66:181–6.

Takasaki H, Okubo Y, Okuyama S. The effect of proprioceptive neuromuscular facilitation on joint position sense: a systematic review. J Sport Rehabil. 2019:1–30. https://doi.org/10.1123/jsr.2018-0498

Tarabichi S, Tarabichi Y, Hawari M. Achieving deep flexion after primary total knee arthroplasty. J Arthroplast. 2010;25(2):219–24.

Vince KG, Kelly MA, Beck J, Insall JN. Continuous passive motion after total knee arthroplasty. J Arthroplast. 1987;2(4):281–4.

Von Eiff MC, von Eiff W, Roth A, Ghanem M. Process optimization in total knee arthroplasty procedures: impact of size-specific instrument sets on costs and revenue. Orthopade. 2019;48(11):963–8.

Wautier D, Thienpont E. Changes in anteroposterior stability and proprioception after different types of knee arthroplasty. Knee Surg Sports Traumatol Arthrosc. 2017;25(6):1792–800.

Wilson CJ, Theodoulou A, Damarell RA, Krishnan J. Knee instability as the primary cause of failure following Total knee arthroplasty (TKA): a systematic review on the patient, surgical and implant characteristics of revised TKA patients. Knee. 2017;24(6):1271–81.

Glossary

Many of the definitions are derived from the AAOS Comprehensive Orthopedic Review, Biomechanics and Biomaterials.

Some definitions are worded to apply specifically to the knee joint.

Where applicable units of measurement are shown next to the term.

Units Units of measurement using the Standard International (SI) System are:

- Length = meter m (or millimeter mm). Mass = Kilogram kg. Time = second s. Force = Newtons N. Pressure = Pascal Pa. N/mm^2.
- 1 inch = 25.4 mm. 1 lb = 0.454 kg. 1 pounds force = 4.45 Newtons. 100 Newtons = 22.5 lbs force. 1 MegaPascal (MPa) = 145 pounds per square inch (psi).
- body weight (BW) typical male 170 lbs approx. 750 Newtons

AAHKS American Association of Hip and Knee Surgeons

AAOS American Academy of Orthopedic Surgeons

Abrasive wear Wear due to an asperity on one surface digging into the opposite surface releasing small particles. Three-body abrasion from loose particles intervening between sliding surfaces.

Acceleration Rate of change of velocity with time

P. S. Walker, *The Artificial Knee*, https://doi.org/10.1007/978-3-030-38171-4

Adhesive wear	Wear at a microscopic location on the surface due to adhesion against the opposite surface, releasing a small wear particle
AJRR	American Joint Replacement Register
All-plastic	A component made completely of polyethylene or another polymer, usually applied to a tibial component
Anatomic axis	A line drawn on a bone in 2D or 3D showing the centerline of the bone based on defined end points
Anterior cruciate	The ligament in the center of the knee which limits the displacement of the femur posteriorly relative to the tibia or of the tibia anteriorly relative to the femur
Anterior displacement	The motion of one bone relative to another, along an axis defined in the anterior direction
Anterior	The front of the knee or in a frontal direction
Arthritis	A painful degenerative condition of the knee where the cartilage bearing surfaces are worn, often accompanied by limb misalignment
Arthroplasty	The surgical repair of a joint which can involve the use of an artificial part or implant
Artificial knee	Implantable device made from synthetic materials to restore function to an arthritic knee. Most commonly referred to a condylar replacement knee (including a unicompartmental) but can include a hinged device
ASTM	American Society for Testing and Materials
Axial force	Vertical force applied in the longitudinal direction of the anatomic axis of a bone such as the femur or tibia
Axis system	*xyz* Cartesian axis system fixed in the femur or tibia defined by bony landmarks or an axis system defined in any body. The axes are mutually perpendicular
Bicruciate retaining (BCR)	An artificial knee design where both of the cruciate ligaments are preserved
Biomechanics	Mechanical principles applied to the musculoskeletal system
Biomimetic	Imitating the structure or function of a biological system. Close to biomimicry

Body	A structure such as a bone, implant, component. Can be depicted for the purpose of analysis
Brittle	The absence of a region of plastic deformation up to the point of fracture
Cam-post	Applied to a posterior stabilized knee where a projecting tibial post fits into a cavity in the center of the femoral component and is interacted on by the cavity to control motion.
Cancellous bone	A network of interconnected bony spicules to resist forces in functional directions, also called spongy or trabecular bone
CAOS	Computer-Assisted Orthopedic Surgery. An international society
CCJR	Current Concepts in Joint Replacement. An educational organization
Ceiling effect	Lack of discriminating ability of the evaluation test to detect clinically relevant changes even if the patient continues to improve
Collateral ligaments	The fibrous tissue structures at the sides of the knee which resist varus and valgus rotations between the femur and the tibia
Compression	The application of a force at a point or over an area of a body
Compressive stress	The force applied over a defined area, divided by the area
Computer-assisted surgery	Surgery where one or more of the surgical instruments or guides uses computer technology, including navigation and robotics
Condylar replacement	Components for resurfacing an arthritic knee. Can cover only one half of the knee (uni) or all of the bearing surfaces (total knee)
Condyles	The regions on the distal femur and proximal tibia which are covered with articular cartilage and which transmit the forces and motions
Congruent	Usually applied to a joint where the opposing bearing surfaces are a close fit, such as the ball and socket of the hip
Constraint	The phenomenon whereby one body is restricted from moving relative to another body or the extent by which it is restricted
Contact area	The area of the contact between two surfaces which are loaded together, such as the contact area in the knee or in an artificial knee

Contact stress The force per unit area on a contact region such as the contact area in the knee

Coordinate system An *xyz* Cartesian axis system fixed in the femur or tibia defined by bony landmarks or an axis system defined in a body, where all axes are mutually at 90 ° to each other

Coronal plane A plane representing the front view of the limb, or knee, or tibia or femur, or the entire body (same as frontal plane)

Cortical bone Solid bone material comprising the tubular diaphyseal sections of the femur and tibia, also located on the outside surfaces of cancellous bone in the metaphysis

CR Type of artificial knee. Designation for a condylar replacement artificial knee where the anterior cruciate is resected but the posterior cruciate is retained

Cross-shear When two opposing sliding surfaces move in slightly different directions in successive motion cycles, causing increased wear

Cruciate ligaments The fibrous tissue bands in the center of the knee which resist relative anterior and posterior displacements between the femur and the tibia

Debridement Removal of damaged cartilage, soft tissue, or bone, from inside the joint to facilitate motion and relieve pain, usually as an arthroscopic procedure

Deformable body An object which changes its shape, or deforms, when forces are applied (see also rigid body)

Degrees of freedom (dof) The number of directions where motion can take place. A body in space has 3 linear and 3 rotational dof

Delamination wear Wear due to the coalescing of subsurface cracks due to subsurface stresses, leading to release of particles or flakes

Dislocation When one surface of a joint crosses the boundaries of the opposite surface such that it reaches an unstable state

Displacement Linear motions between one object and another or the distance between the initial and the final position of an object

Distal	The lower part of the object, e.g., the femur or the tibia
EFORT	European Federation of Orthopedics and Traumatology
Elastic modulus	A material property describing its resistance to change of shape when loaded. Colloquially, the "stiffness" of a material
Elastic	The property of a material that allows it to regain its shape immediately after a force is released
Electrogoniometer	A device that fits around a joint, which has sensors to measure the angle of flexion or other angles of motion.
Electromyography	A diagnostic procedure to assess the health of muscles and the nerve cells that control them
EORS	European Orthopedic Research Society
Equilibrium	A state of a body where the sum of the forces and moments are zero
ESB	European Society of Biomechanics
Euler or Cardan angles	An ordered sequence of 3 rotations of the femur relative to the tibia or tibia relative to femur
Extension	The relative position of the femur and tibia where the bones cannot be further extended (note, the position can vary slightly depending on how much extending moment is applied)
External rotation	Rotation of the femur about the anatomic axis of the tibia such that the medial femoral condyle is moved anteriorly and the lateral condyle posteriorly. Can also be defined as a rotation of the tibia about its anatomic axis such that the medial plateau moves anteriorly and the lateral plateau moves posteriorly
Failure	A fracture of the body or material. Excessive permanent deformation can also be regarded as failure
Fatigue	Eventual failure of a body or material after multiple applications of a force
Finite element analysis	Analysis of the stresses and strains in an object by dividing it into multiple small

	shapes and applying loads and boundary conditions
Fixation peg	One or more pegs on the base of the tibial or femoral component used for enhancing the fixation of the component to the bone
Fixation	The connection of an implant component (e.g., femoral or tibial) to the host bone, typically on a prepared surface exposing cancellous bone
Fluoroscopy	Medical imaging where an x-ray image is continuous, commonly used for studying the motion inside human joints
Force (Newtons)	An entity applied to a body which causes it to move or change its shape. Force has both magnitude and direction
Free body diagram	Depiction of all the forces and moments acting on an object contained within a defined boundary
Fretting	Surface damage at contacting surfaces which experience small relative motions under repetitive loading
Friction coefficient	The ratio of the resistive force to sliding, divided by the force pressing the surfaces together
Friction	The resistive force between the surfaces of two objects in contact when relative sliding occurs
Frontal plane	A plane representing the front view of the limb, or knee, or tibia or femur, or the entire body (same as coronal plane)
Guided Motion Knee	A type of artificial knee where motion is guided or constrained by mechanical means, usually to provide more anatomic motion
Hardness	Resistance to indentation or scratching
ICJR	International Congress for Joint Replacement. An educational organization
Instant center of rotation	The center of rotation on a defined plane between two bodies for a small arc of motion
Intercondylar	The space in between the distal femoral condyles, also called intercondylar notch or fossa
Internal rotation	Rotation of the femur about the anatomic axis of the tibia such that the medial femoral condyle moves posteriorly and the lateral condyle anteriorly. Can also be defined

	as a rotation of the tibia about its anatomic axis such that the medial plateau moves posteriorly and the lateral plateau moves anteriorly
Intramedullary	Inside the hollow tubular diaphyseal portion of the femur or tibia
ISTA	International Society for Technology in Arthroplasty
ISO	International Standards Organisation
Kinematics	A description of the motion of an object without regard for how that motion is produced
Kinetics	A study of the forces that cause motions
KSS	Knee Society Score. One of the most widely used scoring system for evaluating the functional performance of a knee
Lateral collateral ligament	The ligament at the lateral side of the knee which limits the varus rotation between the femur and tibia
Lateral	The outside of the knee
Laxity	The displacements and rotations which occur between the femur and tibia when forces and torques are applied, usually at a fixed angle of flexion
Ligament release	Removing a part of a ligament from its bony attachment or cutting some fibers of the ligament, to reduce the stiffness or tightness
Linearly elastic	A material or body where the deformation is linearly proportional to the applied force
Load	A colloquial term meaning the same as force
Lubrication	Separation of two sliding surfaces by a fluid film or boundary molecules to prevent or minimize the wear of the surfaces
Mass (Kg)	The amount of matter that an object consists of
Maximum flexion	180 ° minus the angle between the anatomic axes of the femur and tibia with the knee maximally flexed
Mechanical axis of the femur	The line joining the center of the femoral head to the center of the distal femur
Mechanical axis of the lower limb	The line joining the center of the femoral head to the center of the ankle at the level of the malleoli

Medial collateral ligament	The ligament at the medial side of the knee which limits the valgus rotation between the femur and tibia
Medial	On the inside of the knee joint, facing the opposite knee
Medial pivot	A type of artificial knee where the medial condyles are congruent and the lateral condyles are incongruent. Such that internal-external rotation pivots on the medial side
Meniscus	Crescent-shaped spacers between the medial and lateral sides of the femur and tibia which make the condyles more congruent
Micromotion	Microscopic (micron ranges) motion between two bodies or surfaces which can cause corrosion or wear particles. Takes place between a plastic tibial insert and the inside base of the metal tibial tray
Mold arthroplasty	The insertion of an inert mobile mold to guide repair between two perfectly shaped joint surfaces
Moment arm	The perpendicular distance between the applied force and a defined point, or between the force and the axis of rotation
Moment	The product of the magnitude of the force (Newtons) and its distance from a defined point (millimeters)
Monoblock	A component which is made from two or more separate parts but is fused together, e.g., a plastic tibial insert fused to a metal baseplate
OREF	Orthopaedic Research and Education Foundation
ORS	Orthopaedic Research Society
Osteotomy	Cutting a wedge-shaped piece of bone from the distal femur or proximal tibia to realign the bone and limb
Oxidation	Oxidation of polyethylene leads to embrittlement and higher rates of wear including delamination
Paradoxical sliding	Abnormal and excessive anterior sliding of the femoral component on the tibial component during a mid-flexion range of motion

Patella flange	The anterior part of a femoral component where the patella articulates during the range of flexion
Patella trochlea	The area covered by articular cartilage on the antero-distal end of the femur where the patella articulates
Patella	The small bone which slides on the anterior femur during flexion-extension and transmits the force between the quadriceps muscle and the proximal tibia
Plastic deformation	Deformation which is not recovered after removal of the force
Plastic insert	The polyethylene tibial component which fits into the metallic tibial tray, a modular construction
Polycentric	A changing center of rotation as one body (e.g., bone) is flexed relative to another body
Posterior cruciate ligament	The ligament in the center of the knee which limits the displacement of the femur anteriorly relative to the tibia, or the displacement of the tibia posteriorly relative to the femur
Posterior tibial slope	In an anatomic knee, the angle between the line from the anterior to the posterior of the proximal tibia and an anterior-posterior horizontal line which is perpendicular to the anatomic axis. Typically 5–7 °
Posterior	The back of the knee or in a backward direction
Pressure	The force per unit area applied by a fluid or the force per unit area applied on a surface
PROM	Patient-reported outcome measure such as KOOS, WOMAC, KSS, to quantify the functional performance and other parameters
Proprioception	The ability to sense position, motion, and equilibrium; has been ascribed to the anterior cruciate and other ligaments
Proximal	At the upper end, usually referred to the position on a bone
PS	Type of artificial knee. Designation for a condylar replacement artificial knee where the anterior and posterior cruciates are

resected, and stability is provided by an intercondylar cam-post

Range of flexion The angular excursion between the femur and tibia between maximally straight and maximally flexed

Resultant force A single force vector representing more than one applied force vector

Resurfacing Replacement components for the bearing surfaces of the knee

Rigid body An object which is considered to be of constant shape even when forces are applied (see deformable body)

Rotation An angular motion (degrees) of a moving body relative to a fixed body about a defined axis in the fixed body

RSA Radiostereometric Analysis, used for determining motion of an artificial knee component relative to the supporting bone, for evaluating fixation

Sagittal radii Usually applied to the radii of the distal femoral condyles seen in the sagittal view, the radius is not constant around the profile

Sagittal The plane describing the side view of the leg or knee

Screw-home The phenomenon where the tibia progressively externally rotates relative to the femur as the tibia is brought into full extension

Shear stress The shear force divided by the area of surface over which the force is applied

Shear A force or stress applied across a surface or across a defined plane in a body

Snap-fit Two components fitted together by a snap mechanism involving temporary elastic deformation of a flexible member, usually applied to a plastic tibial bearing snapping into a metal tibial tray

Soft tissue Tissue excluding bone and cartilage; most often referred to tendon, ligament, muscle, fibrous capsule, synovial membrane

Spongy bone A network of interconnected bony spicules to resist forces in functional directions, also called cancellous or trabecular bone

Stability	In function, there is no subjective feeling of excessive femoral-tibial motion nor any overstressing of soft tissues
Stiffness	Displacement per unit applied force
Strain	Change in length divided by original length or proportionate change in length along a defined line
Stress distribution	The stress pattern across a surface or defined plane, usually denoted with color coding, e.g., red = high stress, blue = low stress
Stress protection	An area of bone which experiences less than its normal stress due to the load being bypassed by an implant component
Stress	Force divided by area, applied to a small element of material, the element located in a body or on a surface
Subluxation	When one surface of a joint reaches the boundaries of the opposite surface but before irreducible dislocation
Survivorship	Probability of an artificial knee surviving successfully for a defined length of time, e.g., 10 and 20 years
TCP	Total Condylar Prosthesis.
Tensile strength	The maximum force or stress a structure can carry before mechanical failure, e.g., a ligament or tendon
Tensile stress	The force applied on a defined area which lengthens the dimension of an object, divided by the area
Three-body abrasion	Wear caused on one or both sliding surfaces due to the presence of a small intervening hard particle
Tibial tray	The metallic tibial component of an artificial knee which houses the plastic bearing surface or plastic insert
Tissue	Materials comprising the human body, including bone, cartilage, tendon, ligament, muscle, synovial fluid
Torque	A twisting action on a body that causes rotation
Total knee arthroplasty	Same as artificial knee
Total knee replacement	Same as artificial knee
Toughness	The amount of energy a material can absorb up to the point of failure

Trabecular bone	A network of interconnected bony spicules to resist forces in functional directions, also called cancellous or spongy bone
Transverse axis	An axis from the medial to the lateral side, usually applied to an axis through the distal femur or across the proximal tibia
Transverse plane	The plane defined by the medial-lateral axis and the anterior-posterior axis of the tibia
Ultracongruent	A condylar replacement artificial knee where the tibial surfaces are almost fully congruent with the femoral bearing surfaces
Unconstrained	Not providing any restraint to motion, can apply to an artificial knee which allows freedom of motion
Unicompartmental knee	An artificial knee consisting of a metal runner for a single femoral condyle and a plastic bearing covering a single tibial plateau
Uphill mechanism	Stability between opposing surfaces of a joint when the surfaces distract relative to each other against the applied force
Valgus	The alignment of the femur on the tibia such that the femoral and tibial condyles are displaced medially creating a "knock-kneed" effect
Varus	The alignment of the femur on the tibia such that the femoral and tibial condyles are displaced laterally creating a "bow-legged" effect
Vector	An entity that has magnitude and direction. Usually applied to a force or a line in space.
Velocity	The rate of positional or angular change of an object's position with time
Viscoelastic	Time-dependent deformation on application of a force. Stress relaxion and creep are associated terms
Vitallium	The trade name for cobalt-chrome-molybdenum alloy which has been widely used for the manufacture of artificial knee components (and other joints)
Wear	Progressive removal of small particles of material from a surface due to sliding of that surface against another surface

Index

P. S. Walker, *The Artificial Knee*, https://doi.org/10.1007/978-3-030-38171-4

MIX
Papier aus verantwortungsvollen Quellen
Paper from responsible sources
FSC® C105338

If you have any concerns about our products,
you can contact us on
ProductSafety@springernature.com

In case Publisher is established outside the EU,
the EU authorized representative is:
Springer Nature Customer Service Center GmbH
Europaplatz 3, 69115 Heidelberg, Germany

Printed by Libri Plureos GmbH
in Hamburg, Germany